American College of
Obstetricians and Gynecologists

MW00837343

ICD-9-CM
ABRIDGED

2010

DIAGNOSTIC
CODING
IN
OBSTETRICS AND
GYNECOLOGY

All diagnostic codes referred to in *ICD-9-CM Abridged: Diagnostic Coding in Obstetrics and Gynecology 2010* were excerpted from the *International Classification of Diseases, 9th Revision, Clinical Modification* (ICD-9-CM), October 2009 revision, published by the United States Government under the auspices of the ICD-9-CM Coordination and Maintenance Committee. Some ICD-9-CM code descriptions have been altered by the American College of Obstetricians and Gynecologists (ACOG) to accommodate the organizational structure of the guide, but this alteration in no way compromises the use of the code.

This guide to ICD-9-CM coding in obstetrics and gynecology is provided by ACOG for educational purposes only. It is not intended to represent the only, or necessarily the best, coding methods for the diagnostic situations discussed, but rather as an approach, view, statement, or opinion that may be helpful to persons responsible for diagnostic coding. ACOG does not necessarily endorse the services described in the guide. The statements made in this publication should not be construed as ACOG policy, recommendations, or guidelines. ACOG makes no representations and/or warranties, expressed or implied, regarding the accuracy of the information contained in this book and disclaims any liability or responsibility for any consequences resulting from or otherwise related to any use of, or reliance on, this book.

ACOG gratefully acknowledges the contribution of the 2009 ACOG Committee on Coding and Nomenclature:

Members:

Gary S. Leiserowitz, MD, Chair
Jon K. Hathaway, MD, Vice Chair
Thaddeus L. Anderson, MD
Traci C. Burgess, MD
Emmanuella Cherisme, MD
Gregory W. DeMeo, DO

Andrea J. Flom, MD
Larry R. Glazerman, MD
Tamara G. Helfer, MD
Kristinell Keil, MD
Robert H. Palmer Jr., MD
Beth W. Rackow, MD

Liaison Members:

James T. Christmas, MD, Society for Maternal-Fetal Medicine
Robert L. Harris, MD, American Urogynecological Society
John T. Queenan Jr, MD, American Society for Reproductive Medicine
William R. Robinson, MD, Society of Gynecologic Oncologists
Craig J. Sobolewski, MD, American Association of Gynecologic Laparoscopists

Ex-Officio Members:

George A. Hill, MD, RBRVS Update Committee Advisor
Barbara S. Levy, MD, Chair of the AMA/Specialty Society, RBRVS Update Committee
Jordan G. Pritzker, MD, MBA, CPT Advisor
Sandra B. Reed, MD, ACOG Representative, RBRVS Update Committee
J. Martin Tucker, MD, Member, CPT Editorial Panel

Past Members/Liaisons:

Michael L. Berman, MD, Society of Gynecologic Oncologists
Kimberly Fischer, MD

Editors:

Savonne Montue, MBA, RHIT, ACS-OB, COBGC
Donna Tyler, CPC, COBGC

Staff:

Albert Strunk, JD, MD
James Scroggs
Anne Diamond

Copyright © 2010 by the American College of Obstetricians and Gynecologists. All rights reserved. No part of this publication may be reproduced, stored in a retrieval system, or transmitted, in any form or by any means, electronic, mechanical, photocopying, recording, or otherwise, without prior written permission from the publisher. Suggestions and comments are welcome and should be addressed to:

ACOG Committee on Coding and Nomenclature
409 12th Street, SW, PO Box 96920, Washington, DC 20090-6920
(202) 863-2498

ISBN 978-1-934946-90-9   12345/32109

CONTENTS

4

INTRODUCTION

In the United States, the *International Classification of Diseases, 9th Revision, Clinical Modification* (ICD-9-CM) is a standard national coding system used to report diagnoses. ICD-9-CM diagnostic codes are used to identify the patient's condition, illness, disease, symptom, or other reasons for seeking medical care. These codes are used in two ways: 1) to report services to insurance carriers for reimbursement and 2) to track disease trends and incidence. Most complete editions of the ICD-9-CM book include the Official Guidelines for Coding and Reporting. These are summarized in the introductions to Volume 1 and Volume 2 of this book. Adherence to the guidelines is required under the Health Insurance Portability and Accountability Act of 1996 (HIPAA).

Because these codes are required for physician reimbursement, it is important that both the physician and his or her staff understand how the ICD-9-CM coding system works. The physician needs to document his or her services using the same terms used in the ICD-9-CM. The staff person needs to be able to interpret the physician's documentation in order to select the appropriate ICD-9-CM diagnostic code or codes. If the documentation is unclear or not specific enough, the staff person should seek additional information from the physician. The ICD-9-CM consists of 3 volumes:

- Volume 1: Diseases: Tabular List
- Volume 2: Diseases: Alphabetic Index
- Volume 3: Procedures: Tabular List and Alphabetic Index

This booklet includes excerpts from Volume 1 and Volume 2, including those codes most often reported by obstetrician–gynecologists. Volume 3, used almost exclusively by hospital medical records departments, is not included.

CHANGES IN ICD-9-CM

ICD-9-CM is not a static document. Revisions, often significant ones, are made each year. Therefore, it is critical that the physician purchase a new book each fall to ensure that he or she is reporting the most current codes. ICD-9-CM books may be purchased through the American College of Obstetricians and Gynecologists (ACOG) Distribution Center (800-762-2264) or from ACOG's online bookstore (sales.acog.org). ICD-9-CM books also are available from many other commercial vendors.

Requests for changes in the ICD-9-CM are reviewed each year by the ICD-9-CM Coordination and Maintenance Committee. These decisions are made each spring and become effective October 1 of the same year.

ACOG Fellows can propose either a revision to a current code or a new diagnostic code. To do so, contact the Committee on Coding and Nomenclature at ACOG, PO Box 96920, 409 12th Street, SW, Washington, DC 20090-6920.

The following guidelines should be used to ensure accurate diagnostic coding:

▨ Do not select a code using only the Alphabetic Index (Volume 2). Sometimes a code listed in the index will appear to be the correct one. However, the Tabular List (Volume 1) may include additional information that indicates another code would be a better, more specific diagnosis. For example, an entry in the Alphabetic Index for "Lesion, vagina" refers the user to code 623.8. However, code 623.8 is defined in the Tabular List as "Other specified noninflammatory disorders of vagina." The user can check the related codes in the same subcategory and may find a more specific code, such as "Vaginal hematoma" (623.6) or "Polyp of vagina" (623.7) that better describes the patient's condition.

▨ Select the most specific code. When the exact diagnostic term is not listed in the Alphabetic Index, the user should look for a more specific term. For example, the term "corpus luteum insufficiency" is not in the Alphabetic Index because it may have several different causes. The user should look up a term in the index that indicates the specific cause of the condition, such as "dysfunction, ovary" or "deficiency, hormone."

▨ Report the code using all the required digits. Diagnoses may have a total of three, four, or five required digits. For example, code 220 (benign neoplasm of ovary) includes only three digits, code 611.0 (inflammatory disease of breast) includes four digits, and code 616.51 (ulceration of vulva in diseases classified elsewhere) includes five digits.

▨ Read any notes or instructions associated with the terms and codes in both Volume 1 and Volume 2.

▨ Do not report a diagnosis as "Rule out," "Probable," or "Suspected." The physician may document a specific condition as a suspected one, but if a definitive diagnosis is not confirmed, only the symptoms are coded on the claim form. Reporting a suspected condition as confirmed can complicate the patient's future insurance coverage.

ICD-9-CM includes a number of coding conventions that assist in the selection of a correct code. The conventions are discussed in the introductions to Volume 1 and Volume 2.

FORMAT AND USE OF THIS BOOK

ICD-9-CM Abridged: Diagnostic Coding in Obstetrics and Gynecology 2010 is a pocket-sized reference to the diagnostic codes most commonly used by obstetrician–gynecologists. It is not a replacement for the complete ICD-9-CM book. As noted previously, it is essential that physicians purchase a new copy of the complete ICD-9-CM every year.

ICD-9-CM Abridged follows the format of the complete ICD-9-CM book. The Alphabetic Index to Diseases and Injuries, which lists terms that identify diseases, conditions, and symptoms, refers the reader to a specific code in the Tabular List of the book. The introductions to the Alphabetic Index to Diseases and Injuries and sections of the Tabular List include brief guidelines on using the information in these sections. Finally, *ICD-9-CM Abridged* includes a section with two supplementary classifications: 1) factors influencing health status and contact with health services (V codes) and 2) external causes of injury and poisoning (E codes). Appendix A lists diagnostic codes for termination of pregnancy. Appendix B lists diagnostic codes for reporting abnormal Pap smear results, cervical dysplasia, and cancer. Appendix C lists diagnostic codes for obstetric ultrasound procedures. Appendix D discusses the ICD-10-CM implementation in the United States.

1

New, Expanded, and Revised ICD-9-CM Codes

New, expanded, and revised ICD-9-CM codes became effective October 1, 2009.

The Health Insurance Portability and Accountability Act of 1996 (HIPAA) requires providers to use the medical code set that is valid at the time the service is provided. Therefore, physicians must begin using the new codes to report their services beginning on the date they became effective.

Following is a list of code changes of interest to obstetrician–gynecologists. New codes or changed wording in existing codes are underlined. Deleted wording has a strikethrough line.

ENDOMETRIAL HYPERPLASIA

Codes in the "disorders of uterus, not elsewhere classified" (621) category were revised and two codes added to capture benign hormonal effects of unopposed estrogen (621.34, benign endometrial hyperplasia) and endometrial precancerous lesions (621.35, endometrial intraepithelial neoplasia [EIN]).

621 Disorders of Uterus, Not Elsewhere Classified
    621.3   Endometrial hyperplasia
           ~~Hyperplasia (adenomatous) (cystic) (glandular) of endometrium~~
           ~~Hyperplastic endometritis~~
    621.30 Endometrial hyperplasia, unspecified
           <u>Hyperplasia (adenomatous) (cystic)</u>
           <u>(glandular) of endometrium</u>
           <u>Hyperplastic endometritis</u>
    621.31 Simple endometrial hyperplasia without atypia
           <u>Excludes: benign endometrial hyperplasia (621.34)</u>
    621.32 Complex endometrial hyperplasia without atypia
           <u>Excludes: benign endometrial hyperplasia (621.34)</u>
    621.33 Endometrial hyperplasia with atypia
           <u>Excludes: endometrial intraepithelial neoplasia [EIN] (621.35)</u>
    <u>621.34 Benign endometrial hyperplasia</u>
    <u>621.35 Endometrial intraepithelial neoplasia [EIN]</u>
           <u>Excludes: malignant neoplasm of endometrium with</u>
           <u>endometrial intraepithelial neoplasia [EIN] (182.0)</u>

MAJOR PUERPERAL INFECTIONS

Category 670 (major puerperal infection) was expanded to capture postpartum infections, such as endometritis, sepsis, and septic pelvic thrombophlebitis with their own unique codes. Prior to this change, code 670.0x (major puerperal infection) included these postpartum infections. The codes in the 670 series require a fifth digit to denote the current episode of care (i.e., unspecified, delivered, or postpartum).

670   Major Puerperal Infection
~~[0,2,4]~~
~~Use 0 as fourth digit for category 670~~
~~Puerperal:~~
~~endometritis~~
~~fever (septic)~~
~~pelvic:~~
~~cellulitis~~
~~sepsis~~
~~peritonitis~~
~~pyemia~~
~~salpingitis~~
~~septicemia~~

670.0   Major puerperal infection, <u>unspecified</u>
[0,2,4]
670.1   Puerperal endometritis
[0,2,4]
670.2   Puerperal sepsis
[0,2,4] Puerperal pyemia
670.3   Puerperal septic thrombophlebitis
[0,2,4]
670.8   Other major puerperal infection
[0,2,4] Puerperal:
     pelvic cellulitis
     peritonitis
     salpingitis

CONGENITAL ANOMALIES OF BREAST

To make it clear that code 757.6 (Specified anomalies of breast) represents abnormalities that were present at birth, the term "congenital" was added.

757   Congenital anomalies of the integument
    757.6 Specified <u>congenital</u> anomalies of breast
        <u>Congenital a</u>Absent breast or nipple
    <u>Excludes: micromastia (611.82)</u>

INCONCLUSIVE MAMMOGRAM

Due to what is termed as dense breasts a routine mammogram may produce inconclusive findings. While dense breasts are not considered an abnormality, it is often the reason further testing is needed in order to confirm that no malignancy is present. A new code was created to explain this circumstance and justify further testing. Further, the title of category 793 was revised to have the term "abnormal" be nonessential which allows the inconclusive test to be coded that is not necessarily abnormal. The term nonessential as it relates to ICD-9-CM is defined on page 5.

793 Nonspecific <u>(abnormal)</u> findings on radiological and other <u>examination</u> of body structure

    793.8 Breast
        <u>793.82 Inconclusive mammogram</u>
            <u>Dense breasts NOS</u>
            <u>Inconclusive mammogram NEC</u>
            <u>Inconclusive mammography due to dense</u>
            <u>breasts</u>
            <u>Inconclusive mammography NEC</u>
      793.89 Other <u>(abnormal)</u> findings on radiological
            examination of breast

FERTILITY PRESERVATION COUNSELING AND PROCEDURE

New codes were developed that recognize that more and more patients are living significant portions of their life following the diagnosis of cancer. Some types of cancer treatment can affect a person's ability to conceive a child or maintain a pregnancy. However, since it may be possible to protect fertility before and after cancer treatments the American Society for Reproductive Medicine (ASRM) in collaboration with ACOG developed codes for encounters to preserve fertility.

The first goal of these codes is to enable coding of visits when the patient is counseled about their fertility preservation options before starting treatment (eg. chemotherapy, surgery, and/or radiation) by their Ob/Gyn or fertility specialist. The second goal is to explain that a procedure (eg, removal and storage of embryos, ova, etc.) is being performed to maintain fertility prior to treatment that may cause infertility.

The use of these codes is not limited to those seeking this advice or procedure prior to cancer treatment. They may be applied to individuals prior to other treatments that could affect fertility.

V26 Procreative management
V26.4 General counseling and advice
V26.42 Encounter for fertility preservation counseling
Encounter for fertility preservation counseling prior to cancer therapy
Encounter for fertility preservation counseling prior to surgical removal of gonads

V26.8 Other specified procreative management
V26.82 Encounter for fertility preservation procedure
Encounter for fertility preservation procedure prior to cancer therapy
Encounter for fertility preservation procedure prior to surgical removal of gonads

2

Alphabetic Index to
Diseases and Injuries

The ICD-9-CM Volume 2: Diseases: Alphabetic Index is usually placed in the front of the ICD-9-CM book before Volume 1. The Alphabetic Index contains terms with subterms, and sub-subterms that identify diseases, conditions, and symptoms. These refer the user to a specific code in Volume 1. Terms in the index can be nouns or adjectives. For example, the main term "Bleeding" has more than 30 subterms indented below it, including "postmenopausal," which refers the user to code 627.1 in the Tabular List. This subterm has an indented sub-subterm "following induced menopause" which refers the user to code 627.4.

ALPHABETIC INDEX (VOLUME 2) CONVENTIONS

Volume 2 conventions relate to nonessential and essential modifiers and the abbreviation NEC (not elsewhere classified). In addition, the index contains three tables with their own rules.

NONESSENTIAL MODIFIERS

Nonessential modifiers are words or phrases in parentheses that may or may not be documented in a patient's record but are designed to assure the user that a code is correct in a specific case. These modifiers are enclosed in parentheses. For example, the index lists:

> Inflammation, inflamed, inflammatory
> labium (majus) (minus) 616.10

The nonessential modifiers "(majus) (minus)" assure the user that 616.10 is reported for an inflammation of the labia, whether it is documented as labium minus, majus, both, or neither.

ESSENTIAL MODIFIERS

Most main terms are followed by indented subterms that describe different conditions or other factors that will determine the correct code in a specific case. These subterms are called "essential modifiers" because the condition must be documented in a patient's record in order for the code to be reported. Sometimes there are several levels of indention. For example, the index lists three columns of indented terms under the main term "Inflammation," including:

> Inflammation, inflamed, inflammatory
> > mammary gland 611.0
> > > puerperal, postpartum 675.2

In order to report code 675.2, the documentation must indicate that the patient has an inflammation of the mammary gland and is in the postpartum period. If she is not in the postpartum period, then code 611.0 is reported.

TABLES

In addition to the listing of terms and subterms, Volume 2 includes 3 tables. The hypertension table and the neoplasm table are listed alphabetically as part of the general Alphabetic Index. The Table of Drugs and Chemicals, not often used by ob-gyns, is not included in this book.

Hypertension Table

The hypertension table lists types of hypertension, many in combination with other conditions, such as hypertension with heart involvement or hypertension affecting a pregnant patient. The table differentiates between malignant, benign, and unspecified hypertension. Users should refer to Volume 1 to ensure that the code listed in the table is the correct one for the specific case.

Neoplasm Table

The neoplasm table lists codes for types of neoplasms by specific anatomic sites. The table differentiates between 3 categories of malignant (primary, secondary, and carcinoma in situ), benign, uncertain behavior, and unspecified neoplasms. These terms are defined in the index immediately preceding the table.

When coding for a neoplasm, users should not immediately turn to the neoplasm table in the index. First, they should look up the term used by the physician to describe the neoplasm (eg, basal cell or epidermoid). The index may either:

- Refer the user to a specific code in Volume 1 OR

- Refer the coder to the neoplasm table in Volume 2 (eg, Lymphoma, benign— see Neoplasm, by site, benign).

In either case, users should refer to Volume 1 to ensure that the code listed is the correct one for the specific case.

ALPHABETIC INDEX

A

Abdomen, acute (*see also* condition) 789.0
Abdominalgia 789.0
Aberrant (congenital) breast 757.6
Ablatio, placentae—*see* Placenta, ablatio
Ablation, uterus 621.8
Abnormal, abnormality, abnormalities
   (*see also* Anomaly)
  acid-base balance 276.4
  amnion 658.9
  autosomes NEC 758.5
    13 758.1
    18 758.2
    21 or 22 758.0
    D_1 758.1
    E_3 758.2
    G 758.0
  basal metabolic rate (BMR) 794.7
  blood pressure
    elevated (without diagnosis of hypertension) 796.2
    low (*see also* Hypotension) 458.9
      reading (nonspecific) 796.3
  blood sugar 790.29
  bowel sounds 787.5
  cervix (acquired) NEC 622.9
    congenital 752.40
    in pregnancy or childbirth 654.6
      causing obstructed labor 660.2
  chest sounds 786.7
  chorion 658.9
  chromosomal NEC 758.89
  clinical findings NEC 796.4
  dynia (*see also* Defect, coagulation)
      286.9
  fat distribution 782.9
  feces 787.7
  findings without manifest disease—*see*
      Findings, abnormal
  fluid
    amniotic 792.3
    peritoneal 792.9
    vaginal 792.9
  function studies, thyroid 794.5
  glucose 790.29
    in pregnancy, childbirth, or puerperium
        648.8
    nonfasting 790.29
  histology NEC 795.4

Abnormal, abnormality, abnormalities—
      (continued)
  increase in
    appetite 783.6
    development 783.9
  karyotype 795.2
  laboratory findings—*see* Findings,
      abnormal
  loss of height 781.91
  loss of weight 783.21
  mammogram—*see* abnormal radiological
      examination, breast
  Mantoux test 795.5
  metabolism (*see also* condition)
      783.9
  Papanicolaou (smear)—*see* Papanicolaou
      smear
  percussion, chest 786.7
  placenta—*see* Placenta, abnormal
  radiological examination 793.99
    abdomen NEC 793.6
    breast 793.89
      mammogram NOS 793.80
      mammographic
        calcification 793.89
        microcalcification 793.81
    gastrointestinal tract 793.4
    genitourinary organs 793.5
    image test inconclusive due to excess
        body fat 793.91
    retroperitoneum 793.6
    skin and subcutaneous tissue
        793.9
  red blood cells (morphology) (volume)
      790.09
  serum enzyme level 790.5
  sperm 792.2
  sputum 786.4
  stool NEC 787.7
    bloody 578.1
      occult 792.1
    bulky 787.7
    color (dark) (light) 792.1
    content (fat) (mucus) (pus) 792.1
  test results without manifest disease—*see*
      Findings, abnormal
  toxicology (findings) NEC 796.0
  ultrasound results—*see* Findings, abnormal,
      structure

Abnormal, abnormality, abnormalities—
(continued)
urination NEC 788.69 (*see also* Urine)
weight
   gain 783.1
     of pregnancy 646.1
      with hypertension—*see* Toxemia,
        of pregnancy
   loss 783.21
ABO, incompatibility reaction 999.6
Aborter, habitual or recurrent NEC
without current pregnancy 629.81
current abortion (*see also* Abortion,
    spontaneous) 634.9
observation in current pregnancy
    646.3
testing male partner of V26.35
Abortion (complete) (incomplete)
failed 638.9
with
   damage to pelvic organ (laceration)
    (rupture) (tear) 638.2
   embolism (air) (amniotic fluid)
    (blood clot) (septic)
    638.6
   genital tract and pelvic infection
    638.0
   hemorrhage, delayed or excessive
    638.1
   metabolic disorder 638.4
   renal failure (acute) 638.3
   sepsis (genital tract) (pelvic organ)
    638.0
    urinary tract 638.7
   shock (postoperative) (septic)
    638.5
   specified complication NEC
    638.7
   toxemia 638.3
   unspecified complication(s)
    638.8
   urinary tract infection 638.7
following threatened abortion—*see*
    Abortion, by type
habitual or recurrent
with
   current abortion (*see also* Abortion,
    spontaneous) 634.9
   current pregnancy 646.3
   without current pregnancy 629.81
induced (legal)—*see* Abortion, legal
late—*see* Abortion, spontaneous

Abortion *(continued)*
legal (legal indication) (medical indication)
    (under medical supervision)
with
   damage to pelvic organ (rupture)
    (tear) 635.2
   embolism (air) (amniotic fluid)
    (blood clot) (pulmonary)
    (septic) 635.6
   genital tract and pelvic infection
    635.0
   hemorrhage, delayed or excessive
    635.1
   metabolic disorder 635.4
   renal failure (acute) 635.3
   sepsis (genital tract) (pelvic organ)
    635.0
    urinary tract 635.7
   shock (postoperative) (septic)
    635.5
   specified complication NEC 635.7
   toxemia 635.3
   unspecified complication(s) 635.8
   urinary tract infection 635.7
missed 632
septic—*see* Abortion, by type, with sepsis
spontaneous 634.9
with
   damage to pelvic organ (rupture)
    (tear) 634.2
   embolism (air) (amniotic fluid)
    (blood clot) (septic) 634.6
   genital tract and pelvic infection
    634.0
   hemorrhage, delayed or excessive
    634.1
   metabolic disorder 634.4
   renal failure 634.3
   sepsis (genital tract) (pelvic organ)
    634.0
    urinary tract 634.7
   shock (postoperative) (septic)
    634.5
   specified complication NEC 634.7
with
   toxemia 634.3
   unspecified complication(s) 634.8
   urinary tract infection 634.7
surgical—*see* Abortion, legal
therapeutic—*see* Abortion, legal
threatened 640.0
tubal—*see* Pregnancy, tubal
Abruption, placenta—*see* Placenta, abruptio

Abscess (acute) (chronic) (*see also* Cellulitis)
  abdomen, abdominal
    cavity—*see* Abscess, peritoneum
    wall 682.2
  abdominopelvic—*see* Abscess, peritoneum
  anorectal 566
  anus 566
  appendix 540.1
  areola (acute) (chronic) (nonpuerperal)
      611.0
    puerperal, postpartum 675.1
  back (any part) 682.2
  Bartholin's gland 616.3
    with or following
      abortion—*see* Abortion, by type,
          with sepsis
        following abortion 639.0
      ectopic or molar pregnancy (*see also*
          categories 633.0–633.9)
          639.0
      complicating pregnancy or puer-
          perium 646.6
  bladder (wall) 595.89
  bowel 569.5
  breast (acute) (chronic) 611.0
    puerperal, postpartum 675.1
  broad ligament (chronic) (*see also*
          Disease, pelvis, inflammatory)
          614.4
    acute 614.3
  buttock 682.5
  cecum 569.5
    with appendicitis 540.1
  cervix (stump) (*see also* Cervicitis)
          616.0
  colon (wall) 569.5
  corpus luteum (*see also* Salpingo-oophoritis)
          614.2
  cul-de-sac (Douglas') (posterior) (*see also*
          Disease, pelvis, inflammatory)
          614.4
    acute 614.3
  extraperitoneal—*see* Abscess, peritoneum
  fallopian tube (*see also* Salpingo-oophoritis)
          614.2
  fecal 569.5
  flank 682.2
  gastric 535.0
  genital organ or tract 616.9
    with or following
      abortion—*see* Abortion, by type,
          with sepsis
        following abortion 639.0

Abscess *(continued)*
  genital organ or tract *(continued)*
    with or following *(continued)*
      ectopic or molar pregnancy (*see also*
          categories 630–633.9)
          639.0
    puerperal, postpartum, childbirth 670.8
  genitourinary system, tuberculous (*see
          also* Tuberculosis) 016.9
  gland, glandular (lymph) (acute) NEC
          683
  gonorrheal NEC (*see also* Gonococcus)
          098.0
  ileocecal 540.1
  iliac (region) 682.2
  inguinal (region) 682.2
    lymph gland or node 683
  intersphincteric (anus) 566
  intestine, intestinal 569.5
    rectal 566
  intra-abdominal (*see also* Abscess, peri-
          toneum) 567.22
    postoperative 998.59
  intraperitoneal—*see* Abscess, peritoneum
  ischiorectal 566
  kidney
    with or following
      abortion—*see* Abortion, by type,
          with urinary tract infection
        following abortion 639.8
      ectopic or molar pregnancy (*see also*
          categories 630–633.9)
          639.8
    complicating pregnancy or puerperium
          646.6
  labium (majus) (minus) 616.4
    complicating pregnancy, childbirth, or
          puerperium 646.6
  lacunar 597.0
  lymph, lymphatic, gland or node (acute)
          683
  marginal (anus) 566
  mesosalpinx (*see also* Salpingo-oophoritis)
          614.2
  milk 675.1
  mons pubis 682.2
  mural 682.2
  nabothian (follicle) (*see also* Cervicitis)
          616.0
  nates 682.5
  navel 682.2
  nipple 611.0
    puerperal, postpartum 675.0

Abscess *(continued)*
omentum—*see* Abscess, peritoneum
operative wound 998.59
ovary, ovarian (corpus luteum) (*see also*
    Salpingo-oophoritis)
    614.2
paravaginal (*see also* Vaginitis) 616.10
pectoral (region) 682.2
pelvis, pelvic (chronic) (*see also* Disease,
    pelvis, inflammatory) 614.4
  acute 614.3
  tuberculous (*see also* Tuberculosis) 016.9
perineum, perineal (superficial) 682.2
  deep (with urethral involvement) 597.0
  urethra 597.0
perirectal (staphylococcal) 566
peritoneum, peritoneal (perforated) (rup-
    tured) 567.22
  with or following
    abortion—*see* Abortion, by type,
        with sepsis
      following abortion 639.0
    appendicitis 540.1
    ectopic or molar pregnancy (*see also*
        categories 630–633.9) 639.0
  pelvic (*see also* Disease, pelvis, inflam-
      matory) 614.4
    acute 614.3
  postoperative 998.59
  puerperal, postpartum, childbirth 670.8
periurethral 597.0
  gonococcal (acute) 098.0
    chronic or duration of 2 months or
        over 098.2
pilonidal 685.0
pubis 682.2
puerperal—*see* Puerperal, abscess, by site
pyemic—*see* Septicemia
pyloric valve 535.0
rectovaginal septum 569.5
rectum 566
retroperineal 682.2
retroperitoneal 567.38
  postprocedural 998.59
round ligament (*see also* Disease, pelvis,
    inflammatory) 614.4
  acute 614.3
sigmoid 569.5
Skene's duct or gland 597.0
stitch 998.59
stomach (wall) 535.0
trunk 682.2
tubal (*see also* Salpingo-oophoritis) 614.2

Abscess *(continued)*
tubo-ovarian (*see also* Salpingo-oophoritis)
    614.2
umbilicus NEC 682.2
urachus 682.2
urethra (gland) 597.0
urinary 597.0
uterus, uterine (wall) (*see also*
    Endometritis) 615.9
  ligament (*see also* Disease, pelvis,
      inflammatory) 614.4
    acute 614.3
  neck (*see also* Cervicitis) 616.0
vagina (wall) (*see also* Vaginitis) 616.10
vaginorectal (*see also* Vaginitis) 616.10
vermiform appendix 540.1
vesical 595.89
vesicouterine pouch (*see also* Disease,
    pelvis, inflammatory) 614.4
vulva 616.4
  complicating pregnancy, childbirth, or
      puerperium 646.6
vulvovaginal gland (*see also* Vaginitis)
    616.3
Absence (organ or part) (complete or partial)
bowel sounds 787.5
breast(s) (acquired) V45.71
  congenital 757.6
broad ligament (congenital) 752.19
cervix (acquired) (uteri) V88.01
  congenital 752.49
  with remaining uterus V88.03
  and uterus V88.01
clitoris (congenital) 752.49
fallopian tube(s) (acquired) V45.77
  congenital 752.19
fibrin 790.92
fibrinogen (congenital) 286.3
  acquired 286.6
labium (congenital) (majus) (minus)
    752.49
ligament, broad (congenital) 752.19
menstruation 626.0
nipple (congenital) 757.6
  acquired V45.71
ovary (acquired) V45.77
  congenital 752.0
red cell 284.9
  acquired (secondary) 284.81
  congenital (hereditary) 284.01
  idiopathic 284.9
sex chromosomes 758.81
thyroid (gland) (surgical) with hypothy-
    roidism 244.0

Absence *(continued)*
  ureter (congenital) 753.4
  urethra (congenital) 753.8
  urinary system, part NEC, (congenital)
      753.8
  uterus (acquired) V88.01
    congenital 752.3
    with remaining cervical stump V88.02
      and cervix V88.01
  vagina, congenital 752.49
    acquired V45.77
  vulva, congenital 752.49
Absorption
  chemical NEC, drug or noxious substance,
      through placenta or breast
      milk
    suspected, affecting management of
      pregnancy 655.5
  uremic—*see* Uremia
Abuse
  adult (spouse) 995.80
    emotional (psychological) 995.82
    multiple forms 995.85
    neglect (nutritional) 995.84
    physical 995.81
    sexual 995.83
  alcohol (*see also* Alcoholism) 305.0
    dependent 303.9
    nondependent 305.0
  child 995.50
    counseling
      perpetrator
        nonparent V62.83
        parent V61.22
        victim V61.21
    emotional (psychological) 995.51
    multiple forms 995.59
    neglect (nutritional) 995.52
    physical 995.54
    sexual 995.53
  drugs, nondependent NEC 305.9
    amphetamine type 305.7
    antidepressants 305.8
    anxiolytic 305.4
    barbiturates 305.4
    caffeine 305.9
    cannabis, marijuana 305.2
    cocaine type 305.6
    hallucinogens (LSD) 305.3
    hashish 305.2
    hypnotic 305.4
    inhalant 305.9
    mixed 305.9

Abuse *(continued)*
  drugs, nondependent *(continued)*
    morphine (opioid) type 305.5
    phencyclidine (PCP) 305.9
    sedative 305.4
    tranquilizers 305.4
    tobacco 305.1
    complicating, pregnancy 649.0
Acantholysis 701.8
Acanthosis (acquired) (nigricans) (adult)
      (juvenile) 701.2
Accessory (congenital) (*see also* Double)
  autosome(s) NEC 758.5
    21 or 22 758.0
  breast tissue, axilla 757.6
  cervix 752.49
  chromosome(s) NEC 758.5
    13–15 758.1
    16–18 758.2
    21 or 22 758.0
    D_1 758.1
    E_3 758.2
    G 758.0
    sex 758.81
  external os 752.49
  fallopian tube (fimbria) (ostium) 752.19
  hymen 752.49
  ligament, broad 752.19
  nipple 757.6
  ovary 752.0
  placental lobe—*see* Placenta, abnormal
  urinary organ or tract NEC 753.8
Accident, accidental (*see also* condition)
  cerebrovascular (current) (CVA)—*see*
      Disease, cerebrovascular,
      acute
Accreta placenta (without hemorrhage)
      667.0
  with hemorrhage 666.0
Acetonemia, diabetic 250.1
Acetonuria 791.6
Achroma, cutis 709.00
Acidosis 276.2
  diabetic 250.1
  lactic 276.2
  metabolic NEC 276.2
    with respiratory acidosis 276.4
  respiratory 276.2
    complicated by
      metabolic acidosis 276.4
      metabolic alkalosis 276.4
Aciduria 791.9
  orotic (congenital) (hereditary) 281.4
Acmesthesia 782.0

Acne (pustular) (vulgaris) 706.1
  erythematosa or rosacea 695.3
  summer 692.72
Acneiform drug eruptions 692.3
Acquired immune deficiency syndrome—
  see Human immunodefi-
  ciency virus (disease)
Acrodermatitis atrophicans (chronica)
  701.8
Acrohyperhidrosis 780.8
Acromastitis 611.0
Acystia 753.8
Addiction (*see also* Dependence)
  alcoholic (ethyl) (methyl) (wood) 303.9
    complicating pregnancy, childbirth, or
      puerperium 648.4
    suspected damage to fetus affecting
      management of pregnancy
      655.4
  drug (*see also* Dependence) 304.9
  heroin 304.0
  morphine (-like substances) 304.0
  nicotine 305.1
  opium 304.0
  tobacco 305.1
  wine 303.9
Addison's
  anemia (pernicious) 281.0
  keloid (morphea) 701.0
Adenitis (*see also* Lymphadenitis)
  acute, unspecified site 683
    epidemic infectious 075
  axillary, acute 683
  Bartholin's gland 616.8
  cervical, acute 683
  chancroid (Ducrey's bacillus) 099.0
  gangrenous 683
  gonorrheal NEC 098.89
  infectious 075
  lymph gland or node, except mesenteric
    acute 683
  phlegmonous 683
  Skene's duct or gland (*see also* Urethritis)
    597.89
  urethral gland (*see also* Urethritis) 597.89
  venereal NEC 099.8
Adenoacanthoma—*see* Neoplasm, by site,
  malignant
Adenocarcinoma (*see also* Neoplasm, by
  site, malignant)
  in adenomatous polyp, polypoid or tubu-
    lar adenoma—*see* Neoplasm,
    by site, malignant

Adenocarcinoma (*(continued)*
  infiltrating duct
    with Paget's disease—*see* Neoplasm,
      breast, malignant
    specified site—*see* Neoplasm, by site,
      malignant
    unspecified site 174.9
  intraductal (noninfiltrating)
    papillary, specified site—*see* Neoplasm,
      by site, in situ
    unspecified site 233.0
  lobular, specified site—*see* Neoplasm, by
    site, malignant
    unspecified site 174.9
  serous, specified site—*see* Neoplasm, by
    site, malignant
    unspecified site 183.0
  signet ring cell—*see* Neoplasm, by site,
    malignant
Adenofibroma
  clear cell—*see* Neoplasm, by site, benign
  endometrioid 220
    borderline malignancy 236.2
    malignant 183.0
  mucinous or serous, specified site—*see*
    Neoplasm, by site, benign
  specified site—*see* Neoplasm, by site,
    benign
  unspecified site 220
Adenofibrosis
  breast 610.2
  endometroid 617.0
Adenomyoma—*see* Neoplasm, by site,
  benign
Adenomyometritis (Adenomyosis)
  (uterus) (internal) 617.0
Adenopathy (lymph gland) 785.6
Adenopharyngitis 462
Adenophlegmon 683
Adenosalpingitis 614.1
Adenosis
  breast (sclerosing) 610.2
  vagina, congenital 752.49
Adherent
  labium (minus) 624.4
  placenta 667.0
    with hemorrhage 666.0
  scar (skin) NEC 709.2
  tendon in scar 709.2
Adhesion(s), adhesive (postinfectional)
  (postoperative)
  abdominal (wall) (*see also* Adhesions,
    peritoneum) 568.0

Adhesion(s), adhesive *(continued)*
   amnion to fetus 658.8
   appendix 543.9
   cervicovaginal 622.3
     congenital 752.49
     postpartal 674.8
      old 622.3
   cervix 622.3
   clitoris 624.4
   intestine (postoperative) (bowel) (omen-
       tum) *(see also* Adhesions,
       peritoneum) 568.0
   labium (majus) (minus), congenital 752.49
   ovary 614.6
     congenital (to cecum, kidney, or
       omentum) 752.0
   pelvic (peritoneal) (postoperative)
      (postinfection) 614.6
     postpartal (old) 614.6
     tuberculous *(see also* Tuberculosis)
      016.9
   peritoneum, peritoneal (fibrous) (post-
      operative) 568.0
     with hernia—*see* Hernia, by site, with
      obstruction
     gangrenous—*see* Hernia, by site, with
      gangrene
     pelvic (postoperative) (postinfective)
      614.6
     to uterus 614.6
   postoperative (gastrointestinal tract) *(see
      also* Adhesions, peritoneum)
     pelvic 614.9
     urethra 598.2
   postpartal, old (vulva, perineum) 624.4
   tubo-ovarian 614.6
   uterus 621.5
     to abdominal wall 614.6
      in pregnancy or childbirth 654.4
   vagina (chronic) (postoperative) (post-
      radiation) 623.2
   vaginitis (congenital) 752.49
Administration, prophylactic
   antibiotics V07.39
   antitoxin, any V07.2
   gamma globulin, RhoGAM V07.2
   other prophylactic chemotherapy V07.39
Admission (encounter) (for)
   adjustment (of) (device)
     breast (implant) (prosthesis) V52.4
      exchange (different material)
       (different size) V52.4
     diaphragm (contraceptive) V25.02

Admission *(continued)*
   adjustment (of) (device) *(continued)*
     intrauterine contraceptive V25.1
     urinary (catheter) V53.6
   artificial insemination V26.1
   attention to artificial opening (of)—*see*
      Attention to artificial opening
   blood typing, Rh V72.86
   breast
     implant exchange (different material)
      (different size) V52.4
     reconstruction following mastectomy
      V51.0
     removal
      prophylactiv V50.41
      tissue expander without synchronous
       insertion of permanent
       implant V52.4
   change of
     catheter in artificial opening—*see*
      Attention to, artificial,
      opening
     dressing (surgical dressing) V58.3
   chemotherapy V58.11
   circumcision, ritual or routine (in absence
      of medical indication) V50.2
   contraceptive—*see* Contraception
   convalescence following V66.9
     chemotherapy V66.2
     radiotherapy V66.1
     surgery V66.0
     treatment (for) NEC V66.5
      combined V66.6
   counseling—*see* Counseling
   desensitization to allergens V07.1
   drug monitoring, therapeutic V58.83
   ear piercing V50.3
   end-of-life care V66.7
   examination—*see* Examination V70.9
   fertility preservation (prior to cancer
     gonads) V26.82
   fitting (of) (device)
     breast (implant) (prosthesis) V52.4
     cystostomy device V53.6
   follow-up examination (routine)—*see*
      Follow-up
   health advice, education, or instruction
     V65.4
   hormone replacement therapy (post-
     menopausal) V07.4
   hospice care V66.7
   issue of
     medical certificate NEC V68.0

Admission *(continued)*
 repeat prescription NEC V68.1
 contraceptive device NEC V25.49
 nonmedical reason NEC V68.89
 observation—*see* Observation
 ovarian removal, prophylactic V50.42
 palliative care V66.7
 Papanicolaou smear—*see* Papanicolaou
   smear
 paternity testing V70.4
 plastic surgery (cosmetic, elective) NEC
   V50.1
  breast reconstruction following mas-
    tectomy V51.0
  following healed injury or operation
    V51.8
 postpartum observation
  immediately after delivery V24.0
  routine follow-up V24.2
 poststerilization (for restoration) V26.0
 prenatal V22.1
  first pregnancy V22.0
  high-risk pregnancy V23.9
  specified problem NEC V23.89
 procreative management V26.9
  specified type NEC V26.8
 prophylactic
  administration of
   antitoxin, any (RhoGAM) V07.2
   antibiotics V07.39
   other chemotherapy V07.39
  organ removal V50.49
   breast V50.41
   ovary V50.42
 radiotherapy V58.0
 removal of
  breast tissue expander without syn-
    chronous insertion of perma-
    nent implant V52.4
  catheter from artificial opening—*see*
    Attention to, artificial, opening
  cystostomy catheter V55.5
  intrauterine contraceptive device V25.42
  subdermal implantable contraceptive
    V25.43
  surgical dressing (sutures) V58.3
  ureteral stent V53.6
 sterilization V25.2
 terminal care V66.7
 tests only—*see* Test
 therapeutic drug monitoring V58.83
 therapy (*see also* Aftercare)
  chemotherapy V58.1

Admission *(continued)*
 therapy *(continued)*
  long-term (current) drug use NEC
    V58.69 (*see also* Drug,
    therapy)
  radiation V58.0
  ultrasound, routine fetal V28.3
 tubal ligation V25.2
 tuboplasty for previous sterilization
   V26.0
 vaccination, prophylactic (against)—*see*
   Vaccination
 vasectomy V25.2
 X-ray of chest
  for suspected tuberculosis V71.2
  routine V72.5
Adrenarche, precocious 259.1
Afibrinogenemia (congenital) 286.3
 acquired 286.6
 postpartum 666.3
Aftercare
 artificial openings—*see* Attention to, artificial, opening
 blood transfusion without reported diagnosis V58.2
 chemotherapy (oral) (intravenous)
   (adjunctive) (maintenance) V58.11
 following surgery (for) (of)
  genital organs or urinary system V58.76
  injury or trauma V58.43
  neoplasm V58.42
  wound closure, planned V58.41
 postpartum
  immediately after delivery V24.0
  routine follow-up V24.2
 postradiation V58.0
 radiation therapy (radiotherapy) V58.0
 removal of dressings (surgical dressings)
   (sutures) V58.3
Agalactia 676.4
Agenesis—*see* Absence, by site, congenital
AIDS (disease) (symptomatic) 042
 Infection—*see* Human immunodeficiency
   virus, infection
AIN I [anal intraepithelial neoplasia I] (histologically confirmed) 569.44
AIN II [anal intraepithelial neoplasia II]
   (histologically confirmed)
   569.44
AIN III [anal intraepithelial neoplasia III]
   230.6
 anal canal 230.5

Air
embolism
with or following
abortion—*see* Abortion, by type,
with embolism
following abortion 639.6
ectopic or molar pregnancy (*see also*
categories 633.0–633.9)
639.6
infusion, perfusion, or transfusion
999.1
due to implanted device—*see*
Complications, due to (presence of) any device, implant,
or graft classified to
996.3–996.5 NEC
in pregnancy, childbirth, or puerperium
673.0
hunger 786.09
Albuminuria (acute) (chronic) (subacute)
791.0
complicating pregnancy, childbirth, or
puerperium 646.2
with hypertension—*see* Toxemia, of
pregnancy
pre-eclamptic (mild) 642.4
severe 642.5
Alcohol, alcoholic (*see also* Alcoholism)
acute intoxication (drunkenness) 305.0
with dependence 303.0
addiction (chronic) 303.9
maternal, with suspected fetal damage
affecting management of
pregnancy 655.4
Alcoholism (chronic) 303.9
acute 303.0
complicating pregnancy, childbirth, or
puerperium 648.4
history V11.3
suspected fetal damage affecting management of pregnancy 655.4
Allen-Masters syndrome 620.6
Allergy, allergic (reaction) 995.3
anaphylactic shock 999.4
angioneurotic edema 995.1
animal (cat) (dog) (epidermal) 477.8
asthma—*see* Asthma
dermatitis (venenata)—*see* Dermatitis
drug, medicinal substance, and biological
(any) (correct medicinal substance properly administered)
(external) (internal) 995.27
eczema—*see* Eczema

Allergy, allergic *(continued)*
gastritis 535.4
pollen (any) (hay fever) 477.0
asthma (*see also* Asthma) 493.0
serum (prophylactic) (therapeutic) 999.5
anaphylactic shock 999.4
skin reaction, specified substance—*see*
Dermatitis, due to
urethritis 597.89
urticaria 708.0
vaccine—*see* Allergy, serum
Allocheiria, allochiria 782.0
Alopecia (pregnancy) (premature) (specific)
704.00
other 704.09
telogen effluvium 704.02
Alzheimer's disease or sclerosis 331.0
Amastia (*see also* Absence, breast) 611.89
Amenorrhea (primary) (secondary)
626.0
due to ovarian dysfunction 256.8
hyperhormonal 256.8
Amputation
cervix (supravaginal) (uteri) (healed) 622.8
in pregnancy or childbirth 654.6
clitoris—*see* Wound, open, clitoris
status (without complication)—*see*
Absence, by site, acquired
genital organ(s) (external) NEC 878.8
complicated 878.9
Amylophagia 307.52
Analgesia (*see also* Anesthesia) 782.0
Anaphylactic shock or reaction—*see* Shock
Anaplasia, cervix 622.1
Anemia (*see also* Sickle Cell, Thalassemia)
280.9
achrestic 281.8
Addison's (pernicious) 281.0
amino acid deficiency 281.4
antineoplastic chemotherapy induced
285.3
due to
antineoplastic chemotherapy 285.3
chemotherapy, antineoplastic 285.3
aplastic 284.9
acquired (secondary) 284.89
congenital 284.01
constitutional 284.01
due to
antineoplastic chemotherapy
284.89
chronic systemic disease 284.89
drugs 284.89

Anemia *(continued)*
    infection 284.89
      radiation 284.89
    idiopathic 284.9
    specified type NEC 284.89
    toxic (paralytic) 284.89
  aregenerative 284.9
    congenital 284.01
  asiderotic 280.9
  blood loss (chronic) (any type) 280.0
    acute 285.1
  chlorotic 280.9
  chronica congenita aregenerativa
      284.01
  chronic simple 281.9
  complicating pregnancy or childbirth
      648.2
  Cooley's (erythroblastic) 282.49
  cytogenic 281.0
  Davidson's (refractory) 284.9
  Diamond-Blackfan (congenital hypoplastic) 284.01
  dimorphic 281.9
  diphasic 281.8
  EPO resistant 285.21
  Erythroblastic, familial 282.49
  Erythropoietin resistant (EPO resistant) 285.21
  Faber's (achlorhydric anemia) 280.9
  factitious (self-induced bloodletting) 280.0
  Fanconi's (congenital pancytopenia) 284.09
  folate (folic acid) deficiency (dietary) (drug-induced) 281.2
  hemorrhagic (chronic) 280.0
    acute 285.1
  hypochromic (idiopathic) 280.9
  hypoplasia, red blood cells 284.81
  in
    chronic illness NEC 285.29
    congenital or familial 284.01
    end-stage renal disease 285.21
    hypoplastic (idiopathic) 284.9
    neoplastic disease 285.22
  Joseph-Diamond-Blackfan (congenital hypoplastic) 284.01
  leptocytosis (hereditary) 282.49
  macrocytic 281.9
    nutritional 281.2
  malabsorption (familial), selective B_{12} with proteinuria 281.1
  malignant (progressive) 281.0

Anemia *(continued)*
  malnutrition 281.9
  megaloblastic 281.9
    combined B_{12} and folate deficiency 281.3
    of or complicating pregnancy 648.2
    refractory 281.3
    specified NEC 281.3
  megalocytic 281.9
  microcytic (hypochromic) 280.9
    familial 282.49
    hypochromic 280.9
  microdrepanocytosis 282.49
  nonregenerative 284.9
  nutritional (deficiency) 281.9
    inadequate dietary iron intake 280.1
    poor iron absorption 280.9
    specified deficiency NEC 281.8
  of chronic illness NEC 285.29
  pernicious 281.0
  pleochromic of sprue 281.8
  posthemorrhagic (chronic) 280.0
    acute 285.1
  postoperative, due to blood loss 285.1
  postpartum 648.2
    malignant (pernicious) 281.0
  puerperal 648.2
  pure red cell 284.81
    congenital 284.01
  refractory (primary), due to
    megaloblastic 281.3
    sideropenic 280.9
  scorbutic 281.8
  secondary (to)
    hemorrhage 280.0
      acute 285.1
    inadequate dietary iron intake 280.1
  semiplastic 284.9
  sickle-cell—*see* Sickle-cell
  sideropenic (refractory) 280.9
  simple chronic 281.9
  target cell (oval) 282.49
  thalassemia 282.49
  thrombocytopenia (*see also* Thrombocytopenia) 287.5
  toxic 284.89
  tropical, macrocytic 281.2
  vegan's 281.1
  vitamin B_{12} deficiency (dietary) 281.1
    pernicious 281.0
  Witts' (achlorhydric anemia) 280.9
  Zuelzer (-Ogden) (nutritional megaloblastic anemia) 281.2
Anesthesia, anesthetic
  complication or reaction NEC (due to)

Anesthesia, anesthetic *(continued)*
 995.2
  correct substance properly administered
   995.2
  overdose or wrong substance given 968.4
 death from
  correct substance properly administered
   995.4
  during delivery 668.9
  overdose or wrong substance given 968.4
 sexual (psychogenic) 302.72
 shock, due to
  correct substance properly administered
   995.4
  overdose or wrong substance given
   968.4
Angina (attack) (syndrome) (vasomotor)
 catarrhal 462
 cruris 443.9
 decubitus 413.0
 erysipelatous 034.0
 erythematous 462
 exudative, chronic 476.0
 infectious 462
 malignant 462
 monocytic 075
 nocturnal 413.0
 Prinzmetal's 413.1
 septic 034.0
 simple 462
 stable NEC 413.9
 staphylococcal 462
 streptococcal 034.0
 variant 413.1
Angiokeratoma—*see* Neoplasm, skin,
  benign
Angioleiomyoma—*see* Neoplasm, connective tissue, benign
Angioma
 malignant—*see* Neoplasm, connective
  tissue, malignant
 placenta—*see* Placenta, abnormal
 serpiginosum 709.1
Angiopathia, angiopathy 459.9
 peripheral 443.9
Anhydration, anhydremia 276.5
 with
  hypernatremia 276.0
  hyponatremia 276.1
Annular (*see also* condition)
 detachment, cervix 622.8
 organ or site, congenital NEC—*see*
  Distortion
Anomaly, anomalous (congenital)
   (unspecified type) (*see also*

Anomaly, anomalous *(continued)*
   Abnormal)
 bladder (neck) (sphincter) (trigone) 753.9
  specified type NEC 753.8
 breast 757.6
  specified type NEC 757.6
 canal of Nuck 752.9
 cervix (uterus) 752.40
  with doubling of vagina and uterus
   752.2
  in pregnancy or childbirth 654.6
   causing obstructed labor 660.2
  specified type NEC 752.49
 chromosomes, chromosomal 758.9
    (*see also* Abnormal, auto-
    somes)
  mitochondrial 758.9
  mosaics 758.89
  sex (complement, XXX) (complement
    XYY) 758.81
   complement, XO or gonadal dysge-
    nesis or Turner's 758.6
  trisomy 21 758.0
 clitoris 752.40
 fallopian tube 752.10
 Gartner's duct 752.41
 hymen 752.40
 kidney(s) (calyx) (pelvis) 753.9
 labium (majus) (minus) 752.40
 ligament
  broad 752.10
  round 752.9
 Müllerian (American Society of
    Reproductive Medicine
    Classifications)
  DES related (report code 760.76 in
    addition to code for anomaly)
 uterus
  aplasia (ASRM Class I) V752.3
  arcuate (ASRM Class VI) V72.3
  bicornuate (complete or partial)
    (ASRM Class IV) 752.3
  didelphus (ASRM Class III)
    752.2
  hypoplasia (ASRM Class I)
    752.3
  septate (ASRM Class V Müllerian
    Anomaly) 752.2
  unicornuate (ASRM Class II)
    752.3
 vagina or cervix
  agenesis (ASRM Class I) 752.49
  hypoplasia (ASRM Class I)
    752.49

Anomaly, anomalous *(continued)*
nipple 757.6
ovary 752.0
paraurethral ducts 753.9
pelvis (bony) complicating delivery 653.0
pigmentation 709.00
rectovaginal (septum) 752.40
renal 753.9
ureter 753.9
obstructive 753.20
specified type NEC 753.4
obstructive 753.29
urethra (valve) 753.9
obstructive 753.6
specified type NEC 753.8
urinary tract or system (any part, except urachus) 753.9
specified type NEC 753.8
uterus 752.3
with only one functioning horn 752.3
in pregnancy or childbirth 654.0
causing obstructed labor 660.2
vagina 752.40
valve formation, ureter 753.29
vesicourethral orifice 753.9
vulva 752.40
Anorexia 783.0
nervosa 307.1
Anovulatory cycle 628.0
Anoxia, cerebral
with or following
abortion—*see* Abortion, by type, with specified complication NEC
following abortion 639.8
ectopic or molar pregnancy (*see also* categories 630–633.9) 639.8
complicating
delivery (cesarean) (instrumental) 669.4
ectopic or molar pregnancy 639.8
obstetric anesthesia or sedation 668.2
during or resulting from a procedure 997.01
Antenatal
care, normal pregnancy V22.1
first V22.0
sampling chorionic villus V28.89
screening—*see* Screening, antenatal
Anteversion
cervix—*see* Anteversion, uterus
uterus, uterine (cervix) (postinfectional) (postpartal, old) 621.6
congenital 752.3

Anomaly, anomalous *(continued)*
in pregnancy or childbirth 654.4
causing obstructed labor 660.2
Antibodies, maternal (blood group) (*see also* Incompatibility) 656.2
anti-D, cord blood 656.1
Anuria 788.5
with or following
abortion—*see* Abortion, by type, with renal failure
following abortion 639.3
ectopic or molar pregnancy (*see also* categories 630–633.9) 639.3
calculus
kidney 592.0
ureter 592.1
due to a procedure 997.5
puerperal, postpartum, childbirth 669.3
sulfonamide, correct substance properly administered 788.5
traumatic (following crushing) 958.5
Anxiety (neurosis) (reaction) (state) 300.00
depression 300.4
generalized 300.02
in
acute stress reaction 308.0
transient adjustment reaction 309.24
panic type 300.01
separation, abnormal 309.21
Aphagia 787.20
psychogenic 307.1
Apnea, apneic (spells) 786.03
sleep NEC (with)
hypersomnia 780.53
hyposomnia, insomnia 780.51
Appendicitis
acute (gangrenous) (inflammatory) (obstructive) 540.9
with perforation, peritonitis, or rupture 540.0
peritoneal abscess 540.1
chronic (recurrent) 542
healed (obliterative) 542
interval 542
obstructive 542
pneumococcal 541
retrocecal 541
subacute (adhesive) 542
Appetite
depraved 307.52
excessive 783.6
psychogenic 307.51

Appetite *(continued)*
  lack or loss *(see also* Anorexia) 783.0
    nonorganic origin 307.59
Arias-Stella phenomenon 621.30
Arrest, arrested
  active phase of labor 661.1
  any plane in pelvis, complicating delivery
      660.1
  cardiac 427.5
    with or following
      abortion—*see* Abortion, by type,
          with specified complication
          NEC
        following abortion 639.8
      ectopic or molar pregnancy *(see also*
          categories 633.0–633.9) 639.8
    complicating
      anesthesia
        correct substance properly admin-
            istered 427.5
        obstetric 668.1
        overdose or wrong substance
            given 968.4
      delivery (cesarean) (instrumental)
          669.4
      surgery 997.1
    personal history V12.53
    postoperative (immediate) 997.1
  development or growth, fetus affecting
      management of pregnancy
      656.5
  transverse (deep) 660.3
Arrhythmia
  postoperative 997.1
  vagal 780.2
Arteriosclerosis, arteriosclerotic 440.9
  renal *(see also* Hypertension, kidney)
      403.90
Arthritis, arthritic (acute) (chronic) (sub-
      acute) 716.9
  meaning Osteoarthritis—*see*
      Osteoarthrosis
  atrophic 714.0
  climacteric NEC 716.3
  deformans *(see also* Osteoarthrosis) 715.9
  degenerative *(see also* Osteoarthrosis)
      715.9
  idiopathic, blennorrheal 099.3
  menopausal NEC 716.3
  nodosa *(see also* Osteoarthrosis) 715.9
  nonpyrogenic NEC 716.9
  primary progressive 714.0
  proliferative 714.0

Arthritis, arthritic *(continued)*
  rheumatic 714.0
  senile or senescent *(see also*
      Osteoarthrosis) 715.9
Arthropathy *(see also* Arthritis) 716.9
Arthrosis *(see also* Osteoarthrosis) 715.9
Artificial
  device (prosthetic)—*see* Fitting, device
  insemination V26.1
  menopause (states) (symptoms) (syndrome)
      627.4
  opening status, vagina V44.7
Ascites 789.5
  abdominal NEC 789.59
  malignant 789.51
ASC-H (atypical squamous cells cannot
      exclude high grade squamous
      intraepithelial lesion)
    anus 796.72
    cervix 795.02
    vagina 795.12
ASC-US (atypical squamous cells of undeter-
      mined significance)
    anus 796.71
    cervix 795.01
    vagina 795.11
Aspermatogenesis 606.0
Aspiration
  acid pulmonary (syndrome) 997.39
  pneumonitis, obstetric 668.0
Asteatosis (cutis) 706.8
Asthenia, asthenic 780.79
Asthenospermia 792.2
Asthma, asthmatic (bronchial) (catarrh)
      (spasmodic) (with) 493.9
  allergic 493.9
    stated cause (external allergen) 493.0
  atopic 493.0
  chronic obstructive pulmonary disease
      (COPD) 493.2
  cough variant 493.82
  endogenous (intrinsic) 493.1
  exercise induced bronchospasm 493.81
  late-onset 493.1
  rhinitis, allergic (hay fever) 493.0
  tuberculous *(see also* Tuberculous,
      pulmonary) 011.9
Atheroma, atheromatous *(see also*
      Arteriosclerosis) 440.9
  skin 706.2
Atonia, atony, atonic
  bladder 596.4
    neurogenic 596.54
  uterus 661.2

Atonia, atony, atonic *(continued)*
  with hemorrhage (postpartum) 666.1
  without hemorrhage
    intrapartum 661.2
    postpartum 669.8
  vesical 596.4
Atresia, atretic (congenital)
  bladder (neck) 753.6
  cervix (acquired) 622.4
    congenital 752.49
    in pregnancy or childbirth 654.6
      causing obstructed labor 660.2
  fallopian tube (acquired) 628.2
    congenital 752.19
  follicular cyst 620.0
  hymen 752.42
    acquired, postinfective 623.3
  ligament, broad 752.19
  ureter 753.29
  ureteropelvic junction 753.21
  ureterovesical orifice 753.22
  urethra (valvular) 753.6
  urinary tract NEC 753.29
  uterus 752.3
    acquired 621.8
  vagina (acquired) 623.2
    congenital 752.49
    postgonococcal (old) 098.2
    postinfectional 623.2
    senile 623.2
  vesicourethral orifice 753.6
  vulva 752.49
    acquired 624.8
Atrophy, atrophic
  appendix 543.9
  blanche (of Milian) 701.3
  breast 611.4
    puerperal, postpartum 676.3
  cervix (mucosa) 622.8
    menopausal 627.8
  colloid, degenerative (senile) 701.3
  diffuse idiopathic, dermatological 701.8
  disuse, pelvic muscles and anal sphincter
    618.83
  emphysema, lung 492.8
  endometrium (senile) 621.8
    cervix 622.8
  fallopian tube (senile), acquired 620.3
  gastritis (chronic) 535.1
  laryngitis, infection 476.0
  myometrium (senile) 621.8
    cervix 622.8
  nasopharynx 472.2

Atrophy, atrophic *(continued)*
  ovary (senile), acquired 620.3
  polyarthritis 714.0
  reticulata 701.8
  rhinitis 472.0
  scar NEC 709.2
  senile, degenerative, of skin 701.3
  skin (patches) (senile) 701.8
  striate and macular 701.3
  subcutaneous 701.9
    due to injection 999.9
  uterus, uterine (acquired) (senile) 621.8
    cervix 622.8
    due to radiation (intended effect) 621.8
  vagina (senile) 627.3
  vulva (primary) (senile) 624.1
Attack
  angina—*see* Angina
  epileptic (*see also* Epilepsy) 345.9
  syncope 780.2
  unconsciousness 780.2
  vasomotor 780.2
  vasovagal (idiopathic) (paroxysmal) 780.2
Attention to artificial opening (of)
  cystostomy V55.5
  nephrostomy V55.6
  ureterostomy V55.6
  urethrostomy V55.6
  urinary tract NEC V55.6
  vagina V55.7
Avulsion (traumatic) (*see also* Wound,
    open, by site) 879.8
  cartilage, symphyseal (inner), complicating
    delivery 665.6
Awareness of heart beat 785.1
Azoospermia 606.0

B
Bacillus (*see also* Infection, bacillus)
  coli
    infection 041.4
      generalized 038.42
    pyemia, septicemia 038.42
Backache (postural) 724.5
Bacteremia 790.7
Bacteriuria, bacteruria 791.9
  with urinary tract infection 599.0
  in pregnancy or puerperium (asympto-
    matic) 646.5
Bartholinitis (suppurating) 616.89
  gonococcal (acute) 098.0
    chronic or duration of 2 months or
      over 098.2

Battered
   adult (spouse) (syndrome) 995.81
   baby or child (syndrome) 995.54
Bedsore (*see also* Ulcer) 707.00
Bereavement V62.82
   as adjustment reaction 309.0
Bicornuate or bicornis uterus 752.3
   in pregnancy or childbirth 654.0
      with obstructed labor 660.2
Bifid—*see* Imperfect, closure
Bifurcation (congenital) (*see also* Imperfect,
            closure)
   ureter 753.4
   urethra 753.8
Bilirubinuria, biliuria 791.4
Biparta, bipartite (*see also* Imperfect,
            closure)
   placenta—*see* Placenta, abnormal
   vagina 752.49
Birth, complications in mother—*see*
            Delivery, complicated
Birthmark 757.32
Black eye NEC 921.0
Blackout 780.2
Bleb(s) 709.8
   emphysematous 492.0
Bleeding (*see also* Hemorrhage) 459.0
   anovulatory 628.0
   atonic, following delivery 666.1
   due to subinvolution 621.1
      puerperal 666.2
   excessive, associated with menopausal
            onset 627.0
   familial (*see also* Defect, coagulation)
            286.9
   following intercourse 626.7
   gastrointestinal 578.9
   hemorrhoids—*see* Hemorrhoids,
            bleeding
   intermenstrual
      irregular 626.6
      regular 626.5
   intraoperative 998.11
   irregular NEC 626.4
   menopausal 627.0
   nipple 611.79
   ovulation 626.5
   postmenopausal 627.1
      following induced menopause 627.4
   postoperative 998.11
   preclimacteric 627.0
   puberty 626.3
      excessive, with onset of menstrual

Bleeding *(continued)*
         periods 626.3
   rectum, rectal 569.3
   tendencies (*see also* Defect, coagulation)
            286.9
   umbilicus 789.9
      cord, complicating delivery 663.8
   unrelated to menstrual cycle 626.6
   vicarious 625.8
Blighted ovum 631
Blind
   sac, fallopian tube (congenital) 752.19
   tract or tube (congenital) NEC—*see*
            Atresia
Bloating 787.3
Block
   kidney (*see also* Disease, renal), postcysto-
            scopic 997.5
   organ or site (congenital) NEC—*see*
            Atresia
   tubal 628.2
Blood (*see also* Dyscrasia)
   mole 631
   occult 792.1
   poisoning (*see also* Septicemia) 038.9
   pressure
      decreased, due to shock following
            injury 958.4
      fluctuating 796.4
      high (*see also* Hypertension) 401.9
         incidental reading (isolated) (non-
            specific), without diagnosis
            of hypertension 796.2
      low (*see also* Hypotension) 458.9
         incidental reading (isolated) (non-
            specific), without diagnosis
            of hypotension 796.3
   spitting (*see also* Hemoptysis) 786.3
   transfusion reaction or complication—*see*
            Complications, transfusion
   vomiting (*see also* Hematemesis) 578.0
Blue
   bloater 491.20
      with exacerbation (acute) 491.21
   dome cyst 610.0
Blushing (abnormal) (excessive) 782.62
Boggy
   cervix 622.8
   uterus 621.8
Boil 680.9
   anus 680.5
   axilla 680.3
   back (any part) 680.2
   breast 680.2

Boil *(continued)*
  buttock 680.5
  labia 616.4
  multiple sites 680.9
  perineum 680.2
  skin NEC 680.9
  specified site NEC 680.8
  umbilicus 680.2
  vulva 616.4
Borderline
  pelvis 653.1
    with obstruction during labor
      660.1
  osteopenia 733.90
Bradycardia 427.89
  chronic (sinus) 427.81
  nodal 427.89
  postoperative 997.1
  sinus 427.89
    with paroxysmal tachyarrhythmia or
      tachycardia 427.81
  tachycardia syndrome 427.81
  vagal 427.89
Bradypnea 786.09
BRBPR (bright red blood per rectum)
  569.3
Breast – see also condition
  buds 259.1
  dense 793.82
  nodule 793.89
Breast feeding difficulties 676.8
Breath, shortness 786.05
Breathing (asymmetrical) (bronchial)
      (labored) (periodic) 786.09
Breech presentation—*see* Delivery
Bronchiolitis (acute) (subacute) (with)
      466.19
  bronchospasm or obstruction 466.19
  catarrhal (acute) (subacute) 466.19
  chronic (obliterative) 491.8
  influenza, flu, or grippe 487.1
Bronchitis (diffuse) (infectious) (inflamma-
      tory) 490
  acute or subacute 466.0
  allergic (acute) (*see also* Asthma) 493.9
  asthmatic (acute) (with) 493.90
    acute exacerbation 493.92
    status asthmaticus 493.91
    chronic 493.2
  catarrhal 490
    acute—*see* Bronchitis, acute
    chronic 491.0
  emphysematous (with) 491.20
    acute bronchitis 491.22

Bronchitis *(continued)*
  exacerbation (acute) 491.21
  exudative 466.0
  fetid (chronic) (recurrent) 491.1
  fibrinous, acute or subacute (with or
      without bronchospasm or
      obstruction) 466.0
  influenzal 487.1
  membranous, acute or subacute (with or
      without bronchospasm or
      obstruction) 466.0
  obliterans 491.8
  obstructive (chronic) (with) 491.20
    acute bronchitis 491.22
    exacerbation (acute) 491.21
  plastic (inflammatory) 466.0
  pneumococcal, acute or subacute (with
      or without bronchospasm or
      obstruction) 466.0
  purulent (chronic) (recurrent) 491.1
    acute or subacute (with or without
      bronchospasm or obstruction)
      466.0
  putrid 491.1
  senile 491.9
  septic, acute or subacute (with or without
      bronchospasm or obstruc-
      tion) 466.0
  smokers' 491.0
  suffocative, acute or subacute 466.0
  tracheitis 490
    acute or subacute 466.0
      with bronchospasm or obstruction
        466.0
    chronic 491.8
  ulcerative 491.8
  viral, acute or subacute 466.0
Bronchoalveolitis 485
Bronchorrhagia 786.3
Bronchorrhea (chronic) (purulent) 491.0
  acute 466.0
Bronchospasm (with)
  asthma—*see* Asthma
  bronchiolitis, acute 466.19
    due to respiratory syncytial virus 466.11
  bronchitis—*see* Bronchitis
  chronic obstructive pulmonary disease
      (COPD) 496
  emphysema—*see* Emphysema
Bruise (skin surface intact) (*see also*
      Contusion)
  with open wound—*see* Wound, open, by
      site

Bruise *(continued)*
  internal organ (abdomen, chest, or
        pelvis)—*see* Injury, internal,
        by site
  umbilical cord 663.6
Bubo
  inguinal NEC 099.8
    chancroidal 099.0
    climatic 099.1
    due to H. ducreyi 099.0
  soft chancre 099.0
  suppurating 683
  syphilitic 091.0
  venereal NEC 099.8
  virulent 099.0
Bulimia 783.6
  nervosa 307.51
Bulla(e) 709.8
Bunion 727.1
Burn
  abdomen, abdominal (muscle) (wall)
        942.03
    with trunk—*see* Burn, trunk, multiple
        sites
    first degree 942.13
    second degree 942.23
    third degree 942.33
      deep 942.43
  anus—*see* Burn, trunk, specified site NEC
  breast(s) 942.01
    with trunk—*see* Burn, trunk, multiple
        sites
    first degree 942.11
    second degree 942.21
    third degree 942.31
      deep 942.41
  cervix (uteri) 947.4
  genitourinary organs
    external (labium, perineum, clitoris)
        942.05
      with trunk—*see* Burn, trunk, multiple
        sites
      first degree 942.15
      second degree 942.25
      third degree 942.35
        deep 942.45
    internal 947.8
  subcutaneous—*see* Burn, by site, third
        degree
  trunk 942.00
    first degree 942.10
    second degree 942.20
    third degree 942.30
      deep 942.40

Burn *(continued)*
  multiple sites 942.09
    first degree 942.19
    second degree 942.29
    third degree 942.39
      deep 942.49
  specified site NEC 942.09
    first degree 942.19
    second degree 942.29
    third degree 942.39
      deep 942.49
  uterus 947.4
  vagina 947.4
  vulva—*see* Burn, genitourinary organs,
        external
Burst stitches or sutures (complication
      of surgery) (external)
      998.32
  internal 998.31

C
Calcification
  breast 793.89
    microcalcification 793.81
  cervix (uteri) 622.8
  fallopian tube 620.8
  ovary 620.8
  subcutaneous 709.3
  uterus 621.8
Calciuria 791.9
Calculus, calculi, calculous
  appendix 543.9
  kidney 592.0
  ureter 592.1
  urinary tract NOS 592.9
  vagina 623.8
Cancer, cancerous—*see* Neoplasm, by site,
      malignant
Candidiasis, candidal 112.9
  specific site NEC 112.89
  urogenital site NEC 112.2
  vagina 112.1
  vulva 112.1
  vulvovaginitis 112.1
Carbuncle—*see* Boil
Carcinoid (tumor)– see Tumor, carcinoid
Carcinoma (*see also* Neoplasm, by site,
      malignant)
  basal cell (pigmented)—*see* Neoplasm,
      skin, malignant
  granulosa cell 183.0
  infiltrating duct
    with Paget's disease—*see* Neoplasm

Carcinoma *(continued)*
   breast, malignant
     unspecified site 174.9
   inflammatory, specified site—*see*
     Neoplasm, by site,
     malignant
     unspecified site 174.9
   in situ (*see also* Neoplasm, by site, in situ)
     epidermoid (*see also* Neoplasm, by site,
      in situ)
      with questionable stromal invasion,
       specified site—*see* Neoplasm,
       by site, in situ
       unspecified site 233.1
     Bowen's type—*see* Neoplasm, skin,
      in situ
     intraductal, specified site—*see*
      Neoplasm, by site, in situ
      unspecified site 233.0
     lobular, specified site—*see* Neoplasm,
      by site, in situ
      unspecified site 233.0
     papillary—*see* Neoplasm, by site, in situ
     squamous cell (*see also* Neoplasm, by
      site, in situ)
      with questionable stromal invasion,
       specified site—*see* Neoplasm,
       by site, in situ
       unspecified site 233.1
     transitional cell—*see* Neoplasm, by site,
      in situ
   intraductal (noninfiltrating)
     papillary, specified site—*see* Neoplasm,
      by site, in situ
      unspecified site 233.0
     specified site—*see* Neoplasm, by site,
      in situ
     unspecified site 233.0
   Leydig cell specified site (*see also* Neoplasm,
     by site, malignant) 183.0
   lobular (infiltrating)
     noninfiltrating, specified site—*see*
      Neoplasm, by site, in situ
      unspecified site 233.0
     specified site—*see* Neoplasm, by site,
      malignant
     unspecified site 174.9
   metastatic—*see* Metastasis, cancer
   papillary
     intraductal (noninfiltrating), specified
      site—*see* Neoplasm, by site,
      in situ
     unspecified site 233.0

Carcinoma *(continued)*
   serous, specified site—*see* Neoplasm, by
     site, malignant
   surface, specified site—*see* Neoplasm,
     by site, malignant
     unspecified site 183.0
   unspecified site 183.0
   secondary—*see* Neoplasm, by site, malig-
     nant, secondary
   serous
     papillary, specified site—*see* Neoplasm,
      by site, malignant
     unspecified site 183.0
     surface, papillary, specified site—*see*
      Neoplasm, by site, malignant
     unspecified site 183.0
   signet ring cell metastatic—*see* Neoplasm,
     by site, secondary
   skin appendage—*see* Neoplasm, skin,
     malignant
   small cell—*see* Neoplasm, by site, malig-
     nant
   squamous (cell)
     intraepidermal, Bowen's type—*see*
      Neoplasm, skin, in situ
     microinvasive, specified site—*see*
      Neoplasm, by site, malignant
     unspecified site 180.9
   theca cell 183.0
   transitional (cell)—*see* Neoplasm, skin,
     malignant
     papillary—*see* Neoplasm, skin, malig-
      nant
   undifferentiated type—*see* Neoplasm, by
     site, malignant
Carcinosarcoma—*see* Neoplasm, by site,
   malignant
Cardiomyopathy
   hypertensive—*see* Hypertension, with
     heart involvement
   peripartum, postpartum 674.5
Cardiopathy (*see also* Disease, heart)
   hypertensive (*see also* Hypertension,
     heart) 402.90
Care (of) (*see also* Admission [for])
   lack of (adult) 995.84
   lactation of mother V24.1
Carpal tunnel syndrome 354.0
Carrier (suspected) of
   bacterial disease (meningococcal, staphy-
     lococcal) NEC V02.59
   cystic fibrosis gene V83.81
   defective gene V83.89

Carrier *(continued)*
   gonorrhea V02.7
   hemophilia A (asymptomatic) V83.01
   hepatitis V02.60
      B V02.61
      C V02.62
      serum V02.61
      specified type NEC V02.69
      viral V02.60
   Staphylococcus NEC V02.59
      methicillin
         resistant Staphylococcus aureus
            V02.54
         susceptible Staphylococcus aureus
            V02.53
   Streptococcus NEC V02.52
      group B V02.51
   venereal disease NEC V02.8
Caruncle (inflamed)
   labium (majus) (minus) 616.89
   urethra (benign) 599.3
   vagina (wall) 616.89
Casts in urine 791.7
Cellulitis (diffuse) (with lymphangitis) *(see also* Abscess)
   abdominal wall 682.2
   anus 566
   areola 611.0
   breast 611.0
      postpartum 675.1
   broad ligament *(see also* Disease, pelvis, inflammatory) 614.4
      acute 614.3
   buttock 682.5
   cervix (uteri) *(see also* Cervicitis) 616.0
   Douglas' cul-de-sac or pouch (chronic) *(see also* Disease, pelvis, inflammatory) 614.4
      acute 614.3
   drainage site (following operation) 998.59
   genital organ—*see* Abscess, genital organ
   gluteal (region) 682.5
   gonococcal NEC 098.0
   labium (majus) (minus) *(see also* Vulvitis) 616.10
   nipple 611.0
   pelvis, pelvic *(see also* Disease, pelvis, inflammatory) 614.4
      with or following
         abortion—*see* Abortion, by type, with sepsis
         following abortion 639.0

Cellulitis *(continued)*
      ectopic or molar pregnancy *(see also* categories 630–633.9) 639.0
   acute 614.3
   puerperal, postpartum, childbirth 670.8
   perineal, perineum 682.2
   perirectal 566
   periurethral 597.0
   periuterine *(see also* Disease, pelvis, inflammatory) 614.4
      acute 614.3
   rectum 566
   retromammary 611.0
   retroperitoneal *(see also* Peritonitis) 567.2
   round ligament *(see also* Disease, pelvis, inflammatory) 614.4
      acute 614.3
   trunk 682.2
   umbilical 682.2
   vaccinal 999.3
   vagina—*see* Vaginitis
   vulva *(see also* Vulvitis) 616.10
Cervical *(see also* condition)
   shortening—*see* Short, cervical
Cervicitis (acute) (chronic) (nonvenereal) (subacute) (with erosion or ectropion) 616.0
   with or following
      abortion—*see* Abortion, by type, with sepsis
      following abortion 639.0
   with or following
      ectopic or molar pregnancy *(see also* categories 630–633.9) 639.0
      ulceration 616.0
   chlamydial 099.53
   complicating pregnancy or puerperium 646.6
   gonococcal (acute) 098.15
      chronic or duration of 2 months or more 098.35
   senile (atrophic) 616.0
   trichomonal 131.09
   tuberculous *(see also* Tuberculosis) 016.7
Cervicocolpitis (emphysematosa) *(see also* Cervicitis) 616.0
Cesarean delivery, operation or section— *see* Delivery
Chancre (any genital site) 091.0
   congenital 090.0
   Ducrey's 099.0

Chancre *(continued)*
    extragenital 091.2
    Hunterian 091.0
    mixed 099.8
    nipple 091.2
    Nisbet's 099.0
    phagedenic 099.0
    Ricord's 091.0
    Rollet's (syphilitic) 091.0
    seronegative or seropositive 091.0
    simple 099.0
    soft 099.0
    urethra 091.0
Change(s) (of) *(see also* Removal of)
    bowel habits 787.99
Checking (of) contraceptive device
            (intrauterine) V25.42
Chemotherapy
    convalescence V66.2
    encounter (for) V58.1
    maintenance V58.1
Chickenpox—*see* Varicella
Childbed fever 670.8
Chill(s) 780.64
    with fever 780.60
    without fever 780.64
    septic—*see* Septicemia
    urethral 599.84
Chlamydia, chlamydial—*see* condition
Chloasma, gravidarum 646.8
Chocolate cyst (ovary) 617.1
Choluria 791.4
Chorioamnionitis 658.4
Choriocarcinoma
    combined with teratoma—*see* Neoplasm,
            by site, malignant
    specified site—*see* Neoplasm, by site,
            malignant
    unspecified site 181
Chorionitis *(see also* Scleroderma) 710.1
Chyluria, nonfilarial 791.1
Cicatrix (adherent) (contracted) (painful)
            709.2
    anus 569.49
    cervix (postoperative) (postpartal) 622.3
        in pregnancy or childbirth 654.6
            causing obstructed labor 660.2
    rectum 569.49
    skin (postinfectional) 709.2
    specified site NEC 709.2
    urethra 599.84
    uterus 621.8
    vagina 623.4
        in pregnancy or childbirth 654.7

Cicatrix *(continued)*
        causing obstructed labor 660.2
CIN I (cervical intraepithelial neoplasia I)
            622.11
CIN II (cervical intraepithelial neoplasia II)
            622.12
CIN III (cervical intraepithelial neoplasia
            III) 233.1
Circulation
    defective 459.9
    failure, peripheral 785.59
Circumcision (ritual) (routine) (male) V50.2
    status (post) female 629.20
Cirrhosis, cirrhotic
    clitoris (hypertrophic) 624.2
    due to cystic fibrosis 277.00
    ovarian 620.8
Claudication, intermittent 443.9
    venous (axillary) 453.89
Closed surgical procedure converted to
            laparoscopy V64.41
Closure
    defective or imperfect NEC—*see*
            Imperfect, closure
    fistula, delayed—*see* Fistula
    hymen 623.3
    vagina 623.2
    vulva 624.8
Clotting defect—*see* Defect, coagulation
Coagulation, intravascular (diffuse)
            (disseminated) *(see also*
            Fibrinolysis) 286.6
Cocciuria 791.9
Coccydynia 724.79
Cold (head) 460
    with influenza, flu, or grippe 487.1
    bronchus or chest—*see* Bronchitis
        with grippe or influenza 487.1
    common (head) 460
        vaccination, prophylactic (against)
            V04.7
Colibacillosis 041.4
    generalized 038.42
Colibacilluria 791.9
Colic (recurrent) 789.0
    abdomen 789.0
    appendix 543.9
    in adult 789.0
    kidney (renal) 788.0
    ureter 788.0
    urethral 599.84
    uterus 625.8
        menstrual 625.3
    virus 460

Colitis, adaptive 564.9
Collapse 780.2
  during or after labor and delivery 669.1
  general 780.2
  postoperative (cardiovascular) 998.0
Collapse *(continued)*
  vascular (peripheral) 785.59
    with or following
      abortion—*see* Abortion, by type,
        with shock
        following abortion 639.5
      ectopic pregnancy (*see also* categories
        633.0–633.9) 639.5
      molar pregnancy (*see also* categories
        630–632) 639.5
    during or after labor and delivery 669.1
Colliculitis urethralis (*see also* Urethritis)
    597.89
Colloid milium 709.3
Colpocele 618.6
Colpocystitis (*see also* Vaginitis) 616.10
Colpospasm 625.1
Comedo, comedones 706.1
Comedocarcinoma (*see also* Neoplasm,
        breast, malignant)
  noninfiltrating
    specified site—*see* Neoplasm, by site,
      in situ
    unspecified site 233.0
Comedomastitis 610.4
Communication, abnormal—*see* Fistula
Complications
  abortion NEC—*see* categories 634–639
  amniocentesis, fetal 679.1
  anesthesia, anesthetic NEC (*see also*
        Anesthesia, complication)
    in labor and delivery 668.9
      cardiac 668.1
      central nervous system 668.2
      pulmonary 668.0
      specific type NEC 668.8
  bleeding (intraoperative) (postoperative)
        998.11
  breast
    implant (prosthetic) 996.79
      infection or inflammation 996.69
      mechanical complication 996.54
    elephantiasis or lymphedema, post-
        mastectomy 457.0
  catheter device
    infection and inflammation due to
      NEC 996.69
    urethral 996.64

Complications *(continued)*
  urinary, indwelling 996.64
  mechanical complication 996.59
    during a procedure 998.2
    urethral, indwelling 996.31
  cesarean section wound 674.3
  contraceptive device, intrauterine NOS
        996.76
    infection or inflammation due to
      996.65
    mechanical complication 996.32
  cystostomy 997.5
  delivery 669.9
    procedure (instrumental) (manual)
      (surgical) 669.4
    specified type NEC 669.8
  ectopic or molar pregnancy NEC 639.9
  fetal, from amniocentesis 679.1
  genitourinary graft, device or implant or
        graft NEC 996.76
    infection due to 996.65
    mechanical complication 996.30
      specified NEC 996.39
    urinary catheter, indwelling 996.64
  hematoma (intraoperative) (postoperative)
        998.12
  hemorrhage (intraoperative) (post-
        operative) 998.11
  infusion 999.88
    blood—*see* Transfusion
    infection, sepsis NEC 999.39
  injection (procedure) 999.9
    drug reaction—*see* Complications,
        vaccination
    infection, sepsis NEC 999.39
    vaccine (any)—*see* Complications,
        vaccination
  in utero procedure
    fetal 679.1
    maternal 679.0
  labor 669.9 (*see also* specified condition
        NEC 669.8)
  perfusion NEC 999.9
  perineal repair (obstetric) 674.3
    disruption 674.2
  pessary (uterus) (vagina)—*see*
        Complications, contraceptive
        device
  postcystoscopic 997.5
  pregnancy NEC 646.9 (*see also*
        Pregnancy)
  puerperium NEC 674.9 (*see also*
        Puerperal)

Complications *(continued)*
  radiotherapy 990
  seroma (intraoperative) (postoperative)
      (noninfected) 998.13
    infected 998.51
  stoma, external, urinary tract 997.5
  surgical procedure complications (postop-
      erative) 998.9
    accidental puncture or laceration
        998.2
    emphysema (surgical) 998.81
    evisceration 998.32
    fistula (persistent postoperative)
        998.6
    foreign body inadvertently left in
        wound (sponge) (suture)
        (swab) 998.4
    gastrointestinal NEC 997.4
    nervous system NEC 997.00
    peripheral vascular NEC 997.2
    respiratory NEC 997.39
    shock (endotoxic) (hypovolemic)
        (septic) 998.0
    stitch abscess 998.59
    urinary NEC 997.5
    wound
      cesarean 674.31
      complication (burst stitches)
          (sutures) (dehiscence)
          (disruption)
        internal 998.31
        external 998.32
      infection 998.59
  therapeutic misadventure NEC 999.9
  surgical treatment 998.9
  transfusion (blood) (lymphocytes)
          (plasma) NEC 999.89
    embolism
      air 999.1
      thrombus 999.2
    hemolysis NEC 999.8
    incompatibility reaction
        ABO 999.6
        minor blood group 999.89
      Rh (factor) 999.7
    infection, sepsis 999.39
    shock or reaction NEC 999.8
    thromboembolism 999.2
  trauma NEC (early) 958.8
  ultrasound therapy NEC 999.9
  ureter 997.5 (*see also* Complications,
      catheter)
    malfunction, ureterostomy 997.5

Complications *(continued)*
    mechanical complication due to graft,
        device, implant, without
        mention of resection 996.39
  urethra 997.5 (*see also* Complications,
      catheter)
    malfunction, urethrostomy 997.5
  vaccination 999.9
    anaphylaxis (shock) NEC 999.4
    cellulitis 999.39
    infection (general) (local) NEC 999.39
    protein sickness 999.5
    reaction (allergic) 999.5
      Herxheimer's 995.0
      serum 999.5
    sepsis 999.3
    serum intoxication, sickness, rash, or
        other serum reaction NEC
        999.5
    vaccinia (generalized) 999.0
      localized 999.39
  vascular
    following infusion, perfusion, or trans-
        fusion 999.2
    infection or inflammation 996.62
    mechanical complication due to graft,
        device or implant 996.1
    postoperative NEC 997.2
      peripheral vessels 997.2
  ventilation therapy NEC 999.9
Compression
  nerve, median (in carpal tunnel) 354.0
  syndrome 958.5
  umbilical cord—*see* Delivery
  urethra—*see* Stricture, urethra
  vein 459.2
Condyloma NEC 078.11
  gonorrheal 098.0
  latum 091.3
  syphilitic 091.3
Conflict
  family V61.9
    specified circumstance NEC V61.8
  interpersonal NEC V62.81
  marital
    involving
      divorce V61.03
      estrangement V61.09
  parent (guardian)-child V61.20
  partner V61.10
Congestion, congestive (chronic) (passive)
  breast 611.79
  catarrhal 472.0

Congestion, congestive *(continued)*
circulatory NEC 459.9
enteritis or gastroenteritis—*see* Enteritis
fibrosis syndrome (pelvic) 625.5
general 799.89
liver 573.0
lung, active or acute (*see also* Pneumonia) 486
ovary 620.8
pelvic 625.5
urethra 599.84
uterus 625.5
with subinvolution 621.1
viscera 799.89
Conjoined twins
causing disproportion (feto-pelvic) 678.1
fetal 678.1
Constipation 564.00
atonic 564.09
drug induced, correct substance properly administered 564.09
neurogenic 564.09
other specified NEC 564.09
outlet dysfunction 564.02
simple 564.00
slow transit 564.01
spastic 564.09
Constriction
organ or site, congenital NEC—*see* Atresia
urethra—*see* Stricture, urethra
Contact with—*see* Exposure to
Contraception, contraceptive and family planning
advice NEC V25.09
family planning V25.09
natural procreative V26.41
to avoid pregnancy V25.04
fitting of diaphragm V25.02
prescribing or use of
oral contraceptive agent V25.01
specified agent NEC V25.02
counseling NEC V25.09 (*see also* Contraception, prescription)
emergency V25.03
fitting of diaphragm V25.02
device (in situ) (status) V45.59
causing menorrhagia 996.76
checking V25.42
complications 996.32
insertion V25.1
intrauterine V45.51
reinsertion V25.42
removal V25.42

Contraception, contraceptive and family planning *(continued)*
subdermal V45.52
fitting of diaphragm V25.02
insertion
intrauterine contraceptive device V25.1
subdermal implantable V25.5
maintenance (examination) V25.40
intrauterine device V25.42
oral contraceptive V25.41
specified method NEC V25.49
subdermal implantable V25.43
management NEC V25.49
prescription
oral contraceptive agent V25.01
emergency V25.03
postcoital V25.03
repeat V25.41
specified agent NEC V25.02
repeat V25.49
sterilization V25.2
surveillance V25.40
intrauterine device V25.42
oral contraceptive agent V25.41
specified method NEC V25.49
subdermal implantable V25.43
Contraction, contracture, contracted
axilla 729.90
Braxton Hicks 644.1
breast implant, capsular 611.83
cervix (*see also* Stricture, cervix) 622.4
congenital 752.49
cicatricial—*see* Cicatrix
organ or site, congenital NEC—*see* Atresia
outlet (pelvis)—*see* Contraction, pelvis
pelvis (acquired) (general) 738.6
complicating delivery 653.1
any type, causing obstructed labor 660.1
generally contracted 653.1
inlet 653.2
midpelvic, midplane 653.8
outlet 653.3
scar—*see* Cicatrix
urethra 599.84
uterus 621.8
abnormal 661.9
clonic, hourglass or tetanic 661.4
dyscoordinate, incoordinate 661.4
hypotonic NEC 661.2
inefficient or poor 661.2
irregular 661.2
vagina (outlet) 623.2

Contusion (skin surface intact)
crush injury—*see* Crush
open wound—*see* Wound, open, by site
abdomen, abdominal (muscle) (wall) 922.2
back 922.31
breast 922.0
buttock 922.32
clitoris 922.4
flank 922.2
internal organs NEC—*see* Injury, internal,
by site
labium (majus) (minus) 922.4
perineum 922.4
pubic region 922.4
trunk 922.9
multiple sites 922.8
specified site—*see* Contusion, by site
vagina 922.4
vulva 922.4
**Conversion of laparoscopic procedure to
open procedure** V64.41
Cough 786.2
with hemorrhage (*see also* Hemoptysis)
786.3
bronchial 786.2
with grippe or influenza 487.1
chronic 786.2
epidemic 786.2
nervous 786.2
smokers' 491.0
Counseling NEC V65.40
without complaint or sickness V65.49
abuse victim NEC V62.89
child V61.21
partner or spouse V61.11
contraceptive—*see* Contraception, counseling
dietary V65.3
exercise V65.41
fertility preservation (prior to cancer
therapy) (prior to surgical
removal of gonads) V26.42
for nonattending third party V65.19
genetic V26.33
health (advice) (education) (instruction)
NEC V65.49
injury prevention V65.43
medical (for) V65.9
feared complaint and no disease found
V65.5
on behalf of another V65.19
paren (guardian)-child conflict V61.20

Counseling *(continued)*
specified problem NEC V61.29
procreative V65.49
sexually transmitted disease NEC
V65.45
gonorrhea V65.45
HIV V65.44
syphilis V65.45
specified reason NEC V65.49
spousal or partner abuse
perpetrator V61.12
victim V61.11
substance use and abuse V65.42
Crabs, meaning pubic lice 132.2
Cramp(s) 729.82
extremity (lower) (upper) NEC
729.82
intestinal, stomach 789.0
uterus 625.8
menstrual 625.3
Crisis
abdomen 789.0
asthmatic—*see* Asthma
emotional NEC 309.29
acute reaction to stress 308.0
hypertensive—*see* Hypertension
sickle cell 282.62
vascular—*see* Disease, cerebrovascular,
acute
Crush, crushed, crushing (injury)
929.9
abdomen 926.19
internal—*see* Injury, internal,
abdomen
breast 926.19
genitalia, external 926.0
internal organ (abdomen, chest, or
pelvis)—*see* Injury, internal,
by site
labium (majus) (minus) 926.0
multiple sites NEC 929.0
syndrome (complication of trauma)
958.5
trunk 926.9
internal organ—*see* Injury, internal, by
site
multiple sites 926.8
specified site NEC 926.19
vulva 926.0
Cryptitis (anal) (rectal) 569.49
Cutis (*see also* condition)
laxa senilis 701.8
marmorata 782.61

Cutis *(continued)*
  osteosis 709.3
  pendula acquired 701.8
  rhomboidalis nuchae 701.8
  verticis gyrata acquired 701.8
Cycle
  anovulatory 628.0
  menstrual, irregular 626.4
Cylindruria 791.7
Cyst (mucus) (retention) (serous)
        (simple)
  amnion, amniotic 658.8
  anus 569.49
  appendix 543.9
  Bartholin's gland or duct 616.2
  blue dome 610.0
  breast (benign) (pedunculated) (solitary)
        (traumatic) 610.0
    involution 610.4
    sebaceous 610.8
  broad ligament (benign) 620.8
    embryonic 752.11
  canal of Nuck (acquired) (serous) 629.1
    congenital 752.41
  carcinomatous—*see* Neoplasm, by site,
        malignant
  cervix 622.8
    embryonic 752.41
    nabothian (gland) 616.0
  chorion 658.8
  clitoris 624.8
  dermoid (*see also* Neoplasm, by site,
        benign)
    with malignant transformation 183.0
    implantation
      external area or site (skin) NEC
        709.8
      vagina 623.8
      vulva 624.8
  embryonal, genitalia, external 752.41
  endometrial 621.8
    ectopic 617.9
  epidermoid (inclusion) (*see also* Cyst,
        skin) 706.2
    not of skin—*see* Cyst, by site
  epithelial (inclusion) (*see also* Cyst, skin)
        706.2
  fallopian tube 620.8
    congenital 752.11
  fimbrial (congenital) 752.11
  follicle (atretic) (graafian) (ovarian) 620.0
    nabothian (gland) 616.0
  Gartner's duct 752.11

Cyst *(continued)*
  graafian follicle 620.0
  granulosal lutein 620.2
  hydatid, fallopian tube 752.11
  hymen 623.8
    embryonal 752.41
  implantation (dermoid)
    external area or site (skin) NEC 709.8
    vagina 623.8
    vulva 624.8
  inclusion (epidermal) (mucous) (squa-
        mous) (*see also* Cyst, skin)
        706.2
    not of skin—*see* Neoplasm, by site,
        benign
  keratin 706.2
  labium (majus) (minus) (sebaceous)
        624.8
  lutein 620.1
  malignant—*see* Neoplasm, by site,
        malignant
  milk 611.5
  Müllerian duct
    cervix (embyonal) 752.41
    fallopian tube 752.11
    vagina (embryonal) 752.41
  myometrium 621.8
  nabothian (follicle) (ruptured) 616.0
  neoplastic (*see also* Neoplasm, by site,
        unspecified nature)
    benign—*see* Neoplasm, by site, benign
    uterus 621.8
  nipple 610.0
  omentum (lesser) 568.89
  ovary, ovarian (twisted) 620.2
    adherent 620.2
    chocolate 617.1
    congenital 752.0
    corpus
      albicans 620.2
      luteum 620.1
    dermoid 220
    developmental 752.0
    due to failure of involution NEC 620.2
    endometrial 617.1
    follicular (atretic) (graafian) (hemor-
        rhagic) 620.0
    hemorrhagic 620.2
    in pregnancy or childbirth 654.4
      causing obstructed labor 660.2
    multilocular 239.5
    pseudomucinous, retention, serous or
        theca lutein 620.2

Cyst *(continued)*
   tuberculous *(see also* Tuberculosis)
      016.6
     unspecified 620.2
   para ovarian 752.11
   paratubal (fallopian) 620.8
   paraurethral duct 599.89
   pelvis, in pregnancy or childbirth
      654.4
     causing obstructed labor 660.2
   peritoneum 568.89
   pilonidal (infected) (rectum)
     with abscess 685.0
     malignant 173.5
   placenta (amniotic)—*see* Placenta, abnormal
   pudenda (sweat glands) 624.8
     sebaceous 624.8
   rectum (epithelium) (mucous) 569.49
   retention (ovary) 620.2
   retroperitoneal 568.89
   sebaceous (duct) (gland) 706.2
     breast 610.8
     genital organ 629.8
   serous (ovary) 620.2
   Skene's gland 599.89
   skin 706.2
     breast 610.8
     genital organ 629.8
   suburethral 599.89
   theca-lutein (ovary) 620.2
   tubo-ovarian 620.8
     inflammatory 614.1
   ureterovesical orifice
     congenital 753.4
   urethra 599.84
   uterine
     ligament 620.8
       embryonic 752.11
     tube 620.8
   uterus (body) (corpus) (recurrent) 621.8
     embryonal 752.3
   vagina, vaginal (squamous cell) (wall)
      623.8
     embryonal 752.41
     implantation, inclusion 623.8
   vulva (sweat glands) 624.8
     congenital 752.41
     implantation, inclusion 624.8
     sebaceous gland 624.8
     vulvovaginal gland 624.8
Cystadenocarcinoma—*see* Carcinoma
Cystadenofibroma
   clear cell—*see* Neoplasm, by site, benign
   endometrioid 220

Cystadenofibroma *(continued)*
   borderline malignancy 236.2
   malignant 183.0
   mucinous or serous
     specified site—*see* Neoplasm, by site,
       benign
     unspecified site 220
   specified site—*see* Neoplasm, by site,
      benign
   unspecified site 220
Cystadenoma *(see also* Neoplasm, by site,
     benign)
   malignant—*see* Neoplasm, by site,
     malignant
   mucinous, papillary, pseudomucinous or
     serous
     borderline malignancy
       specified site—*see* Neoplasm, uncer-
         tain behavior
       unspecified site 236.2
     specified site—*see* Neoplasm, by site,
       benign
     unspecified site 220
Cystic *(see also* condition)
   breast, chronic (disease) 610.1
   corpora lutea 620.1
   mass—*see* Cyst
   mastitis, chronic 610.1
   ovary 620.2
Cystitis (bacillary) (diffuse) (septic)
     595.9
   with or following
     abortion—*see* Abortion, by type, with
       urinary tract infection
     following abortion 639.8
     ectopic or molar pregnancy *(see also*
       categories 633.0–633.9)
       639.8
     fibrosis 595.1
     leukoplakia, malakoplakia 595.1
     metaplasia 595.1
   acute 595.0
   allergic 595.89
   blennorrhagic (acute) 098.11
     chronic or duration of 2 months or
       more 098.31
   bullous 595.89
   chlamydial 099.53
   chronic 595.2
     interstitial 595.1
   complicating pregnancy, childbirth, or
     puerperium 646.6
   cystic(a) 595.81

Cystitis *(continued)*
  emphysematous 595.89
  encysted 595.81
  gangrenous 595.89
  glandularis 595.89
  gonococcal (acute) 098.11
    chronic or duration of 2 months or
      more 098.31
  incrusted 595.89
  interstitial 595.1
  irritation 595.89
  malignant 595.89
  monilial 112.2
  panmural 595.1
  polyposa 595.89
  Reiter's (abacterial) 099.3
  specified NEC 595.89
  subacute 595.2
  submucous 595.1
  trichomoniasis 131.09
  tuberculous *(see also* Tuberculosis)
    016.1
  ulcerative 595.1
Cystocele (-rectocele) (without uterine
    prolapse) 618.01
  in pregnancy or childbirth 654.4
    causing obstructed labor 660.2
  lateral 618.02
  midline 618.01
  paravaginal 618.02
    with uterine prolapse 618.4
      complete 618.3
      incomplete 618.2
Cystosarcoma phyllodes 238.3
  benign 217
  malignant—*see* Neoplasm, breast,
    malignant
Cystostomy (status) V44.50
  with complication 997.5
Cystourethritis (*see also* Urethritis)
    597.89
Cystourethrocele (*see also* Cystocele) (with-
    out uterine prolapse)
    618.09
  with uterine prolapse 618.4
    complete 618.3
    incomplete 618.2

D

Damage
  coccyx, complicating delivery 665.6
  pelvic
    joint or ligament, during delivery 665.6

Damage *(continued)*
  with or following
    abortion—*see* Abortion, by type,
      with damage to pelvic
      organs following abortion
      639.2
    ectopic or molar pregnancy (*see also*
      categories 630–633.9)
      639.2
    during delivery 665.5
Death
  after delivery (cause not stated) (sudden)
    674.9
  anesthetic
    due to
      correct substance properly adminis-
        tered 995.4
      overdose or wrong substance given
        968.4
    during delivery 668.9
  fetus, fetal—*see* Pregnancy
  from pregnancy NEC 646.9
  sudden (cause unknown)
    during delivery 669.9
    under anesthesia NEC 668.9
    puerperal, during puerperium 674.9
Deciduitis (acute)
  with or following
    abortion—*see* Abortion, by type, with
      sepsis
    following abortion 639.0
    ectopic or molar pregnancy (*see also*
      categories 630–633.9)
      639.0
  in pregnancy 646.6
  puerperal, postpartum 670.1
Deciduoma malignum 181
Decrease, decreased
  blood
    platelets 287.5
    pressure 796.3
      due to shock following
        injury 958.4
        operation 998.0
  estrogen 256.39
    postablative 256.2
  fetal movements 655.7
  function, ovary in hypopituitarism 253.4
  glucose 790.29
  libido 799.81
  respiration due to shock following injury
    958.4
Decubitus (ulcer) 707.00

Defect, defective
chromosome—*see* Anomaly, chromosome
circulation (acquired) 459.9
coagulation (factor) (*see also* Deficiency,
 coagulation factor) 286.9
 with
  abortion—*see* Abortion, by type,
   with hemorrhage
  ectopic or molar pregnancy (*see also*
   categories 634–638) 639.1
  acquired (any) 286.7
  antepartum or intrapartum 641.3
  causing hemorrhage of pregnancy or
   delivery 641.3
  postpartum 666.3
  specified type NEC 286.9
congenital, organ or site NEC—*see*
 Anomaly
developmental—*see* Anomaly, by site
fibrin polymerization 286.3
filling (bladder) (kidney) (ureter) 793.5
gene, carrier (suspected) of V83.89
platelet (qualitative), constitutional
 286.4
renal pelvis 753.9
 obstructive 753.29
ureter 753.9
 obstructive 753.29
vascular (acquired) (local) 459.9
Deficiency, deficient
anemia—*see* Anemia, deficiency
calcium metabolism
 hypercalcemia 275.42
 hypocalcemia 275.41
 other disorders 275.49
 unspecified 275.40
coagulation defects (*see also* Defect, coagulation) 286.9
 acquired 286.7
 congenital
  factor VIII disorder 286.0
  factor IX disorder 286.1
  factor XI deficiency 286.2
  other clotting factors 286.3
 defibrination syndrome 286.6
 hemorrhagic disorder due to circulating
  anticoagulants 286.5
 von Willeberand's disease 286.4
hormones
 follicle-stimulating (FSH) 253.4
 luteinizing 253.4
 melanocyte-stimulating 253.4
 prolactin 253.4

Deficiency, deficient *(continued)*
intrinsic (urethral) sphincter (ISD) 599.82
ovarian 256.39
placenta—*see* Placenta, insufficiency
salt 276.1
thrombopoietin 287.3
urine 788.5
vascular 459.9
Deformity
anus (acquired) 569.49
breast (acquired) 611.89
 congenital 757.6
 reconstructed 612.0
canal of Nuck 752.9
cervix (acquired) (uterus) 622.8
 congenital 752.40
cicatricial—*see* Cicatrix
clitoris (congenital) 752.40
 acquired 624.8
fallopian tube (congenital) 752.10
 acquired 620.8
fetal—*see* Pregnancy, complicated by
hymen (congenital) 752.40
labium (majus) (minus) (congenital)
 752.40
 acquired 624.8
nipple (congenital) 757.6
 acquired 611.89
ovary (congenital) 752.0
 acquired 620.8
pelvis, pelvic (acquired) (bony) 738.6
 with disproportion—*see* Pregnancy
rectovaginal septum (congenital)
 752.40
 acquired 623.8
rectum (acquired) 569.49
sebaceous gland (acquired) 706.8
ureter (opening) (congenital) 753.9
urethra (valve) (congenital) 753.9
 acquired 599.84
urinary tract or system (congenital)
 753.9
uterus (congenital) 752.3
 acquired 621.8
vagina (congenital) 752.40
 acquired 623.8
vulva (congenital) 752.40
 acquired 624.8
Degeneration, degenerative
breast—*see* Disease, breast
cervix, due to radiation (intended effect,
 adverse effect or misadven-
 ture) 622.8

Degeneration, degenerative *(continued)*
cutis 709.3
nipple 611.9
ovary 620.8
cystic, microcystic 620.2
peritoneum 568.89
placenta—*see* Placenta, abnormal
skin (colloid) 709.3
uterus (cystic) 621.8
Dehiscence
cesarean wound 674.1
episiotomy 674.2
operation wound 998.32
deep 998.31
extenal 998.32
internal 998.31
superficial 998.33
perineal wound (postpartum) 674.2
traumatic injury wound repair 998.33
uterine wound 674.1
Dehydration (cachexia) (with) 276.5
hypernatremia 276.0
hyponatremia 276.1
Delay, delayed
delivery—*see* Delivery
development, sexual 259.0
menarche 256.39
due to pituitary hypofunction
253.4
menstruation (cause unknown) 626.8
puberty 259.0
vaccination V64.00
Delirium, delirious
exhaustion (*see also* Reaction, stress,
acute) 308.9
puerperal 293.9
uremic—*see* Uremia
Delivery
cesarean (for) 669.7
abnormal—*see* Delivery, complicated
by abnormal
elective 669.7
complicated (by) NEC 669.9 (*see also*
Delivery, labor)
abnormal, abnormality of pelvic organs
or tissues (maternal)
654.9
bladder, dilation 654.4
abnormality causing obstructed
labor 660.2
cervix 654.6
abnormality causing obstructed
labor 660.2
annular detachment 665.3

Delivery *(continued)*
complicated (by) *(continued)*
abnormal *(continued)*
cervix *(continued)*
anteversion 654.4
cicatrix 654.6
edema 654.6
lateroversion 654.4
polyp 654.6
retroversion 654.3
rigid 654.6
scar 654.6
stenosis 654.6
cystocele 654.4
abnormality causing obstructed
labor 660.2
hymen, persistent 654.8
kidney, ectopic 654.4
pelvis, pelvic
abnormality causing obstructed
labor 660.1
contraction 653.1
general 653.1
inlet 653.2
midpelvic 653.8
midplane 653.8
outlet 653.3
cretin (dwarf type) 653.1
floor 654.4
Nagele's pelvis 653.0
Robert's pelvis 653.0
scoliotic 653.0
spondylolisthesis 653.3
spondylolysis 653.3
tipping 653.0
tumor 654.9
perineum, scar 654.8
rectocele 654.4
soft parts (of pelvis) 654.9
abnormality causing obstructed
labor 660.2
uterus (formation) 654.0
abnormality causing obstructed
labor 660.2
adhesions (to abdominal wall)
654.4
anteversion 654.4
bicornis or bicornuate uterus
654.0
displacement 654.4
double (congenital) 654.0
fibroid (tumor) (fibromyomata)
654.1

Delivery *(continued)*
  complicated (by) *(continued)*
    abnormal *(continued)*
      incarcerated 654.3
      infantile genitalia or uterus 654.4
      lateroversion 654.4
      prolapse 654.4
      retroversion 654.3
      sacculation 654.4
      scar 654.9
        due to previous cesearean
          delivery 654.2
      vagina 654.7
        abnormality causing obstructed
          labor 660.2
        cyst (Gartner's duct) 654.7
        rigid 654.7
        scar 654.7
        septate 654.7
        stenosis 654.7
      vulva 654.8
        abnormality causing obstructed
          labor 660.2
        rigid 654.8
        scar 654.8
    amnion, amniotic fluid
      amnionitis 658.4
      dropsy amnion 657.0
      effusion, amniotic fluid 658.1
      embolism, amniotic fluid 673.1
      hydramnios, polyhydramnios 657.0
      oligohydramnios 658.0
    anesthetic death 668.9
    bleeding (*see also* Delivery, complicated
      by hemorrhage) 641.9
    disproportion NEC 653.9
      abnormality causing obstructed
        labor 660.1
      cephalopelvic disproportion (nor-
        mally formed fetus) 653.4
    embolism (pulmonary) 673.2
      air 673.0
      amniotic fluid 673.1
      blood-clot 673.2
      cerebral 674.0
      fat 673.8
      pyemic 673.3
      septic 673.3
    fetal conditions
      abnormality causing obstructed
        labor 660.1
      acid–base balance 656.8
      death (near term) (stillbirth) NEC 656.4

Delivery *(continued)*
  complicated (by) *(continued)*
    fetal conditions *(continued)*
      early (before 22 completed weeks
        gestation) 632
      deformity 653.7
      depressed fetal heart tones 659.7
      distress 656.8
      excessive growth (size of fetus)
        653.5
      heart rate or rhythm 659.7
      hydrocephalic 653.6
      hydrops fetalis 653.7
      locked mates 660.5
      meconium in liquor 656.8
      myelomeningocele 653.7
      nonviable 656.4
      sacral teratomas 653.7
    hematoma
      broad ligament 665.7
      ischial spine 665.7
      pelvic 665.7
      perineum 664.5
      soft tissues 665.7
      subdural 674.0
      umbilical cord 663.6
      vagina 665.7
      vulva 664.5
    hemorrhage (uterine) (antepartum)
      (intrapartum) 641.9
      accidental 641.2
      associated with afibrinogenemia or
        coagulation defect 641.3
      cerebral 674.0
      due to
        placental condition—*see* Delivery,
          placenta
        trauma 641.8
        uterine leiomyoma 641.8
      marginal sinus rupture 641.2
      postpartum (atonic) (immediate)
        (within 24 hours) 666.1
        delayed or secondary 666.2
        third stage 666.0
    labor (abnormal) 661.9
      arrested active phase 661.1
      atony (hypotonic) (inertia)
        661.2
        with hemorrhage 666.1
        other uterine inertia 661.2
      primary 661.0
      secondary 661.1

Delivery *(continued)*
  complicated (by) *(continued)*
    labor *(continued)*
      dilation, cervix, incomplete or slow
        661.0
      dystocia
        cervical 661.2
        positional 652.8
        shoulder girdle 660.4
      early onset (22–36 weeks gestation)
        644.2
      failed, failure
        fetal head to enter pelvic brim
          652.5
        induction 659.1
          mechanical or surgical 659.0
          medical 659.1
        trial (vaginal delivery) 660.6
      false 644.1
      incoordinate 661.4
      obstructed (due to) 660.0
        abnormality of pelvic organs or
          tissues 660.2
        deep transverse arrest 660.3
        impacted shoulders 660.4
        locked twins 660.5
        malposition and malpresentation
          of fetus 660.0
        persistent occipitoposterior 660.3
        shoulder dystocia 660.5
      precipitate 661.3
      premature
        before 37 completed weeks
          gestation 644.2
        threatened 644.2
      prolonged 662.1
        active stage 661.2
        first stage 662.0
        second stage 662.2
        due to
          cervical dystocia 661.2
          contraction ring (Bandl's)
            661.4
          latent phase 661.0
          tetanic uterus 661.4
          uterine inertia 661.2
            primary 661.0
            secondary 661.1
      slow slope active phase 661.2
    laceration (rupture) 664.9
      anus (sphincter) 664.2
        with mucosa 664.3
        old, healed 654.8

Delivery *(continued)*
  complicated (by) *(continued)*
    laceration *(continued)*
      not associated with third-degree
        perineal laceration 664.6
      bladder (urinary) 665.5
      bowel 665.5
      cervix 665.3
      fourchette 664.0
      hymen 664.0
      labia (majora) (minora) 664.0
      pelvic
        floor 664.1
        organ NEC 665.5
      perineum, perineal 664.4
        central 664.4
        extensive NEC 664.4
        first degree 664.0
        fourth degree 664.3
        muscles 664.1
        second degree 664.1
        skin 664.0
        slight 664.0
        third degree 664.2
      peritoneum 665.5
      periurethral tissue 664.8
      rectovaginal (septum) (without
        perineal lacerations) 665.4
      with perineum 664.2
      with anal or rectal mucosa 664.3
      threatened NEC 644.1
      urethra 665.5
      uterus 665.1
        before labor 665.0
      vagina (deep) (without perineal lac-
        eration) 665.4
      with perineum 664.0
      muscles, with perineum 664.1
      vulva 664.0
      undelivered 644.1
    maternal conditions
      distress 669.0
      eclampsia 642.6
      elderly
        multigravida 659.6
        primigravida 659.5
      fever during labor 659.2
      injury NEC 665.9
      maternal hypotension syndrome 669.2
      multiparity (grand) 659.4
      sudden death, unknown cause
        669.9
      young maternal age 659.8

Delivery *(continued)*
  complicated (by) *(continued)*
    missed (at or near term) 656.4
    multiple gestation NEC 651.9
      conjoined (Siamese) twins 653.7
      causing obstructed labor 660.1
      delayed delivery (one or more
        mates) 662.3
      locked mates 660.5
      more than 4 fetuses 651.8
        with fetal loss and retention of
          one or more fetus(es) 651.6
      quadruplet NEC 651.2
        with fetal loss and retention of
          one or more fetus(es) 651.5
      triplets NEC 651.1
        with fetal loss and retention of
          one or more fetus(es) 651.4
      twins NEC 651.0
        with fetal loss and retention of
          one or more fetus(es) 651.3
    placenta, placental
      ablatio or abruptio 641.2
      abnormality 656.7
        with hemorrhage 641.2
      accreta 667.0
        with hemorrhage 666.0
      adherent (without hemorrhage)
        667.0
        with hemorrhage 666.0
      apoplexy 641.2
      disease 656.7
      hemorrhage NEC 641.9
      increta (without hemorrhage)
        667.0
        with hemorrhage 666.0
      low (implantation) 641.1
        without hemorrhage 641.0
      malposition 641.1
        without hemorrhage 641.0
      marginal sinus rupture 641.2
      percreta 667.0
        with hemorrhage 666.0
      premature separation 641.2
      previa (central) (lateral) (marginal)
        (partial) 641.1
        without hemorrhage 641.0
      retained (trapped) (with hemorrhage)
        666.0
        without hemorrhage 667.0
      vicious insertion 641.1
    presentation or position of fetus NEC
      652.9

Delivery *(continued)*
  complicated (by) *(continued)*
    presentation or position of fetus
      (continued)
      abnormal (breech), with version
        successful version 652.1
        unsuccessful (attempted) version
          652.2
      abnormal position causing obstructed
        labor 660.0
      acromion 652.8
      brow 652.4
      chin 652.4
      compound 652.8
      crossbirth 652.3
      face 652.4
      in multiple gestation 652.6
      mal lie 652.9
      mentum 652.4
      oblique 652.3
      prolapse (fetal)
        arm or hand 652.7
        extremity 652.8
        foot or leg 652.8
        umbilical cord 663.0
      shoulder 652.8
      transverse 652.3
      unstable lie 652.0
    previous
      cesarean delivery 654.2
      premature delivery V23.41
      surgery
        any previous surgery, causing
          obstructed labor 660.2
        bariatric 649.2
        cervix 654.6
        gynecological NEC 654.9
        pelvic soft tissues NEC 654.9
        perineum or vulva 654.8
        rectum 654.8
        uterus NEC 654.9
          from previous cesarean delivery
            654.2
        vagina 654.7
        vulva 654.8
    rupture *(see also* Delivery, trauma,
        laceration)
      marginal sinus 641.2
      membranes
        artificial with delayed delivery 658.3
        spontaneous with delayed delivery
          658.2
        premature 658.1
    Siamese twins 678.1

Delivery *(continued)*
  complicated (by) *(continued)*
    trauma, obstetric *(see also* Delivery, specific condition)
      diastasis recti 665.8
      inversion, uterus 665.2
      penetration, pregnant uterus by instrument 665.1
      separation, pubic bone or symphysis pubis 665.6
      shock (birth) (obstetric) (puerperal) 669.1
      trauma NEC 665.9
    umbilical cord 663.9
      around neck, tightly or with compression 663.1
        without compression 663.3
      bruising 663.6
      complication NEC 663.9
        specified type NEC 663.8
      compression NEC 663.2
      entanglement NEC 663.3
        with compression 663.2
      marginal attachment 663.8
      prolapse (complete) (occult) (partial) 663.0
      short (short cord syndrome) 663.4
      thrombosis (vessels) 663.6
      vascular lesion 663.6
      vasa previa 663.5
      velamentous insertion 663.8
    vacuum extractor NEC 669.5
Dependence
  alcohol, alcoholic (ethyl) (methyl) (wood) 303.9
    maternal, with suspected fetal damage affecting management of pregnancy 655.4
  drug NEC 304.9
    analgesic NEC 304.6
      synthetic with morphine-like effect 304.0
    amphetamine(s) (type) 304.4
    Angel dust 304.6
    anxiolytic 304.1
    barbiturate(s) (compounds) 304.1
    cocaine 304.2
    codeine 304.0
    combination (excluding morphine or opioid type drug) NEC 304.8
      morphine or opioid type drug with any other drug 304.7

Dependence *(continued)*
  drug *(continued)*
    complicating pregnancy, childbirth, or puerperium 648.3
    Demerol 304.0
    hallucinogenic 304.5
    hashish 304.3
    heroin 304.0
    hypnotic NEC 304.1
    inhalant 304.6
    lysergic acid (amide) 304.5
    marihuana 304.3
    mescaline 304.5
    methadone 304.0
    methamphetamine(s) 304.4
    morphine (sulfate) (sulfite) (type) 304.0
    narcotic NEC 304.9
    nonbarbiturate sedatives and tranquilizers with similar effect 304.1
    opium (alkaloids) (derivatives) (tincture) 304.0
    PCP (phencyclidine) 304.6
    Percodan 304.0
    phenobarbital 304.1
    psychostimulant NEC 304.4
    sedative 304.1
    soporific NEC 304.1
    specified type NEC 304.6
    speed 304.4
    suspected damage to fetus affecting management of pregnancy 655.5
    synthetic, with morphine-like effect 304.0
    tranquilizing 304.1
    Valium 304.1
  glue (airplane) (sniffing) 304.6
  tobacco 305.1
    complicating pregnancy, childbirth, or puerperium 649.0
Depletion
  potassium 276.8
  salt or sodium 276.1
  volume (extracellular fluid) (plasma) 276.5
Depraved appetite 307.52
Depression 311
  acute *(see also* Psychosis, affective) 296.2
    recurrent episode 296.3
    single episode 296.2
  anaclitic 309.21
  anxiety 300.4

Depression *(continued)*
basal metabolic rate (BMR) 794.7
nervous 300.4
neurotic 300.4
postpartum 648.4
psychogenic, psychoneurotic 300.4
reactive 300.4
situational (acute) (brief) 309.0
prolonged 309.1
Depressive reaction
acute (transient) 309.0
with anxiety 309.28
prolonged 309.1
situational (acute) 309.0
prolonged 309.1
Deprivation
affecting adult 995.82
emotional V62.89
sleep V69.4
Dermatitis (allergic) (contact) (occupational)
(venenata) 692.9
ab igne 692.82
acneiform 692.9
actinic—*see* Dermatitis, due to sun
anaphylactoid NEC 692.9
atrophicans 701.8
diffusa 701.8
maculosa 701.3
autoimmune progesterone 279.49
berlock, berloque 692.72
blister beetle 692.89
caterpillar 692.89
diabetic 250.8
due to
acetone 692.2
acids 692.4
alcohol (skin contact) (substances classifiable to 980.0–980.9)
692.4
allergy NEC 692.9
ammonia (household) (liquid) 692.4
arnica 692.3
arsenic 692.4
cantharides 692.3
carbon disulphide 692.2
caustics 692.4
chemical(s) NEC 692.4
chlorocompounds 692.2
cold weather 692.89
cosmetics 692.81
cyclohexanes 692.2
deodorant 692.81
detergents 692.0

Dermatitis *(continued)*
due to *(continued)*
dichromate 692.4
drugs and medicinals (correct substance properly administered)
external (in contact with skin) 692.3
dyes 692.89
hair 692.89
epidermophytosis—*see*
Dermatophytosis
external irritant NEC 692.9
specified agent NEC 692.89
fungicides 692.3
furs 692.89
greases NEC 692.1
infrared rays, except from sun 692.82
ingested substance 693.9
specified substance NEC 693.8
insecticides 692.4
internal agent 693.9
iodine 692.3
irradiation 692.82
jewelry 692.83
keratolytics 692.3
mercury, mercurials 692.3
metals 692.83
Neomycin 692.3
nylon 692.4
oils NEC 692.1
paint solvent 692.2
pediculocides 692.3
petroleum products (substances classifiable to 981) 692.4
phenol 692.3
plants NEC 692.6
plastic 692.4
poisonous plant (ivy) 692.6
preservatives 692.89
rubber 692.4
solvents (any) (substances classifiable
to) (982.0–982.8) 692.2
specified agent NEC 692.89
sun 692.70
acute 692.72
chronic NEC 692.74
specified NEC 692.79
sunburn 692.71
tanning bed 692.82
topical medications 692.3
ultraviolet rays, except from sun
692.82
X-rays 692.82
dysmenorrheica 625.8

Dermatitis *(continued)*
eczematoid NEC, eczematous NEC
692.9
friction 709.8
gestationis 646.8
gonococcal 098.89
heat 692.89
hiemalis 692.89
hypostatic, hypostatica 454.1
with ulcer 454.2
lichenified NEC 692.9
lichenoid, chronic 701.0
lichenoides purpurica pigmentosa 709.1
meadow 692.6
nummular NEC 692.9
osteatosis, osteatotic 706.8
papillaris capillitii 706.1
perioral 695.3
perstans 696.1
pigmented purpuric lichenoid 709.1
pruritic NEC 692.9
psoriasiform nodularis 696.2
repens 696.1
sensitization NEC 692.9
septic *(see also* Septicemia) 686.00
gonococcal 098.89
stasis 454.1
due to
postphlebitic syndrome 459.12
with ulcer 459.13
varicose veins—*see* Varicose
ulcerated or with ulcer (varicose) 454.2
varicose 454.1
with ulcer 454.2
xerotic 706.8
Dermatolysis (congenital) (exfoliativa) 701.8
Dermatomegaly NEC 701.8
Dermatophytosis
fingernails, toenails 110.1
perianal (area) 110.3
vulva 110.8
Dermatosclerosis *(see also* Scleroderma)
710.1
localized 701.0
Dermatosis 709.9
Bowen's—*see* Neoplasm, skin, in situ
gonococcal 098.89
menstrual NEC 709.8
papulosa nigra 709.8
pigmentary NEC 709.00
progressive 709.09
Schamberg's 709.09
senile NEC 709.3

Dermoid (cyst) *(see also* Neoplasm, by site,
benign)
with malignant transformation 183.0
Dermopathy, senile NEC 709.3
Desensitization to allergens V07.1
Deviation
organ or site, congenital NEC—*see*
Malposition, congenital
ureter (congenital) 753.4
Diabetes, diabetic (mellitus) 250.0
with
coma (with ketoacidosis) 250.3
due to secondary diabetes 249.3
hyperosmolar (nonketotic) 250.2
due to secondary diabetes 249.2
complication NEC 250.9
due to secondary diabetes 249.9
specified NEC 250.8
due to secondary diabetes 249.8
hyperosmolarity 250.2
due to secondary diabetes 249.9
ketosis, ketoacidosis 250.1
due to secondary diabetes 249.1
specified manifestations NEC 250.8
due to secondary diabetes 249.8
asymptomatic 790.29
gestational
complicating pregnancy, childbirth, or
puerperium (maternal) (conditions classifiable to
790.21–790.29) 648.8
nongestational
complicating pregnancy, childbirth, or
puerperium (maternal) (conditions classifiable to 249 and
250) 648.0
Pre-diabetes 790.29
Diaphoresis (excessive) NEC *(see also*
Hyperhidrosis) 780.8
Diarrhea, diarrheal (acute) (chronic) 787.91
dietetic 787.91
due to *Bacillus coli* or *Escherichia coli*—*see*
Enteritis, *E. coli*
dyspeptic 787.91
fermentative 787.91
functional 564.5
following gastrointestinal surgery 564.4
inflammatory 787.91
Difficulty
feeding, breast 676.8
swallowing *(see also* Dysphagia) 787.2
Dilatation (Dilated) (Dilation)
appendix (cystic) 543.9

Dilatation *(continued)*
  bladder (sphincter)
    in pregnancy or childbirth 654.4
      causing obstructed labor 660.2
  cervix (uteri)—*see* Incompetency, cervix
  mammary duct 610.4
  organ or site, congenital NEC—*see*
        Distortion
  urethra (acquired) 599.84
Discharge
  anal NEC 787.99
  breast or nipple 611.79
  excessive urine 788.42
  umbilicus 789.9
  urethral 788.7
    bloody 599.84
  vaginal 623.5
Discomfort, chest 786.59
Discrepancy, uterine size-date 649.6
Disease, diseased *(see also* Syndrome)
  Albarrán's (colibacilluria) 791.9
  Albright (-Martin) (-Bantam) 275.49
  angiopastic, angiospasmodic 443.9
  antral (chronic) 473.0
    acute 461.0
  anus NEC 569.49
  autoimmune NEC 279.49
  appendix 543.9
  bacterial NEC 040.89
  Baerensprung's (eczema marginatum)
        110.3
  Bannister's 995.1
  Bateman's 078.0
  Biermer's (pernicious anemia) 281.0
  bleeder's 286.0
  Bloodgood's 610.1
  Bouveret (-Hoffmann) (paroxysmal
        tachycardia) 427.2
  Bowen's—*see* Neoplasm, skin, in situ
  bowel, functional 564.9
  breast 611.9
    cystic or fibrocystic (chronic) 610.1
    inflammatory 616.9
    Paget's 174.0
    puerperal, postpartum NEC 676.
    specified NEC 611.89
  Breisky's (kraurosis vulvae) 624.09
  Bright's, arteriosclerotic *(see also*
        Hypertension, kidney)
        403.90
  broad ligament, noninflammatory
        620.9
    specified NEC 620.8

Disease, diseased *(continued)*
  Brocq's meaning prurigo 698.2
  Buschke's 710.1
  cardiac—*see* Disease, heart
  cardiovascular (arteriosclerotic) hyperten-
        sive—*see* Disease, heart
  cellular tissue NEC 709.9
  cerebrovascular NEC 437.9
    acute 436
    postpartum 674.0
  cervix (uteri)
    inflammatory 616.0
    noninflammatory 622.9
      specified NEC 622.8
  Christmas 286.1
  circulatory (system) NEC 459.9
  climatic bubo (Durand–Nicolas–Favre)
        (Frei's) 099.1
  colon, functional 564.9
  Concato's (pericardial polyserositis), peri-
        toneal 568.82
  Cooper's 610.1
  Csillag's (lichen sclerosus et atrophicus)
        701.0
  Down's (mongolism) 758.0
  Ducrey's (bacillus) (chancre) 099.0
  Fahr-Volhard (malignant nephrosclerosis)
        403.00
  fallopian tube, noninflammatory 620.9
    specified NEC 620.8
  Fanconi's (congenital pancytopenia)
        284.09
  Favre–Racouchot (elastoidosis cutanea
        nodularis) 701.8
  fibrocystic—*see* Fibrocystic, disease
  Filatoff's, Filatov's (infectious mononu-
        cleosis) 075
  Fordyce–Fox (apocrine miliaria) 705.82
  frontal sinus (chronic) 473.1
    acute 461.1
  genital organs NEC 629.9
    specified NEC 629.8
  Gougerot's (trisymptomatic) 709.1
  Hageman (congenital factor XII deficiency)
        286.3
  Hallopeau's (lichen sclerosus et atrophicus)
        701.0
  heart (organic) with *(see also* Pericarditis)
    acute pulmonary edema *(see also*
        Failure, ventricular, left),
        hypertensive 402.91
    arteriosclerotic or sclerotic—*see*
        Arteriosclerosis, coronary
    functional 427.9

Disease, diseased *(continued)*
 heart *(continued)*
  postoperative 997.1
  hypertensive *(see also* Hypertension,
   heart) 402.90
   benign 402.10
   malignant 402.00
  postpartum 674.8
  sclerotic—*see* Arteriosclerosis,
   coronary
 Hebra's prurigo 698.2
 hemoglobin (Hb)—*see* Sickle-cell
 Herxheimer's (diffuse idiopathic cutaneous
  atrophy) 701.8
 high fetal gene or hemoglobin thalassemia
  282.49
 Huchard's (continued arterial hypertension) 401.9
 Huguier's (uterine fibroma) 218.9
 hunger 251.1
 Hutchinson's, meaning angioma serpiginosum 709.1
 kissing 075
 labia
  inflammatory 616.10
  noninflammatory 624.9
   specified NEC 624.8
 Lewandowski–Lutz (epidermodysplasia
  verruciformis) 078.19
 Lipschütz's 616.50
 liver 573.9
  drug induced 573.3
  organic 573.9
 lung
  nonspecific, chronic 496
  obstructive (chronic) (COPD) (with)
   496
   acute
    bronchitis 491.22
    exacerbation NEC 491.21
   asthma (chronic) (obstructive)
    493.2
   bronchiectasis 494.0
   bronchitis (chronic) 491.20
   emphysema NEC 492.8
   diffuse (with fibrosis) 496
   polycystic asthma (chronic) (obstruc-
    tive) 493.2
 malignant *(see also* Neoplasm, by site,
  malignant)
  previous, affecting management of
   pregnancy V23.89
 microvascular 413.9

Disease, diseased *(continued)*
 musculoskeletal system 729.9
 nipple 611.9
  Paget's 174.0
 ovary (noninflammatory) NEC 620.9
  cystic 620.2
  polycystic 256.4
  specified NEC 620.8
 Paget's—*see* Paget's disease
 parametrium 629.9
 Parkinson's 332.0
 pelvis, pelvic NEC 629.9
  gonococcal—*see* Gonorrhea
  infection *(see also* Disease, pelvis,
   inflammatory) 614.9
  inflammatory (PID) 614.9
   with or following
    abortion—*see* Abortion, by type,
     with sepsis
     following abortion 639.0
    ectopic or molar pregnancy *(see
     also* categories 633.0–633.9)
     639.0
   acute 614.3
   chronic 614.4
   complicating pregnancy 646.6
   peritonitis (acute) 614.5
    chronic NEC 614.7
   puerperal, postpartum, childbirth
    670.8
   specified NEC 614.8
  peritoneum NEC 629.9
  specified NEC 629.8
 perineum
  inflammatory 616.9
   specified NEC 616.8
  noninflammatory 624.9
   specified NEC 624.8
 peripheral, arterial or vascular 443.9
 peritoneum 568.9
  pelvic 629.9
   specified NEC 629.8
 Phocas' 610.1
 placenta, complicating pregnancy or
  childbirth 656.7
 Pollitzer's (hidradenitis suppurativa) 705.83
 Preiser's (osteoporosis) 733.09
 Reclus' (cystic) 610.1
 rectum NEC 569.49
 renal (functional) (pelvis) 593.9
  acute 584.9
  complicating pregnancy or puerperium
   NEC 646.2

Disease, diseased *(continued)*
 renal *(continued)*
  with hypertension—*see* Toxemia, of
   pregnancy
  hypertensive *(see also* Hypertension,
   kidney) 403.90
  tubular *(see also* Nephrosis, tubular)
   584.5
  renovascular (arteriosclerotic) *(see also*
   Hypertension, kidney) 403.90
 respiratory (tract)
  acute or subacute (upper) NEC 465.9
   multiple sites NEC 465.8
   streptococcal 034.0
  obstructive 496
 Schimmelbusch's 610.1
 sebaceous glands NEC 706.9
 serum NEC 999.5
 Sheehan's (postpartum pituitary necrosis)
  253.2
 sickle-cell—*see* Sickle Cell
 trophoblastic—*see* Hydatidiform mole
 tubo-ovarian
  inflammatory *(see also* Salpingo-
   oophoritis) 614.2
  noninflammatory 620.9
   specified NEC 620.8
 uterus (organic) 621.9
  infective, inflammatory *(see also*
   Endometritis) 615.9
  noninflammatory 621.9
   specified type NEC 621.8
 vagina, vaginal
  inflammatory 616.10
  noninflammatory 623.9
   specified NEC 623.8
 Valsuani's (progressive pernicious anemia,
  puerperal) 648.2
  complicating pregnancy or puerperium
   648.2
 vascular 459.9
  arteriosclerotic—*see* Arteriosclerosis
  hypertensive—*see* Hypertension
  obliterative peripheral 443.9
  occlusive 459.9
  peripheral (occlusive) 443.9
 venereal
  chlamydial NEC 099.50
   anus 099.52
   bladder 099.53
   cervix 099.53
   genitourinary NEC 099.55

Disease, diseased *(continued)*
 venereal *(continued)*
  chlamydial *(continued)*
   lower 099.53
   specified NEC 099.54
   pelvic inflammatory disease 099.54
   peritoneum 099.56
   rectum 099.52
   vagina 099.53
   vulva 099.53
  fifth or sixth 099.1
  complicating pregnancy, childbirth, or
   puerperium 647.2
  specified nature or type NEC 099.8
 virus (filterable) NEC
  complicating pregnancy, childbirth, or
   puerperium 647.6
  contact (with) V01.79
  exposure to V01.7
  maternal, with fetal damage affecting
   management of pregnancy
   655.3
  vaccination, prophylactic (against)
   V04.89
 vulva
  inflammatory 616.10
  noninflammatory 624.9
Disfigurement (due to scar) 709.2
Disorder *(see also* Disease)
 anxiety—*see* Anxiety
 autoimmune NEC 279.49
 bladder, functional NEC 596.59
 coagulation (factor)—*see* Defect, coagulation
 coccyx 724.70
  specified NEC 724.79
 depressive—*see* Depression
 eating NEC 307.50
 electrolyte NEC 276.9
  with or following
   abortion—*see* Abortion, by type,
    with metabolic disorder
   following abortion 639.4
   ectopic or molar pregnancy *(see also*
    categories 633.0–633.9)
    639.4
  acidosis 276.2
  alkalosis 276.3
 emancipation as adjustment reaction
  309.22
 factitious (with combined psychological
  and physical signs and symptoms) 300.19

Disorder *(continued)*
genitourinary system, psychogenic
306.50
hemorrhagic NEC due to intrinsic circulating anticoagulants 286.5
hemostasis (*see also* Defect, coagulation)
286.9
intestinal, functional NEC 564.9
lactation 676.9
menopausal 627.9
specified NEC 627.8
menstrual 626.9
psychogenic 306.52
specified NEC 626.8
metabolism NEC
with or following
abortion—*see* Abortion, by type,
with metabolic disorder
following abortion 639.4
ectopic or molar pregnancy (*see also*
categories 633.0–633.9)
639.4
basal 794.7
calcium 275.40
in labor and delivery 669.0
sodium 276.9
micturition—*see* Urine
panic 300.01
postmenopausal 627.9
specified type NEC 627.8
premenstrual dysphoric (PMDD) 625.4
sexual
desire, hypoactive 302.71
function, psychogenic 302.70
skin NEC 709.9
specified type NEC 709.8
vascular 709.1
social, of childhood and adolescence
specified NEC 780.59
soft tissue 729.9
stress (*see also* Reaction, stress, acute)
308.9
suspected—*see* Observation
Displacement, displaced
cervix—*see* Displacement, uterus
device, implant, or graft—*see*
Complications, mechanical
epithelium
columnar of cervix 622.10
cuboidal, beyond limits of external os
(uterus) 752.49
fallopian tube (acquired) 620.4
congenital 752.19

Displacement, displaced *(continued)*
opening (congenital) 752.19
hymen (congenital) (upward) 752.49
intrauterine device 996.32
organ or site, congenital NEC—*see*
Malposition, congenital
ovary (acquired) 620.4
congenital 752.0
free in peritoneal cavity (congenital)
752.0
into hernial sac 620.4
ureter or ureteric opening or orifice
(congenital) 753.4
uterine opening of oviducts or fallopian
tubes 752.19
uterus, uterine (*see also* Malposition,
uterus) 621.6
congenital 752.3
Disproportion 653.9 (*see also* Delivery,
complicated by)
breast, reconstructed 612.1
between native and reconstructed
612.1
Disruption
family V61.09
due to
child in
care of non-parental family member V61.06
death of family member V61.07
extended absence of family member NEC V61.08
foster care V61.06
welfare custody V61.05
divorce V61.03
estrangement V61.09
parent-child V61.04
family member
on military deployment V61.01
return from military deployment
V61.02
legal separation V61.03
marital V61.10
involving
divorce V61.03
estrangement V61.09
sleep-wake cycle (24-hour) 780.55
wound—*see* Complication, Surgical,
Procedures, Wound
Distention
abdomen (gaseous) 787.3
liver 573.9
uterus 621.8

Distortion (congenital)
  bladder 753.8
  cervix (uteri) 752.49
  clitoris 752.49
  hymen 752.49
  labium (majus) (minus) 752.49
  lumbar spine with disproportion
        (fetopelvic) 653.0
    causing obstructed labor 660.1
  ovary 752.0
  oviduct 752.19
  ureter 753.4
    causing obstruction 753.20
  urethra 753.8
    causing obstruction 753.6
  uterus 752.3
  vagina 752.49
  vulva 752.49
Distress
  abdomen 789.0
  colon, intestinal 564.9
  epigastric 789.0
  fetal (syndrome) affecting management
        of pregnancy or childbirth
        656.8
  intrauterine—*see* Distress, fetal
  maternal 669.0
  respiratory 786.09
Disturbance (*see also* Disease or Disorder)
  acid-base equilibrium 276.9
  circulatory 459.9
  electrolyte—*see* Electrolyte imbalance
  equilibrium 780.4
  innervation uterus, sympathetic, parasym-
        pathetic 621.8
  nervous functional 799.2
  situational (transient) (*see also* Reaction,
        adjustment), acute 308.3
  sleep—*see* Sleep
Diuresis 788.42
Diverticula, diverticulosis, diverticulum
        (acute) (multiple) (ruptured)
  appendix (noninflammatory) 543.9
  bladder (acquired) (sphincter) 596.3
  broad ligament 620.8
  fallopian tube 620.8
  organ or site, congenital NEC—*see*
        Distortion
  urethra (acquired) 599.2
    congenital 753.8
Division
  cervix uteri 622.8
  external (cervical) into two openings by

Division *(continued)*
    frenum 752.49
  hymen 752.49
  labia minora (congenital) 752.49
  vein 459.9
Dizziness 780.4
Double (*see also* Accessory)
  bladder 753.8
  clitoris 752.49
  organ or site NEC—*see* Accessory
  pelvis (renal) with double ureter
        753.4
  ureter (one or both sides) 753.4
  urethra 753.8
  urinary meatus 753.8
  uterus (any degree) 752.2
    with doubling of cervix and vagina
        752.2
    in pregnancy or childbirth 654.0
  vagina 752.49
    with doubling of cervix and uterus
        752.2
  vulva 752.49
Down's disease or syndrome (mongolism)
        758.0
Drop, hemoglobin 790.01
Dropsy, dropsical (*see also* Edema) 782.3
  abdomen 789.5
  amnion (*see also* Hydramnios) 657
  ovary 620.8
  uremic—*see* Uremia
Drug (*see also* condition)
  addiction, dependence, habit (*see also*
        Dependence) 304.9
  adverse effect NEC, correct substance
        properly administered 995.2
  therapy (maintenance) status NEC V58.1
    long-term (current) use V58.69
      antibiotics V58.62
      anticoagulants V58.61
      anti-inflammatories, non-steroidal
        (NSAID) V58.64
      antiplatelets or antithrombotics
        V58.63
      aspirin V58.66
      high-risk medications NEC V58.69
      insulin V58.67
      methadone V58.69
      opiate analgesic V58.69
      steroids V58.65
Drunkenness (*see also* Abuse, drugs, non-
        dependent) 305.0
  alcoholism—*see* Alcoholism

Duplication—*see* Accessory, Double
Dwarf, dwarfism, ovarian 758.6
Dyschromia 709.00
Dyscrasia
blood
with antepartum hemorrhage 641.3
puerperal, postpartum 666.3
ovary 256.8
Dysequilibrium 780.4
Dysesthesia 782.0
Dysfibrinogenemia (congenital) (*see also* Defect, coagulation) 286.3
Dysfunction
bleeding, uterus 626.8
colon 564.9
endometrium 621.8
hepatic or hepatocellular 573.9
liver 573.9
ovary, ovarian 256.9
hyperfunction 256.1
estrogen 256.0
hypofunction 256.39
postablative 256.2
specified NEC 256.8
placental—*see* Placenta, insufficiency
psychosexual (with) 302.70
dyspareunia (functional) (psychogenic) 302.76
inhibition
orgasm 302.73
sexual
desire 302.71
excitement 302.72
sexual aversion 302.79
specified disorder NEC 302.79
vaginismus 306.51
rectum 564.9
sexual 302.70
sinoatrial node 427.81
somatic 739.9
abdomen 739.9
pelvic 739.5
specified site NEC 739.9
uterus, complicating delivery—*see* Delivery
Dysgenesis
gonadal (due to chromosomal anomaly) 758.6
pure 752.7
ovarian 758.6
tidal platelet 287.3

Dysgerminoma
specified site—*see* Neoplasm, by site, malignant
unspecified site 183.0
Dyskeratosis (*see also* Keratosis)
cervix 622.10
uterus NEC 621.8
Dysmenorrhea (primary) (secondary) 625.3
psychogenic 306.52
Dysmetabolic syndrome X 277.7
Dysorexia 783.0
Dyspareunia 625.0
psychogenic 302.76
Dysphagia 787.2
sideropenic 280.8
Dysplasia (*see also* Anomaly)
anus 569.44
intraepithelial neoplasia I [AIN I] (histologically confirmed) 569.44
intraepithelial neoplasia II [AIN II] (histologically confirmed) 569.44
intraepithelial neoplasia III [AIN III] 230.6
anal canal 230.5
mild (histologically confirmed) 569.44
moderation (histologically confirmed) 569.44
severe 230.6
anal canal 230.5
cervix (uteri) 622.10
cervical intraepithelial neoplasia I (CIN I) 622.11
cervical intraepithelial neoplasia II (CIN II) 622.12
cervical intraepithelial neoplasia III (CIN III) 233.1
mild 622.11
moderate 622.12
severe 233.1
epithelial, uterine cervix 622.10
mammary (benign) (gland) 610.9
cystic 610.1
specified type NEC 610.8
skin 709.8
vagina 623.0
mild 623.0
moderate 623.0
severe 233.31
vulva 624.8
intraepithelial neoplasia I (VIN I) 624.01
intraepithelial neoplasia II (VIN II) 624.02

Dysplasia *(continued)*
vulva *(continued)*
intraepithelial neoplasia III (VIN III)
233.32
mild 624.01
moderate 624.02
severe 233.32
Dyspnea (nocturnal) (paroxysmal) 786.09
asthmatic (bronchial) *(see also* Asthma)
493.9
with bronchitis *(see also* Asthma) 493.9
chronic 493.2
hyperventilation 786.01
uremic—*see* Uremia
Dystocia—*see* Delivery, labor
Dystrophy, dystrophia 783.9
ovarian 620.8
pigmentary *(see also* Acanthosis) 701.2
skin NEC 709.9
vulva 624.09
Dysuria 788.1
psychogenic 306.53

E
Eclampsia, eclamptic (coma) (convulsions)
(delirium) 780.39
not associated with pregnancy or childbirth 780.39
pregnancy, childbirth, or puerperium 642.6
with pre-existing hypertension 642.7
Ectasia, ectasis breast (duct) 610.4
Ectopic, ectopia (congenital)
auricular beats 427.61
beats 427.60
breast tissue 757.6
endometrium 617.9
kidney, in pregnancy or childbirth 654.4
causing obstructed labor 660.2
organ or site NEC—*see* Malposition,
congenital
pregnancy—*see* Pregnancy, ectopic
Ectropion
anus 569.49
cervix 622.0
with mention of cervicitis 616.0
rectum 569.49
urethra 599.84
Eczema (acute) (chronic)
atopic 691.8
asteatotic 706.8
hypertrophicum 701.8
hypostatic—*see* Varicose, vein
marginatum 110.3

Eczema *(continued)*
stasis (lower extremity) 454.1
ulcerated 454.2
vaccination, vaccinatum 999.0
varicose (lower extremity)—*see* Varicose,
vein
Edema, edematous 782.3
angioneurotic (any site) (with urticaria)
995.1
angiospastic 443.9
cervix (acute) (uteri) 622.8
puerperal, postpartum 674.8
circumscribed, acute 995.1
complicating pregnancy (gestational) 646.1
with hypertension—*see* Toxemia, of
pregnancy
connective tissue 782.3
due to
lymphatic obstruction—*see* Edema,
lymphatic
salt retention 276.0
essential, acute 995.1
genital organs 629.8
infectious 782.3
localized 782.3
due to venous obstruction (lower
extremity) 459.2
lymphatic, due to mastectomy operation
457.0
periodic 995.1
salt 276.0
traumatic NEC 782.3
vulva (acute) 624.8
Edwards' syndrome 758.2
Effect, adverse NEC *(see also* Complications)
anesthesia, unspecified 995.22
anesthetic, in labor and delivery NEC
668.9
drugs and medicinals NEC 995.2
correct substance properly administered 995.2
fluoroscopy NEC 990
implantation (removable) of isotope or
radium NEC 990
ingestion or injection of isotope (therapeutic) NEC 990
insulin 995.23
lack of care (adult) 995.84
radiation (diagnostic) (therapeutic)
(X-ray) NEC 990
maternal with suspected damage to
fetus affecting management
of pregnancy 655.6
serum (prophylactic) (therapeutic) NEC

Effect, adverse NEC *(continued)*
    999.5
  specified NEC 995.89
Effects, late—*see* Late, effect (of)
Effusion
  amniotic fluid (*see also* Rupture, membranes, premature) 658.1
  peritoneal (chronic) 568.82
EIN (endometrial intraepithelial neoplasia) 621.35
Elastosis (atrophicans) (senilis) 701.8
Electrolyte imbalance 276.9
  with or following
    abortion—*see* Abortion, by type, with metabolic disorder
      following abortion 639.4
    ectopic or molar pregnancy (*see also* categories 633.0–633.9) 639.4
    hyperemesis gravidarum (before 22 completed weeks gestation) 643.1
Elevation (*see also* Findings, abnormal)
  acid phosphatase 790.5
  amylase 790.5
  basal metabolic rate (BMR) 794.7
  blood pressure (*see also* Hypertension) 401.9
    reading (incidental) (nonspecific), no diagnosis of hypertension 796.2
  blood sugar 790.29
  body temperature (of unknown origin) (*see also* Pyrexia) 780.60
  Rh titer 999.7
  tumor markers—*see* Tumor, markers
  transaminase 790.4
Elongation, elongated (congenital) (*see also* Distortion)
  cervix (uteri) 752.49
    acquired 622.6
    hypertrophic 622.6
  labia minora, acquired 624.8
Embolism
  any type, with or following (*see also* Embolism, obstetric)
    abortion—*see* Abortion, by type, with embolism
      following abortion 639.6
  any type, with or following *(continued)*
    ectopic or molar pregnancy (*see also* categories 633.0–633.9) 639.6
  due to (presence of) any device, implant, or graft classifiable to 996.3–

Embolism *(continued)*
    996.5—*see* Complications
  fat (cerebral) (pulmonary) (systemic) 958.1
  following infusion, perfusion, or transfusion
    air 999.1
    thrombus 999.2
  obstetrical (pulmonary) 673.2
    air 673.0
    amniotic fluid (pulmonary) 673.1
    blood-clot 673.2
    cardiac 674.8
    fat 673.8
    septic 673.3
    specified NEC 674.8
  postoperative NEC 997.2
    cerebral 997.02
    peripheral vascular 997.2
  pyemic (multiple) 038.9
    Aerobacter aerogenes 038.49
    enteric gram-negative bacilli 038.40
    Enterobacter aerogenes 038.49
    Escherichia coli 038.42
    Hemophilus influenzae 038.41
    pneumococcal 038.2
    Proteus vulgaris 038.49
    Pseudomonas (aeruginosa) 038.43
    Serratia 038.44
    specified organism NEC 038.8
    staphylococcal 038.10
      aureus 038.11
      specified organism NEC 038.19
    streptococcal 038.0
  septicemic—*see* Embolism, pyemic
  spinal cord (nonpyogenic) in pregnancy or puerperium 671.5
  thrombus (thromboembolism) following infusion, perfusion, or transfusion 999.2
  vein (deep)
    with inflammation or phlebitis—*see* Thrombophlebitis
    lower extremity (distal) 453.42
      deep 453.40
      acute 453.40
      chronic 453.50
    specified NEC 453.8
Emesis (*see also* Vomiting)
  bilious 787.04
  gravidarum—*see* Hyperemesis, gravidarum
Emphysema (chronic) (diffuse) (essential) (obstructive) 492.8

Emphysema *(continued)*
  with bronchitis
    chronic (with) 491.20
      acute bronchitis 491.22
      exacerbation (acute) 491.21
  cellular, connective or laminated tissue
    (surgical) 998.81
  obstructive diffuse with fibrosis
    492.8
  subcutaneous (surgical) 998.81
  surgical 998.81
Empyema (general) (pleura) (streptococcal)
  accessory sinus (chronic) (*see also*
    Sinusitis) 473.9
  antrum (chronic) (*see also* Sinusitis, maxil-
    lary) 473.0
  frontal (sinus) (chronic) (*see also* Sinusitis,
    frontal) 473.1
Encephalitis, encephalomyelitis (chronic)
  (granulomatous)
  postchickenpox 052.0
Encephalopathy (acute) (due to)
  hypoglycemic 251.2
  influenza (virus) 487.8
  serum (nontherapeutic) (therapeutic)
    999.5
Encounter for (*see also* Admission, for)
  administrative purpose only V68.9
    referral of patient without examination
      or treatment V68.81
    specified purpose NEC V68.89
End-of-life care V66.7
Endocervicitis (*see also* Cervicitis) 616.0
  due to intrauterine (contraceptive) device
    996.65
  gonorrheal (acute) 098.15
    chronic or duration of 2 months or
      over 098.35
  hyperplastic 616.0
  trichomonal 131.09
  tuberculous (*see also* Tuberculosis) 016.7
Endocrine—*see* condition
Endometrioma 617.9
Endometriosis 617.9
  appendix 617.5
  bladder 617.8
  bowel 617.5
  broad ligament 617.3
  cervix 617.0
  colon 617.5
  cul-de-sac (Douglas') 617.3
  exocervix 617.0
  fallopian tube 617.2

Endometriosis *(continued)*
  genital organ NEC 617.8
  in scar of skin 617.6
  internal 617.0
  intestine 617.5
  lung 617.8
  myometrium 617.0
  ovary 617.1
  parametrium 617.3
  pelvic peritoneum 617.3
  rectovaginal septum 617.4
  rectum 617.5
  round ligament 617.3
  skin 617.6
  specified site NEC 617.8
  umbilicus 617.8
  uterus 617.0
  vagina 617.4
  vulva 617.8
Endometritis (nonspecific) (purulent) (septic) (suppurative) 615.9
  with or following
    abortion—*see* Abortion, by type, with
      sepsis
      following abortion 639.0
    ectopic or molar pregnancy (*see also* cate-
      gories 633.0–633.9) 639.0
  acute 615.0
  blennorrhagic 098.16
    acute 098.16
    chronic or duration of 2 months or
      over 098.36
  cervix, cervical (*see also* Cervicitis) 616.0
    hyperplastic 616.0
  chronic 615.1
  complicating pregnancy 670.1
    septic 670.2
  decidual 615.9
  gonorrheal (acute) 098.16
    chronic or duration of 2 months or
      over 098.36
  hyperplastic (*see also* Hyperplasia,
    endometrium) 621.30
    cervix 616.0
  polypoid—*see* Endometritis, hyperplastic
  puerperal, postpartum, childbirth 670.1
    septic 670.2
  senile (atrophic) 615.9
  subacute 615.0
  tuberculous (*see also* Tuberculosis)
    016.7
Endosalpingioma 236.2
Endotoxic shock 785.52

Engorgement, breast 611.79
  puerperal, postpartum 676.2
Enlargement, enlarged (*see also*
      Hypertrophy)
  abdomen 789.3
  organ or site, congenital NEC—*see*
      Anomaly, specified type NEC
  thyroid (gland) (*see also* Goiter) 240.9
Entanglement, umbilical cord(s) 663.3
  with compression 663.2
  around neck with compression
    663.1
  twins in monoamniotic sac 663.2
Enteritis (acute) (chronic) (diarrheal)
  adaptive 564.9
  influenzal 487.8
  membraneous 564.9
  mucous 564.9
  myxomembraneous 564.9
  neurogenic 564.9
  spasmodic 564.9
Enteroarticular syndrome 099.3
Enterocele (*see also* Hernia)
  pelvis, pelvic (acquired) (congenital)
    618.6
  vagina, vaginal (acquired) (congenital)
    618.6
Enuresis 788.30
  nocturnal 788.36
Epidermodysplasia verruciformis
    078.19
Epidermoid inclusion (*see also* Cyst, skin)
    706.2
Epilepsy, epileptic (idiopathic) 345.9
  climacteric 345.9
  convulsions 345.9
  generalized 345.9
    convulsive 345.1
    flexion 345.1
    nonconvulsive 345.0
  grand mal (idiopathic) 345.1
    petit mal 345.0
  seizure 345.9
  status (grand mal) 345.3
    petit mal 345.2
  symptomatic 345.9
Epispadias, female 753.8
Epistaxis (multiple) 784.7
  vicarious menstruation 625.8
Epstein-Barr infection (viral) 075
Erosion
  cervix (uteri) (acquired) (chronic)
    (congenital) 622.0

Erosion (*continued*)
  with mention of cervicitis
    616.0
  gastric, stomach 535.4
  urethra 599.84
  uterus 621.8
Eructation 787.3
Eruption
  skin (*see also* Dermatitis) 782.1
  vesicular 709.8
Erythroblastopenia (acquired) 284.89
  congenital 284.01
Erythroblastophthisis 284.01
Erythromelia 701.8
Esthiomene 099.1
Estrangement V61.0
Estrogen receptor status V86
Eversion
  cervix (uteri) 622.0
    with mention of cervicitis 616.0
  urethra (meatus) 599.84
  uterus 618.1
    complicating delivery 665.2
    puerperal, postpartum 674.8
Evidence
  of malignancy
    cytologic
      without histologic confirmation
        anus 796.76
        cervix 795.06
        vagina 795.16
Evisceration, operative wound 998.32
Examination (general) (routine) (of) (for)
    V70.9
  annual V70.0
  antibody response V72.61
  cervical Papanicolaou smear—*see*
      Papanicolaou smear
  following
    accident (motor vehicle) V71.4
    inflicted injury (victim or culprit) NEC
      V71.6
    rape or seduction, alleged (victim or
      culprit) V71.5
    involving high-risk medication NEC
      V67.51
    specified condition NEC V67.59
  follow-up (routine)—*see* Follow-up
  gynecological V72.31
    for contraceptive maintenance V25.40
      intrauterine device V25.42
      pill V25.41
      specified method NEC V25.49

Examination *(continued)*
    laboratory V72.60
        ordered as part of a routine general
            medical examination V72.62
        pre-operative/ V72.63
        pre-procedural V72.63
        specified NEC V72.69
    lactating mother V24.1
    medical (for) (of) V70.9
        donor (potential) V70.8
        general V70.9
            routine V70.0
            specified reason NEC V70.8
        medicolegal reasons V70.4
        specified reason NEC V70.8
    pelvic (annual) (periodic) V72.31
        Medicare patient V76.2, V76.47 or
            V76.49, V72.31
            high risk V15.89
    periodic (annual) (routine) V70.0
    postpartum
        immediately after delivery V24.0
        routine follow-up V24.2
    pregnancy (unconfirmed) (possible) V72.40
        negative result V72.41
        positive result V72.42
    prenatal V22.1
        first pregnancy V22.0
        high-risk pregnancy V23.9
        specified problem NEC V23.89
    preoperative specified NEC V72.83
    prior to chemotherapy V72.83
    radiological NEC V72.5
    screening—*see* Screening
    special V72.9
    specified type or reason NEC V72.85
        preoperative V72.83
            specified NEC V72.83
    vaginal Papanicolaou smear—*see*
            Papanicolaou smear
    Welcome to Medicare physical V70.0
Exanthem, exanthema (*see also* Rash) 782.1
Excess, excessive, excessively
    alcohol level in blood 790.3
    development, breast 611.1
    diaphoresis (*see also* Hyperhidrosis) 780.8
    drinking (alcohol) NEC (*see also* Abuse,
            drugs, nondependent) 305.0
        continual or habitual (*see also*
            Alcoholism) 303.9
    eating 783.6
    fat 278.00
        causing inconclusive findings, radio-

Excess, excessive, excessively *(continued)*
        logic test 793.91
    gas 787.3
    large, organ or site, congenital NEC—*see*
            Anomaly, specified type NEC
    long
        organ or site, congenital NEC—*see*
            Anomaly, specified type NEC
        umbilical cord (entangled), in preg-
            nancy or childbirth 663.3
            with compression 663.2
    menstruation 626.2
    nutrients (dietary) NEC 783.6
    potassium (K) 276.7
    secretion (*see also* Hypersecretion)
        milk 676.6
        sputum 786.4
        sweat (*see also* Hyperhidrosis) 780.8
    short
        organ or site, congenital NEC—*see*
            Anomaly, specified type
            NECskin NEC 701.9
    sodium (Na) 276.0
    thirst 783.5
    tissue in reconstructed breast 612.0
    weight 278.00
        gain 783.1
            of pregnancy 646.1
        loss 783.21
Exhaustion, exhaustive (physical NEC)
            780.79
    delirium (*see also* Reaction, stress, acute)
            308.9
    maternal, complicating delivery 669.8
    postinfectional NEC 780.79
    psychosis (*see also* Reaction, stress, acute)
            308.9
Exposure to
    AIDS virus V01.79
    anthrax V01.81
    communicable disease V01.9
    Escherichia coli (E. coli) V01.83
    German measles V01.4
    gonorrhea V01.6
    human immunodeficiency virus (HIV)
            V01.79
    rubella V01.4
    SARS-associated coronavirus V01.82
    syphilis V01.6
    tuberculosis V01.1
    varicella V01.71
    venereal disease V01.6
    viral disease NEC V01.79

Extroversion
uterus 618.1
    complicating delivery 665.2
    postpartal (old) 618.1
Extrusion
breast implant (prosthetic) 996.54
device, implant, or graft—*see*
        Complications, mechanical

F

Failure, failed
attempted abortion—*see* Abortion,
        failed
cardiorespiratory, specified during or due
        to a procedure 997.1
cervical dilatation in labor 661.0
circulation, circulatory 799.89
    peripheral 785.50
conscious sedation, during procedure
        995.24
device, implant, or graft—*see*
        Complications
heart (acute) (sudden)
    with or following
        abortion—*see* Abortion, by type,
            with specified complication
            NEC
        ectopic or molar pregnancy (*see also*
            categories 633.0–633.9)
            639.8
    arteriosclerotic 440.9
    complicating
        delivery (cesarean) (instrumental)
            669.4
        obstetric anesthesia or sedation
            668.1
        surgery 997.1
    hypertensive 402.91
        benign 402.11
        malignant 402.01
    postoperative (immediate) 997.1
    specified during or due to a procedure
        997.1
induction (of labor) 659.1
    abortion (*see also* Abortion, failed)
        638.9
    by oxytocic drugs 659.1
    instrumental (mechanical) 659.0
    medical 659.1
    surgical 659.0
kidney—*see* Failure, renal
medullary 799.89
moderate sedation, during procedure
    995.24

Failure, failed (*continued*)
ovarian (primary) 256.39
    iatrogenic 256.2
    postablative 256.2
    postirradiation 256.2
    postsurgical 256.2
ovulation 628.0
renal (kidney)
    with or following
        abortion—*see* Abortion, by type,
            with renal failure
            following abortion 639.3
        crushing 958.5
        ectopic or molar pregnancy (*see also*
            categories 633.0–633.9)
            639.3
        hypertension (*see also* Hypertension,
            kidney) 403.91
        labor and delivery (acute) 669.3
    due to a procedure 997.5
    hypertensive (*see also* Hypertension,
        kidney) 403.91
    puerperal, postpartum 669.3
to progress 661.2
to thrive (adult) 783.7
trial of labor NEC 660.6
tubal ligation 998.89
ventouse NEC 660.7
ventricular (*see also* Failure, heart)
    hypertensive (*see also* Hypertension,
        heart) 402.91
        benign 402.11
        malignant 402.01
Fainting (fit) (spell) 780.2
Falciform hymen 752.49
Fallopian insufflation
fertility testing V26.21
following sterilization reversal
    V26.22
False (*see also* condition)
labor (pains) 644.1
positive
    serological test for syphilis 795.6
    Wassermann reaction 795.6
pregnancy 300.11
Family, familial (*see also* condition)
affected by
    family member
        currently on deployment (military)
            V61.01
        returned from deployment (military)
            (current or past conflict)
            V61.02

Family, familial *(continued)*
disruption *(see also* Disruption, family)
V61.09
estrangement V61.09
problem V61.9
specified circumstances NEC
V61.8
Fasciitis 729.4
Fat
embolism (cerebral) (pulmonary) (systemic) 958.1
with or following
abortion—*see* Abortion, by type,
with embolism
following abortion 639.6
ectopic or molar pregnancy *(see also*
categories 630–633.9)
639.6
complicating delivery or puerperium
673.8
in pregnancy, childbirth, or the puerperium 673.8
excessive 278.00
general 278.00
in stool 792.1
necrosis *(see also* Fatty, degeneration)
breast (aseptic) (segmental) 611.3
mesentery, omentum 567.8
Fatigue 780.79
chronic, syndrome 780.71
during pregnancy 646.8
general 780.79
muscle 729.89
postural, posture 729.89
syndrome chronic 780.71
undue 780.79
Feared complaint unfounded V65.5
Feigned illness V65.2
Fever 780.60
with chills 780.60
catarrhal (acute) 460
chronic 472.0
childbed 670.8
continued 780.60
during labor 659.2
ephemeral (of unknown origin) *(see also*
Pyrexia) 780.60
glandular 075
hay (allergic) (with rhinitis) 477.9
with asthma (bronchial) *(see also*
Asthma) 493.0
due to
pollen, any plant or tree 477.0

Fever *(continued)*
specified allergen other than pollen
477.8
intermittent (bilious) of unknown origin
(see also Pyrexia) 780.6
milk 672
persistent (of unknown origin) 780.6
postoperative 998.89
due to infection 998.59
puerperal, postpartum 672
pyemic or septic—*see* Septicemia
unknown origin 780.6
uremic—*see* Uremia
Fibrillation
atrial (established) (paroxysmal)
427.31
cardiac (ventricular) 427.41
postoperative 997.1
ventricular 427.41
Fibrinogenopenia (congenital) (hereditary)
(see also Defect, coagulation)
286.3
acquired 286.6
Fibrinolysis (acquired) (hemorrhagic)
(pathologic) 286.6
with or following
abortion—*see* Abortion, by type, with
hemorrhage, delayed or
excessive
following abortion 639.1
ectopic or molar pregnancy *(see also* categories 633.0–633.9)
639.1
antepartum or intrapartum 641.3
postpartum 666.3
Fibrinopenia (hereditary) *(see also* Defect,
coagulation) 286.3
acquired 286.6
Fibroadenosis, breast (chronic) (cystic)
(diffuse) (periodic) 610.2
Fibrocystic disease 277.00
breast 610.1
Fibroid (tumor) *(see also* Neoplasm, connective tissue, benign)
in pregnancy or childbirth 654.1
causing obstructed labor 660.2
uterus *(see also* Leiomyoma, uterus)
218.9
Fibromatosis—*see* Neoplasm, connective
tissue, uncertain behavior
Fibromyalgia 729.1
Fibromyoma *(see also* Neoplasm, connective tissue, benign)
uterus (corpus)—*see* Leiomyoma, uterus

Fibromyositis (*see also* Myositis) 729.1
Fibrosclerosis, breast 610.3
Fibrosis, fibrotic
  amnion 658.8
  anal papillae 569.49
  anus 569.49
  appendix, appendiceal, noninflammatory
      543.9
  bladder (interstitial) (localized submucosal)
      595.1
  breast 610.3
  cervix 622.8
  chorion 658.8
  cystic (of pancreas) (with) (due to) 277.00
    manifestations
      gastrointestinal 277.03
      pulmonary 277.02
      specified NEC 277.09
    meconium ileus 277.01
    presence of any device, implant, or
        graft—*see* Complications
    pulmonary exacerbation 277.02
  muscle, iatrogenic (from injection) 999.9
  ovary 620.8
  perineum, in pregnancy or childbirth 654.8
    causing obstructed labor 660.2
  placenta—*see* Placenta, abnormal
  radiation—*see* Effect, adverse, radiation
  rectal sphincter 569.49
  skin NEC 709.2
  submucous NEC 709.2
  syncytium—*see* Placenta, abnormal
  urethra 599.84
  uterus (nonneoplastic) 621.8
    neoplastic (*see also* Leiomyoma, uterus)
        218.9
  vagina 623.8
  vesical 595.1
Fibrositis (periarticular) (rheumatoid) 729.0
Fifth disease (eruptive), venereal 099.1
Filling defect
  bladder 793.5
  gastrointestinal tract (intestine)
      (stomach) 793.4
  ureter 793.5
Fimbrial cyst (congenital) 752.11
Fimbriated hymen 752.49
Findings, (abnormal), without diagnosis
      (examination) (laboratory
      test) 796.4
  17-ketosteroids, elevated 791.9
  acetonuria 791.6
  acid phosphatase 790.5
  albuminuria 791.0

Findings, abnormal, without diagnosis
      (continued)
  alcohol in blood 790.3
  alkaline phosphatase 790.5
  amniotic fluid 792.3
  amylase 790.5
  anal—*see* Papanicolaou smear
  antenatal screening 796.5
  anisocytosis 790.09
  antibody titers, elevated, antigen-anti-
        body reaction 795.79
  bacteriuria 791.9
  bicarbonate 276.9
  bile in urine 791.4
  bleeding time (prolonged) 790.92
  blood culture, positive 790.7
  blood gas level (arterial) 790.91
  C-reactive protein (CRP) 790.95
  calcium 275.40
  carbonate 276.9
  casts, urine 791.7
  catecholamines 791.9
  cells, urine 791.7
  cervical—*see* Papanicolaou smear
  chloride 276.9
  chromosome analysis 795.2
  chyluria 791.1
  coagulation study 790.92
  cytology specified site NEC 796.9
  echogram NEC—*see* Findings, abnormal,
        structure
  electrolyte level, urinary 791.9
  enzymes, serum NEC 790.5
  fibrinogen titer coagulation study 790.92
  filling defect—*see* Filling defect
  function study, thyroid 794.5
  glucose 790.29
    elevated
        fasting 790.21
        tolerance test 790.22
    low 251.2
  glycosuria 791.5
  hematinuria 791.2
  hematocrit drop (precipitous) 790.01
  hematuria 599.70
  hemoglobinuria 791.2
  histological NEC 795.4
  human immunodeficiency virus (HIV) V08
  immunoglobulins, elevated 795.79
  indolacetic acid, elevated 791.9
  karyotype 795.2
  ketonuria 791.6
  lactic acid dehydrogenase (LDH) 790.4
  lipase 790.5

Findings, abnormal, without diagnosis
(continued)
mammogram
    dense breasts 793.82
    inconclusive 793.82
myoglobinuria 791.3
oxygen saturation 790.91
Papanicolaou (smear)—*see* Papanicolaou
    smear
peritoneal fluid 792.9
pleural fluid 792.9
poikilocytosis 790.09
potassium
    deficiency 276.8
    excess 276.7
PPD 795.5
proteinuria 791.0
prothrombin time (prolonged) (partial)
    (PT) (PTT) 790.92
radiologic (X-ray) 793.9
    abdomen 793.6
    breast 793.89
        abnormal mammogram NOS
            793.80
        mammographic calcification 793.89
        mammographic microcalcification
            793.81
    gastrointestinal tract 793.4
    genitourinary organs 793.5
    inconclusive due to excess body fat
        793.91
    placenta 793.99
    retroperitoneum 793.6
    skin 793.9
    subcutaneous tissue 793.9
red blood cell (count) (morphology)
    (volume) 790.09
scan, thyroid 794.5
sedimentation rate, elevated 790.1
serological (for)
    human immunodeficiency virus (HIV)
        inconclusive 795.71
        positive V08
    syphilis
        false positive 795.6
        positive
            finding only—*see* Syphilis, latent
            follow-up of latent syphilis—*see*
                Syphilis, latent
serum, enzymes NEC 790.5
SGOT, SGPT 790.4
sickling of red blood cells 790.09
skin test, positive 795.79

Findings, abnormal, without diagnosis
(continued)
    tuberculin (without active tuberculosis)
        795.5
sperm 792.2
stool NEC 792.1
    bloody 578.1
    occult 792.1
    color 792.1
    culture, positive 792.1
structure, body (ultrasound) (X-ray)—*see*
        Findings, abnormal radio-
        logic
thyroid (function) (metabolism rate)
        (scan) (uptake) 794.5
tuberculin skin test (without active tuber-
        culosis) 795.5
ultrasound—*see* Findings, abnormal,
        structure
urine, urinary constituents
    culture, positive 791.9
    blood 599.70
vaginal—*see* Papanicolaou smear
vaginal fluid 792.9
vanillylmandelic acid (VMA), elevated
        791.9
Wassermann reaction
    false positive 795.6
    positive
        finding only—*see* Syphilis, latent
        follow-up of latent syphilis—*see*
                Syphilis, latent
xerography 793.89
Fissure, fissured
anus, anal, postanal 565.0
clitoris (congenital) 752.49
nipple 611.2
    puerperal, postpartum 676.1
rectum 565.0
skin 709.8
Fistula (sinus)
abdomen (wall) to uterus 619.2
anorectal 565.1
anus, anal (infectional) (recurrent) 565.1
appendix, appendicular 543.9
Bartholin's gland 619.8
breast 611.0
    puerperal, postpartum 675.1
cervicosigmoidal 619.1
cervicovesical 619.0
cervix 619.8
colostomy 569.69
colovaginal (acquired) 619.1

Fistula *(continued)*
   congenital, NEC—*see* Anomaly, specified
         type NEC
   cul-de-sac, Douglas' 619.8
   entero-uterine 619.1
      congenital 752.3
   enterovaginal 619.1
      congenital 752.49
   fallopian tube (external) 619.2
   frontal sinus (*see also* Sinusitis, frontal) 473.1
   horseshoe 565.1
   in ano 565.1
   intestinouterine 619.1
   intestinovaginal 619.1
      congenital 752.49
   labium (majus) (minus) 619.8
   nipple—*see* Fistula, breast
   oro-antral (*see also* Sinusitis, maxillary)
         473.0
   perianal 565.1
   perineum, perineal (with urethral involve-
         ment) NEC 599.1
   perirectal 565.1
   peritoneum (*see also* Peritonitis) 567.2
   periurethral 599.1
   postoperative, persistent 998.6
   rectolabial 619.1
   rectourethral 599.1
      congenital 753.8
   rectouterine 619.1
      congenital 752.3
   rectovaginal (old, postpartal) 619.1
      congenital 752.49
   rectovesical (congenital) 753.8
   rectovesicovaginal 619.1
   rectum (to skin) 565.1
   sigmoidovaginal 619.1
      congenital 752.49
   skin, vagina 619.2
   umbilico-urinary 753.8
   ureterovaginal 619.0
   urethra 599.1
      congenital 753.8
      tuberculous 016.3
   urethroperineal 599.1
   urethrorectal 599.1
      congenital 753.8
   urethrovaginal 619.0
   urethrovesicovaginal 619.0
   urinary (persistent) (recurrent) 599.1
   uteroabdominal (anterior wall) 619.2
      congenital 752.3
   uterofecal 619.1

Fistula *(continued)*
   uteroureteric 619.0
   uterovesical 619.0
      congenital 752.3
   vagina (wall) (postpartal, old) 619.8
   vaginocutaneous (postpartal) 619.2
   vaginoileal (acquired) 619.1
   vaginoperineal 619.2
   vesicocervicovaginal 619.0
   vesicometrorectal 619.1
   vesicosigmoidovaginal 619.1
   vesicoureterovaginal 619.0
   vesicovaginal 619.0
   vulvorectal 619.1
      congenital 752.49
Fit
   epileptic (*see also* Epilepsy) 345.9
   fainting 780.2
Fitting (of)
   artificial
      breast V52.4
         implant exchange (different mate-
               rial) (different size) V52.4
   cystostomy device V53.6
   diaphragm (contraceptive) V25.02
   intrauterine contraceptive V25.1
   urinary device V53.6
Flatus 787.3
   vaginalis 629.8
Fleshy mole 631
Fluid
   abdomen 789.5
   loss (acute) (with) 276.5
      hypernatremia 276.0
      hyponatremia 276.1
   peritoneal cavity 789.5
   retention 276.6
Fluor (albus) (vaginalis) 623.5
   trichomonal (*Trichomonas vaginalis*)
         131.00
Flushing 782.62
   menopausal 627.2
Flutter
   atrial or auricular 427.32
   heart (ventricular) 427.42
   postoperative 997.1
Follicle
   cervix (nabothian) (ruptured) 616.0
   graafian, ruptured, with hemorrhage
         620.0
Folliculitis
   decalvans 704.09
   gonorrheal (acute) 098.0

Folliculitis *(continued)*
    chronic or duration of 2 months or
        more 098.2
    keloid, keloidalis 706.1
    ulerythematosa reticulata 701.8
Follow-up (examination) (routine) (follow-
        ing) V67.9
    chemotherapy (cancer) V67.2
    high-risk medication V67.51
    injury NEC V67.59
    postpartum
        immediately after delivery V24.0
        routine V24.2
    radiotherapy V67.1
    specified condition NEC V67.59
    specified surgery NEC V67.09
    surgery V67.00
        vaginal pap smear V67.01
    treatment V67.9
Foreign body
    accidentally left during a procedure
        998.4
    entering through orifice (current)
        (old)
        anus 937
        cervix (canal) uterine 939.1
        genitourinary tract 939.9
        rectosigmoid (junction) 937
        rectum 937
        ureter 939.0
        urethra 939.0
        uterus (any part) 939.1
        vagina 939.2
        vulva 939.2
    granuloma (old)
        skin, soft tissue NEC, subcutaneous
            tissue 709.4
    in open wound (*see also* Wound, open, by
        site complicated)
        soft tissue (residual) 729.6
    internal organ, not entering through an
        orifice—*see* Injury, internal,
        by site, with open wound
    old or residual
        skin, soft tissue, subcutaneous tissue
        729.6
        with granuloma 709.4
    operation wound, left accidentally
        998.4
Formation, ureter (congenital) 753.29
Formication 782.0
Freckle 709.09
    malignant melanoma in—*see* Melanoma

Freckle *(continued)*
    melanotic (of Hutchinson)—*see*
        Neoplasm, skin, in situ
Frenum, external os 752.49
Frequency (urinary) NEC 788.41
    micturition 788.41
    nocturnal 788.43
    polyuria 788.42
    psychogenic 306.53
Friedländer's
    B (bacillus) NEC (*see also* condition)
        041.3
        sepsis or septicemia 038.49
    disease (endarteritis obliterans)—*see*
        Arteriosclerosis
Frommel's disease 676.6
Frommel–Chiari syndrome 676.6
Frozen pelvis 620.8
Fugue reaction to exceptional stress
    (transient) 308.1
Furuncle 680.9
    anus 680.5
    axilla 680.3
    breast 680.2
    labium (majus) (minus) 616.4
    multiple sites 680.9
    perineum 680.2
    skin NEC 680.9
    specified site NEC 680.8
    umbilicus 680.2
    vulva 616.4
Fusion, fused (congenital)
    hymen 752.42
    hymeno-urethral 599.89
        causing obstructed labor 660.1
    labium (majus) (minus) 752.49
    organ or site NEC—*see* Anomaly, speci-
        fied type NEC
    urethral-hymenal 599.89
    vagina 752.49
    vulva 752.49

G
Galactocele (breast) (infected) 611.5
    puerperal, postpartum 676.8
Galactophoritis 611.0
    puerperal, postpartum 675.2
Galactorrhea 676.6
    not associated with childbirth 611.6
Galacturia 791.1
Gangrene, gangrenous (anemia) (skin)
    (ulcer)
    adenitis 683

Gangrene, gangrenous *(continued)*
 anus 569.49
 appendix—*see* Appendicitis, acute
 bladder 595.89
 gas (bacillus)
  with or following
   abortion—*see* Abortion, by type,
    with sepsis
    following abortion 639.0
   ectopic or molar pregnancy (*see also*
    categories 633.0–633.9)
    639.0
   puerperal, postpartum, childbirth
    670.8
  hernia—*see* Hernia, by site, with gangrene
  obstruction (*see* Obstruction, intestine)
 liver 573.8
 ovary (*see also* Salpingo-oophoritis) 614.2
 rectum 569.49
 rupture—*see* Hernia, by site, with
  gangrene
 uterus (*see also* Endometritis) 615.9
 vulva (*see also* Vulvitis) 616.10
Gartner's duct or cyst (persistent) 752.11
Gastritis 535.5
 acute 535.0
 alcoholic 535.3
 allergic 535.4
 antral 535.4
 atrophic-hyperplastic 535.1
 catarrhal 535.0
 chronic (atrophic) 535.1
 cirrhotic 535.4
 follicular 535.4
  chronic 535.1
 glandular 535.4
  chronic 535.1
 sclerotic 535.4
 subacute 535.0
 suppurative 535.0
 toxic 535.4
Gastroduodenitis (*see also* Gastritis) 535.5
 catarrhal or infectional 535.0
Gastrorrhagia, Gastrostaxis 578.0
Genetic susceptibility to (*see also*
    Screening, genetic)
 neoplasm, malignant of
  breast V84.01
  endometrium V84.04
  other V84.09
  ovary V84.02
 other disease V84.89

Genital warts 078.11
Giant urticaria 995.1
Globinuria 791.2
Glycopenia 251.2
Glycosuria 791.5
Goiter 240.9
 complicating pregnancy, childbirth, or
    puerperium 648.1
 simple 240.0
Gonadoblastoma
 specified site—*see* Neoplasm, by site
    uncertain behavior
 unspecified site 236.2
Gonococcus, gonococcal (disease) (infec-
    tion) (*see also* condition)
    098.0
 anus 098.7
 dermatosis 098.89
 genitourinary (acute) (organ) (system)
    (*see also* Gonorrhea) 098.0
  lower 098.0
   chronic 098.2
  upper 098.10
   chronic 098.30
 lymphatic (gland) (node) 098.89
 peritonitis 098.86
 pyosalpinx (chronic) 098.37
  acute 098.17
 rectum 098.7
 septicemia 098.89
 skin 098.89
 specified site NEC 098.89
Gonorrhea (acute) 098.0
 Bartholin's gland (acute) 098.0
  chronic or duration of 2 months or
    over 098.2
 bladder (acute) 098.11
  chronic or duration of 2 months or
    over 098.31
 carrier (suspected of) V02.7
 cervix (acute) 098.15
  chronic or duration of 2 months or
    over 098.35
 chronic 098.2
 complicating pregnancy, childbirth, or
    puerperium 647.1
 contact or exposure to V01.6
 fallopian tube (chronic) 098.37
  acute 098.17
 ovary (acute) 098.19
  chronic or duration of 2 months or
    over 098.39
 pelvis (acute) 098.19
  chronic or duration of 2 months or

Gonorrhea *(continued)*
    over 098.39
  urethra (acute) 098.0
    chronic or duration of 2 months or
      over 098.2
  vagina (acute) 098.0
    chronic or duration of 2 months or
      over 098.2
  vulva (acute) 098.0
    chronic or duration of 2 months or
      over 098.2
Grand
  mal (idiopathic) *(see also* Epilepsy) 345.1
  multipara
    affecting management of labor and
      delivery 659.4
    status only (not currently pregnant)
      V61.5
Granuloma NEC
  abdomen (wall) 568.89
    skin (pyogenicum) from residual for-
      eign body 709.4
  anus 569.49
  appendix 543.9
  exuberant 701.5
  faciale 701.8
  foreign body (in soft tissue) NEC
    in operative wound 998.4
    skin, subcutaneous tissue 709.4
  inguinale (Donovan) 099.2
    venereal 099.2
  operation wound 998.59
    foreign body 998.4
    stitch (external) (internal wound) 998.89
    talc 998.7
  peritoneum 568.89
  pudendorum (ulcerative) 099.2
  rectum 569.49
  skin (pyogenicum) from foreign body or
    material 709.4
  urethra 599.84
  vagina 099.2
  venereum 099.2
Granulomatosis, disciformis chronica et
    progressiva 709.3
Green sickness 280.9
Gynandroblastoma
  specified site—*see* Neoplasm, by site,
    uncertain behavior
  unspecified site 236.2
Gynandromorphism 752.7
Gynatresia (congenital) 752.49
Gynecological examination V72.31
  for contraceptive maintenance V25.40

Gynecomastia 611.1

H
Habit, habituation
  drug *(see also* Dependence) 304.9
  laxative *(see also* Abuse, drugs, nondepen-
    dent) 305.9
  use of nonprescribed drugs *(see also*
    Abuse, drugs, nondependent)
    305.9
Headache (due to) 784.0
  allergic or cluster 339.00
  associated with sexual activty 339.82
  menstrual 346.4
  orgasmic 339.82
  premenstrual 346.4
  preorgasmic 339.82
Headache *(continued)*
  spinal anesthesia complicating labor and
    delivery 668.8
    postpartum 668.8
  vascular 784.0
Heartburn 787.1
Heberden's syndrome (angina pectoris)
    413.9
HELLP 642.5
Hematemesis 578.0
  with ulcer—*see* Ulcer, by site, with
    hemorrhage
Hematinuria *(see also* Hemoglobinuria)
    791.2
Hematocele (congenital) (diffuse) (idio-
    pathic) 629.0
  broad ligament 620.7
  canal of Nuck 629.0
  fallopian tube 620.8
  ovary 629.0
  pelvis, pelvic 629.0
    with ectopic pregnancy *(see also*
      Pregnancy, ectopic) 633.90
    with intrauterine pregnancy 633.91
  periuterine, retrouterine 629.0
  traumatic—*see* Injury, internal, pelvis
  uterine ligament 629.0
  uterus 621.4
  vagina 623.6
  vulva 624.5
Hematoma (skin surface intact) (trau-
    matic) *(see also* Contusion)
  any site, traumatic (internal)—*see* Injury,
    internal
  with
    open wound—*see* Wound, open, by site
    skin surface intact—*see* Contusion

Hematoma *(continued)*
  abdomen (wall)—*see* Contusion, abdomen
  amnion 658.8
  breast (nontraumatic) 611.89
  broad ligament (nontraumatic) 620.7
    complicating delivery 665.7
  cesarean section wound 674.3
  chorion—*see* Placenta, abnormal
  complicating delivery (perineum) (vulva)
        664.5
    pelvic 665.7
    vagina 665.7
  corpus luteum (nontraumatic) (ruptured)
        620.1
  fallopian tube 620.8
  genital organ (nontraumatic) NEC 629.8
    traumatic (external site) 922.4
  graafian follicle (ruptured) 620.0
  internal organs (abdomen, chest, or
        pelvis)—*see* Injury, internal,
        by site
  labia (nontraumatic) 624.5
  liver (subcapsular) 573.8
  obstetrical surgical wound 674.3
  ovary (corpus luteum) (nontraumatic)
        620.1
  pelvis (nontraumatic) 629.8
    complicating delivery 665.7
  perineal wound (obstetrical) 674.3
    complicating delivery 664.5
  placenta—*see* Placenta, abnormal
  postoperative 998.12
  retroperitoneal (nontraumatic) 568.81
  umbilical cord 663.6
  uterine ligament (nontraumatic) 620.7
  uterus 621.4
  vagina (nontraumatic) (ruptured) 623.6
    complicating delivery 665.7
    traumatic 922.4
  vulva (nontraumatic) 624.5
    complicating delivery 664.5
    traumatic 922.4
Hematometra 621.4
Hematosalpinx 620.8
  with ectopic or molar pregnancy (*see also*
        categories 633.0–633.9)
        639.2
  infectional (*see also* Salpingo-oophoritis)
        614.2
Hematuria (benign) (essential) (idiopathic)
        (intermittent) (paroxysmal)
        599.70
  gross 599.71
  microscopic 599.72

Hemoglobinemia, due to blood transfu-
        sion NEC 999.8
Hemoglobinuria, hemoglobinuric 791.2
Hemolysis
  intravascular (disseminated) NEC 286.6
    with or following
        abortion—*see* Abortion, by type,
              with hemorrhage, delayed or
              excessive
          following abortion 639.1
          ectopic or molar pregnancy (*see also*
                categories 633.0–633.9)
                639.1
          hemorrhage of pregnancy 641.3
    transfusion NEC 999.89
Hemoperitoneum 568.81
  infectional (*see also* Peritonitis) 567.2
  traumatic—*see* Injury, internal, peritoneum
Hemophilia (familial) (hereditary)
  A, carrier (asymptomatic) V83.01
  acquired 286.5
  B (Leyden) 286.1
  C 286.2
  calcipriva (*see also* Fibrinolysis) 286.7
  nonfamilial 286.7
  secondary 286.5
  vascular 286.4
Hemophilus influenzae NEC 041.5
  bronchopneumonia 482.2
  infection NEC 041.5
  meningitis 320.0
  pneumonia (broncho-) 482.2
Hemoptysis 786.3
Hemorrhage, hemorrhagic (nontraumatic)
        (*see also* Bleeding) 459.0
  abdomen 459.0
  accidental (antepartum) 641.2
  anemia (chronic) 280.0
    acute 285.1
  antepartum—*see* Hemorrhage, pregnancy
  anus (sphincter) 569.3
  brain (miliary) (nontraumatic)
    postoperative 997.02
    puerperal, childbirth 674.0
  breast 611.79
  cervix (stump) (uteri) 622.8
  cesarean section wound 674.3
  complicating
    delivery—*see* Delivery, complication
    surgical procedure 998.11
  concealed NEC 459.0
  corpus luteum (ruptured) 620.1
  cutaneous 782.7
  cystitis—*see* Cystitis

Hemorrhage, hemorrhagic *(continued)*
delayed
   with or following
      abortion—*see* Abortion, by type,
         with hemorrhage, delayed or
         excessive
         following abortion 639.1
      ectopic or molar pregnancy (*see also*
         categories 633.0–633.9)
         639.1
   postpartum 666.2
due to
   any device, implant, or graft (presence
      of) classifiable to 996.3–
      996.5—*see* Complications
   intrinsic circulating anticoagulant 286.5
episiotomy 674.3
external 459.0
fallopian tube 620.8
fibrinogenolysis, fibrinolytic (acquired)
   (*see also* Fibrinolysis) 286.6
intermenstrual (irregular) 626.6
   regular 626.5
internal (organs) 459.0
intestine 578.9
intraabdominal 459.0
   during or following surgery 998.11
intracranial, puerperal, postpartum, childbirth 674.0
intrapartum—*see* Hemorrhage, complicating delivery
intrapelvic 629.8
intraperitoneal 459.0
intrauterine (*see also* Hemorrhage, pregnancy and Hemorrhage,
   postpartum) 621.4
ligature, vessel 998.11
lower extremity NEC 459.0
mole 631
mucous membrane NEC 459.0
omentum 568.89
ovary 620.1
perineal wound (obstetrical) 674.3
peritoneum, peritoneal 459.0
petechial 782.7
placenta NEC 641.9
   from surgical or instrumental damage
      641.8
   previa 641.1
postpartum—*see* Pregnancy, complication
pregnancy—*see* Pregnancy, complication
purpura (primary) (*see also* Purpura,

Hemorrhage, hemorrhagic *(continued)*
      thrombocytopenic) 287.3
   retroperitoneal 459.0
   retroplacental (*see also* Placenta, separa-
      tion) 641.2
   secondary (nontraumatic) 459.0
      following initial hemorrhage at time of
         injury 958.2
   skin 782.7
   spontaneous NEC 459.0
      petechial, subcutaneous 782.7
   third stage 666.0
   traumatic—*see* nature of injury
      recurring or secondary (following ini-
         tial hemorrhage at time of
         injury) 958.2
   ulcer—*see* Ulcer, by site, with hemor-
      rhage
   urethra (idiopathic) 599.84
   uterus, uterine (abnormal) 626.9
      climacteric 627.0
      complicating delivery—*see* Delivery,
         complicated by
      due to intrauterine contraceptive
         device 996.76
         perforating uterus 996.32
      functional or dysfunctional 626.8
      postmenopausal 627.1
      prepubertal 626.8
      pubertal 626.3
      unrelated to menstrual cycle 626.6
   vagina 623.8
      functional 626.8
   vasa previa 663.5
   viscera 459.0
   vulva 624.8
Hemorrhoids (anus) (rectum) (without
      complication) 455.6
   complicated NEC 455.8
   complicating pregnancy and puerperium
      671.8
   external 455.3
      with complication NEC 455.5
      bleeding, prolapsed, strangulated, or
         ulcerated 455.5
      thrombosed NEC 455.7
   internal 455.0
      with complication NEC 455.2
      bleeding, prolapsed, strangulated, or
         ulcerated 455.2
      thrombosed 455.1
   residual skin tag 455.9

Hepatitis 573.3
  autoimmune 571.42
  drug-induced 573.3
  infectious hepatitis virus—*see* Hepatitis,
    viral, type A
  inoculation—*see* Hepatitis, viral
  serum—*see* Hepatitis, viral
  Type A—*see* Hepatitis, viral, type A
  Type B—*see* Hepatitis, viral, type B
  viral (acute) (chronic) (sub-acute) 070.9
    specified type NEC 070.59
      with hepatic coma 070.49
    type A 070.1
      with hepatic coma 070.0
    type B (acute) 070.30
      with hepatic coma 070.20
      carrier status V02.61
      chronic (with) 070.32
        hepatic coma 070.22
          with hepatitis delta 070.23
        hepatitis delta 070.33
          with hepatic coma 070.23
      hepatitis delta 070.31
        with hepatic coma 070.21
    type C (acute) 070.51
      with hepatic coma 070.41
      carrier status V02.62
      chronic 070.54
        with hepatic coma 070.44
      in remission 070.54
    type delta (with hepatitis B carrier
      state) (with) 070.52
      active hepatitis B disease—*see*
        Hepatitis, viral, type B
      hepatic coma 070.42
    type E 070.53
      with hepatic coma 070.43
    vaccination and inoculation (prophy-
      lactic) V05.3
Hermaphroditism (true) 752.7
  with specified chromosomal anomaly—
    see Anomaly, chromosomes,
    sex
Hernia, hernial (acquired) (recurrent) with
  bladder (sphincter) (*see also* Cystocele)
    618.01
  fallopian tube 620.4
  inguinal (with) 550.9
    gangrene (obstructed) 550.0
    obstruction 550.1
      and gangrene 550.0
  ovary 620.4
  rectovaginal 618.6

Hernia, hernial *(continued)*
  uterus 621.8
    pregnant 654.4
  vaginal (posterior) 618.6
  vesical (*see also* Cystocele) 618.01
Herpes, herpetic
  auricularis (zoster) 053.71
  genital, genitalis 054.10
    specified site NEC 054.19
  gestationis 646.8
  otitis externa (zoster) 053.71
  perianal 054.10
  vulva 054.12
  vulvovaginitis 054.11
  zoster 053.9
    complicated 053.8
      specified NEC 053.79
HGSIL (high grade squamous intraepithe-
    lial lesion) (cytologic finding)
    (Pap smear finding)
  anus 796.74
  cervix 795.04
    biopsy finding—code to CIN II or
      CIN III
  vagina 795.14
Hidradenitis (axillaris) (suppurative)
    705.83
Hidradenoma (nodular)—*see* Neoplasm,
    skin, benign
High
  basal metabolic rate (BMR) 794.7
  blood pressure (*see also* Hypertension)
    401.9
    incidental reading (isolated) (nonspe-
      cific), no diagnosis of hyper-
      tension 796.2
  compliance bladder 596.4
  head at term 652.5
  risk
    behavior—*see* Problem
    human papillomavirus (HPV) DNA
      test positive
      anal 796.75
      cervical 795.05
      vaginal 795.15
    patient taking drugs (prescribed)
      V67.51
      nonprescribed (*see also* Abuse, drugs,
        nondependent) 305.9
    pregnancy V23.9
      inadequate prenatal care V23.7
      specified problem NEC V23.89
Hirsutism (*see also* Hypertrichosis) 704.1

History, family (of)
anemia V18.2
cardiac death V17.41
diabetes mellitus V18.0
disease (of)
  bronchus V16.1
  cystic fibrosis V18.1
  cardiovascular V17.4
  coronary artery V17.3
  digestive system V18.5
    colonic polyps V18.51
  endocrine system V18.1
  genitourinary system NEC V18.7
  lung V16.1
estrogen therapy V87.43
eye disorder V19.0
hearing loss V19.2
leukemia V16.6
malignant neoplasm
  anorectal V16.0
  anus V16.0
  appendix V16.0
  breast V16.3
  cervix V16.49
  fallopian tube V16.41
  intestine V16.0
  ovary V16.41
  rectum V16.0
  stomach V16.0
  testes V16.1
  trachea V16.1
  urinary organs V16.59
  uterus V16.49
  vagina V16.49
  vulva V16.49
mental retardation V18.4
polycystic kidney V18.61
metabolic disease NEC V18.1
skin condition V19.4
History, personal (of)
abuse
  child V15.41
  emotional V15.42
  neglect V15.42
  physical V15.41
  sexual V15.41
affective psychosis V11.1
alcoholism V11.3
  specified as drinking problem (*see also*
    Abuse, drugs, nondepen-
    dent) 305.0
allergy to
  analgesic agent NEC V14.6

History, personal (of) *(continued)*
  anesthetic NEC V14.4
  antibiotic agent NEC V14.1
  anti-infective agent NEC V14.3
  drug, specified type NEC V14.8
  narcotic agent NEC V14.5
  penicillin V14.0
  serum V14.7
  sulfa or sulfonamides V14.2
  vaccine V14.7
arthritis V13.4
cardiac death, successfully resuscitated
    V12.53
chemotherapy, antineoplastic V87.41
cigarette smoking V15.82
contraception V15.7
disease (of)
  affecting management of pregnancy
    V23.1
  digestive system (polyps, colonic)
    V12.72
  Hodgkin's V10.72
  infectious V12.00
    malaria V12.03
    parasitic V12.00
    poliomyelitis V12.02
    specified NEC V12.09
    tuberculosis V12.01
  skin V13.3
  trophoblastic V13.1
  ulcer (peptic) V12.71
disorder (of)
  endocrine system V12.2
  genital system V13.29
  immunity V12.2
  specified type NEC V11.8
  metabolic V12.2
  obstetric V13.29
    affecting management of current
      pregnancy V23.49
    pre-term labor V23.41
    pre-term labor (patient not preg-
      nant) V13.21
  urinary system V13.00
    calculi V13.01
    specified NEC V13.09
drug use, nonprescribed (*see also* Abuse,
    drugs, nondependent) 305.9
dysplasia, cervical V13.22
embolism (pulmonary) V12.51
failed conscious sedation V15.80
moderate sedation V15.80
health hazard V15.9

History, personal (of) *(continued)*
  injury NEC V15.59
  insufficient prenatal care V23.7
  in utero procedure
    during pregnancy V15.21
    while a fetus V15.22
  irradiation V15.3
    leukemia V10.60
    lymphoid V10.61
    monocytic V10.63
    myeloid V10.62
    specified type NEC V10.69
  malignant neoplasm (of)
    anus V10.06
    bladder V10.51
    bone V10.81
    breast V10.3
    bronchus V10.11
    cervix uteri V10.41
    colon V10.05
    fallopian tube V10.44
    genital organ V10.40
    specified site NEC V10.44
    kidney V10.52
    liver V10.07
    lung V10.11
    lymph glands or nodes NEC V10.79
      lymphosarcoma V10.71
    ovary V10.43
    perineum V10.89
    placenta V10.44
    rectum, rectosigmoid junction
      V10.06
    renal pelvis V10.53
    skin V10.83
      melanoma V10.82
      specified site NEC V10.89
    trachea V10.12
    ureter V10.59
    urethra V10.59
    urinary organ V10.50
    uterus V10.42
      adnexa V10.44
      corpus V10.42
    vagina V10.44
    vulva V10.44
  mental disorder
    affective type V11.1
    manic-depressive V11.1
    neurosis V11.2
    schizophrenia V11.0
    specified type NEC V11.8
  noncompliance with medical treatment
    V15.81

History, personal (of) *(continued)*
  nutritional deficiency V12.1
  poor obstetric V13.29
    affecting management of current preg-
      nancy V23.49
    pre-term labor V23.41
    pre-term labor (patient not pregnant)
      V13.21
  rape V15.41
  surgery to
    heart V15.1
    organs NEC V15.29
  therapy
    antineoplastic drug V87.41
    drug NEC V87.49
    estrogen V87.43
    immunosuppression V87.46
    monoclonal drug V87.42
  thrombophlebitis V12.52
  thrombosis V12.51
Hives (bold) *(see also* Urticaria) 708.9
Hooded clitoris 752.49
Hospice care V66.7
Hourglass contraction, contracture,
    uterus 661.4
Human immunodeficiency virus (disease)
    (illness) 042
  infection V08
    with symptoms, symptomatic 042
Human immunodeficiency virus-2
    infection 079.53
Human papillomavirus 079.4
  high risk, DNA test positive
    anal 796.75
    cervical 795.05
    vaginal 795.15
  low risk, DNA test positive
    anal 796.79
    cervical 795.09
    vaginal 795.19
Human T-cell lymphotrophic virus I
    infection (HTLV-I) 079.51
Human T-cell lymphotrophic virus II
    infection (HTLV-II) 079.52
Human T-cell lymphotropic virus-III
    (HTLV-III)—*see* Human
    immunodeficiency virus
Hydatid cyst or tumor, fallopian tube
    752.11
Hydatidiform mole (benign) (complicating
    pregnancy) 630
  invasive 236.1
  malignant 236.1

Hydatidiform mole *(continued)*
  previous, affecting management of pregnancy V23.1
Hydradenitis 705.83
Hydradenoma—*see* Hidradenoma
Hydramnios 657
Hydroa gestationis 646.8
Hydroadenitis 705.83
Hydrocele
  canal of Nuck 629.1
  round ligament 629.8
  vulva 624.8
Hydrocephalic fetus
  affecting management or pregnancy 655.0
  causing disproportion 653.6
    with obstructed labor 660.1
Hydrocolpos (congenital) 623.8
Hydrometra 621.8
Hydrometrocolpos 623.8
Hydronephrosis, hydroureteronephrosis 591
Hydroperitoneum 789.5
Hydrops 782.3
  abdominis 789.5
  amnii (complicating pregnancy) (*see also* Hydramnios) 657
Hydrorrhea, gravidarum 658.1
Hydrosalpinx (fallopian tube) (follicularis) 614.1
Hydrourethra 599.84
Hyperactive, hyperactivity
  basal cell, uterine cervix 622.10
  bladder 596.51
  bowel (syndrome) 564.9
    sounds 787.5
Hyperamylasemia 790.5
Hyperaphia 782.0
Hyperazotemia 791.9
Hypercalcemia, hypercalcemic (idiopathic) 275.42
Hypercalcinuria 275.40
Hyperchloremia 276.9
Hyperelectrolytemia 276.9
Hyperemesis, gravidarum
  gravidarum (mild) (before 22 completed weeks gestation) 643.0
    with
  carbohydrate depletion 643.1
  dehydration 643.1
  electrolyte imbalance 643.1
  metabolic disturbance 643.1
  severe (with metabolic disturbance) 643.1

Hyperemia (acute)
  anal mucosa 569.49
  liver (active) (passive) 573.8
  ovary 620.8
Hyperheparinemia (*see also* Circulating anticoagulants) 286.5
Hyperinsulinism (ectopic) (functional) (organic) NEC 251.1
  iatrogenic 251.0
  reactive or spontaneous 251.2
  therapeutic misadventure (from administration of insulin) 962.3
Hyperiodemia 276.9
Hyperkalemia 276.7
Hyperkeratosis (*see also* Keratosis)
  cervix 622.10
  coccyx 724.71
  senile (with pruritus) 702.0
  vagina 623.1
  vulva 624.0
Hyperlipidemia 272.4
Hypermobility
  colon 564.9
  urethra 599.81
Hyperplasia, hyperplastic
  appendix (lymphoid) 543.0
  breast (*see also* Hypertrophy, breast) 611.1
    ductal 610.8
      atypical 610.8
  cervical gland 785.6
  cervix (uteri) 622.10
    basal cell 622.10
    congenital 752.49
    endometrium 622.10
    polypoid 622.10
  clitoris, congenital 752.49
  endocervicitis 616.0
  endometrium, endometrial (adenomatous) (cystic) (glandular) (polypoid) 621.30
    benign 621.34
      with atypia 621.33
      without atypia (complex) (simple) 621.32
    cervix 622.10
  epithelial 709.89
    nipple 611.89
    skin 709.8
    vaginal wall 623.0
  glandularis (cystica uteri) (endometrium) (interstitialis uteri) 621.30
  hymen, congenital 752.49

Hypertension Table

	Malignant	Benign	Unspecified
Hypertension, hypertensive (crisis) (disease) (essential) (primary) (systemic) (uncontrolled)	401.0	401.1	401.9
with			
heart involvement (conditions classifiable to 429.2 due to hypertension) (*see also* Hypertension, heart)	402.00	402.10	402.90
renal (kidney) involvement (*see also* Hypertension, kidney)	403.00	403.10	403.90
renal sclerosis or failure			
with heart involvement—*see* Hypertension, cardiorenal			
failure (and sclerosis (*see also,* Hypertension, kidney)	403.01	403.11	403.91
sclerosis without failure (*see also* Hypertension, kidney)	403.00	403.10	403.90
accelerated—*see* Hypertension, by type, malignant	401.0		
antepartum—*see* Hypertension, complicating pregnancy, childbirth, or the puerperium			
cardiovascular (arteriosclerotic) (sclerotic)	402.00	402.10	402.90
with			
heart failure	402.01	402.11	402.91
complicating pregnancy, childbirth, or the puerperium	642.2	642.0	642.9
with			
albuminuria (and edema) (mild)	—	—	642.4
severe	—	—	642.5
edema (mild)	—	—	642.4
severe	—	—	642.5
heart disease	642.2	642.2	642.2
and renal disease	642.2	642.2	642.2
chronic	642.2	642.0	642.0
with pre-eclampsia or eclampsia	642.7	642.7	642.7
essential	—	642.0	642.0
with pre-eclampsia or eclampsia	—	642.7	642.7
gestational	—	—	642.3
pre-existing	642.2	642.0	642.0
with pre-eclampsia or eclampsia	642.7	642.7	642.7
secondary to renal disease	642.1	642.1	642.1
with pre-eclampsia or eclampsia	642.7	642.7	642.7
transient	—	—	642.3
gestational (transient) NEC	—	—	642.3

(continued)

Hypertension Table *(continued)*

	Malignant	Benign	Unspecified
Hypertension, hypertensive *(continued)*			
heart (disease) (conditions classifiable to 429.2 due to hypertension)	402.00	402.10	402.90
with heart failure	402.01	402.11	402.91
kidney	403.00	403.10	403.90
necrotizing	401.0	—	—
postoperative	—	—	997.91
renal (disease) *(see also* Hypertension, kidney)	403.00	403.10	403.90
transient	—	—	796.2
of pregnancy	—	—	642.3
venous, chronic (asymptomatic) (idiopathic) due to			
deep vein thrombosis *(see also* Syndrome, postphlebitic)	—	—	459.10

Hyperplasia, hyperplastic *(continued)*
lymph node (gland) 785.6
lymphoid (diffuse) (nodular) 785.6
appendix 543.0
myometrium, myometrial 621.2
organ or site, congenital NEC—*see*
Anomaly, specified type
NEC
ovary 620.8
thyroid (*see also* Goiter) 240.9
urethrovaginal 599.89
uterus, uterine (myometrium) 621.2
endometrium—*see* Hyperplasia,
endometrium
vulva 624.3
Hyperpnea (*see also* Hyperventilation)
786.01
Hyperpotassemia 276.7
Hypersecretion
androgens (ovarian) 256.1
estrogen 256.0
hormone, ovarian androgen 256.1
insulin—*see* Hyperinsulinism
milk 676.6
Hypersensitive, hypersensitiveness, hyper-
sensitivity (*see also* Allergy)
colon 564.9
drug (*see also* Allergy, drug) 995.2
reaction (*see also* Allergy) 995.3
Hypersomnia 780.54
with sleep apnea 780.53
Hypersteatosis 706.3
Hyperthecosis, ovary 256.8
Hypertransaminemia 790.4
Hypertrophy, hypertrophic
anal papillae 569.49
apocrine gland 705.82
arthritis (chronic) (*see also*
Osteoarthrosis) 715.9
Bartholin's gland 624.8
breast 611.1
cystic, fibrocystic 610.1
massive pubertal 611.1
puerperal, postpartum 676.3
senile (parenchymatous) 611.1
cardiac (chronic) with hypertensive (*see*
also Hypertension, heart)
402.90
cervix (uteri) 622.6
congenital 752.49
elongation 622.6
clitoris (cirrhotic) 624.2
congenital 752.49

Hypertrophy, hypertrophic *(continued)*
endometrium (uterus) (*see also*
Hyperplasia, endometrium)
621.30
gland, glandular (general) NEC 785.6
hymen, congenital 752.49
labium (majus) (minus) 624.3
lymph gland 785.6
myometrium 621.2
nipple 611.1
organ or site, congenital NEC—*see*
Anomaly, specified type NEC
ovary 620.8
rectum, rectal sphincter 569.49
scar 701.4
skin condition NEC 701.9
thyroid (gland) (*see also* Goiter) 240.9
urethra 599.84
uterus 621.2
puerperal, postpartum 674.8
vagina 623.8
vulva 624.3
Hyperventilation (tetany) 786.01
Hypocalcemia 275.41
Hypochloremia 276.9
Hypocythemia (progressive) 284.9
Hypoestrinism, hypoestrogenism 256.39
Hypoferremia 280.9
due to blood loss (chronic) 280.0
Hypofibrinogenemia 286.3
acquired 286.6
congenital 286.3
Hypofunction, ovary 256.39
postablative 256.2
Hypoglycemia (spontaneous) 251.2
coma 251.0
diabetic 250.3
due to secondary diabetes 249.3
diabetic 250.8
due to secondary diabetes 249.8
due to insulin 251.0
familial (idiopathic) 251.2
reactive 251.2
specified NEC 251.1
Hypogonadism, ovarian (primary) 256.39
Hypoplasia, hypoplasis
bladder 753.8
breast (areola) 611.82
cervix (uteri) 752.49
endometrium 621.8
fallopian tube 752.19
hymen 752.49
labium (majus) (minus) 752.49

Hypoplasia, hypoplasis *(continued)*
  megakaryocytic 287.3
  ovary 752.0
  ureter 753.29
  uterus 752.3
  vagina 752.49
  vulva 752.49
Hypotension (arterial) (constitutional) 458.9
  chronic 458.1
  iatrogenic 458.29
  maternal, syndrome (following labor and
      delivery) 669.2
  of hemodialysis 458.21
  permanent idiopathic 458.1
  postoperative 458.29
  specified type NEC 458.8
  transient 796.3
Hypothyroidism (acquired)
  complicating pregnancy, childbirth, or
      puerperium 648.1
  due to
    ablation 244.1
      radioactive iodine 244.1
      surgical 244.0
    iodine (administration) (ingestion) 244.2
    irradiation therapy 244.1
    p-aminosalicylic acid (PAS) 244.3
    phenylbutazone 244.3
    resorcinol 244.3
  iatrogenic NEC 244.3
Hypotonia, hypotonicity, hypotony
  bladder 596.4
  uterus, uterine (contractions)—*see*
      Inertia, uterus
Hypoventilation 786.09
Hypovolemia 276.5
  surgical shock 998.0
  traumatic (shock) 958.4
Hysteralgia, pregnant uterus 646.8

I
Ichthyosis (acquired)
  gravis (*see also* Necrosis, liver)
    complicating pregnancy 646.7
  infectious (catarrhal) (epidemic) 070.1
    with hepatic coma 070.0
Ileus, postoperative 997.4
Imbalance, electrolyte—*see* Electrolyte
Immaturity
  fetus or infant light-for-dates—*see* Light-
      for-dates
  organ or site NEC—*see* Hypoplasia
  sexual 259.0

Immunization—*see* Incompatibility
Immunotherapy, prophylactic V07.2
Impacted, intrauterine device (IUD)
      996.32
Impaired, impairment (function)
  cognitive, mild 331.83
  glucose
    fasting 790.21
    tolerance test (oral) 790.22
  liver 573.8
  rectal sphincter 787.99
Imperfect
  closure (congenital)
    genitalia, genital organs
      clitoris 752.49
      external 752.49
      organ or site NEC—*see* Anomaly,
          specified type, by site
      ureter 753.4
      uterus (with communication to blad-
          der, intestine, or rectum)
          752.3
    development—*see* Anomaly, by site
Imperforate (congenital)—*see* Atresia
Implant, endometrial 617.9
Implantation
  anomalous—*see* Anomaly, specified type,
      by site
    ureter 753.4
  cyst or dermoid
    external area or site (skin) NEC 709.8
    vagina 623.8
    vulva 624.8
  placenta, low or marginal—*see* Placenta
      previa
Inadequate, inadequacy
  development
    fetus, affecting management of preg-
        nancy 656.5
    genitalia, after puberty NEC 259.0
    organ or site NEC—*see* Hypoplasia, by
        site
  nervous system 799.2
  prenatal care in current pregnancy V23.7
  pulmonary function 786.09
  respiration 786.09
  sample
    cytology
      anal 796.78
      cervical 795.08
      vaginal 795.18
Incarceration, incarcerated
  fallopian tube 620.8

Incarceration, incarcerated (*continued*)
hernia—*see* Hernia, by site, with obstruction
   tion
   gangrenous—*see* Hernia, by site, with
      gangrene
uterus 621.8
   gravid 654.3
      causing obstructed labor 660.2
Incompatibility
ABO or blood (group) NEC
   affecting management of pregnancy
      656.2
   infusion or transfusion reaction 999.6
Rh (blood group) (factor) (Rhesus)
   affecting management of pregnancy
      656.1
   infusion or transfusion reaction 999.7
Incompetency, incompetence, incompetent
cervix, cervical (os) 622.5
   in pregnancy 654.5
pelvic fundus
   pubocervical tissue 618.81
   rectovaginal tissue 618.82
vein, venous (saphenous) (varicose) (*see
     also* Varicose, vein) 454.9
Incomplete (*see also* condition)
bladder emptying 788.21
Inconclusive
image test due to excess body fat 793.91
mammogram, mammography 793.82
   due to dense breasts 793.8
Incontinence (urinary) 788.30
without sensory awareness 788.34
anal sphincter 787.6
continuous leakage 788.37
due to
   cognitive impairment 788.91
   severe physical disability 788.91
   immobility 788.91
feces 787.6
mixed (urge and stress) 788.33
neurogenic 788.39
overflow 788.38
paradoxical 788.39
specified NEC 788.39
stress 625.6
urethral sphincter 599.84
urge 788.31
   and stress 788.33
Indolent bubo NEC 099.8
Induced
abortion—*see* Abortion, induced
delivery—*see* Delivery
labor—*see* Delivery

Induration, indurated
breast (fibrous) 611.79
   puerperal, postpartum 676.3
broad ligament 620.8
chancre 091.0
   anus 091.1
   extragenital NEC 091.2
liver (chronic) (acute) 573.8
phlebitic—*see* Phlebitis
skin 782.8
Inertia
bladder 596.4
   neurogenic 596.54
uterus, uterine 661.2
   primary 661.0
   secondary 661.1
Infantile (*see also* condition)
genitalia, genitals 259.0
   in pregnancy or childbirth NEC
      654.4
      causing obstructed labor 660.2
os, uterus 259.0
pelvis 738.6
   with disproportion (fetopelvic)
      653.1
      causing obstructed labor 660.1
uterus (*see also* Infantile, genitalia)
      259.0
vulva 752.49
Infantilism, sexual (with obesity) 259.0
Infarct, infarction
hepatic 573.4
specified site 410.8
unspecified site 410.9
Infection, infected, infective
      (opportunistic)
with lymphangitis—*see* Lymphangitis
abortion—*see* Abortion, by type, with
      sepsis
abscess (skin)—*see* Abscess, by site
Aerobacter aerogenes NEC 041.85
amniotic fluid or cavity 658.4
anus or anal canal (papillae) (sphincter)
      569.49
axillary gland 683
Bacillus NEC 041.89
   coli—*see* Infection, Escherichia coli
   coliform NEC 041.85
bacterial NEC 041.9
   specified NEC 041.89
      anaerobic NEC 041.84
      gram-negative NEC 041.85
         anaerobic NEC 041.84

Infection, infected, infective *(continued)*
Bacteroides (fragilis) (melaninogenicus)
(oralis) NEC 041.82
Bartholin's gland 616.8
Bedsonia 079.98
specified NEC 079.88
bladder *(see also* Cystitis) 595.9
breast 611.0
puerperal, postpartum 675.2
with nipple 675.9
specified type NEC 675.8
nonpurulent 675.2
purulent 675.1
bronchus *(see also* Bronchitis) 490
Candida—*see* Candidiasis
cellulitis—*see* Cellulitis, by site
cervical gland 683
cervix *(see also* Cervicitis) 616.0
cesarean section wound 674.3
Chlamydia 079.98
specified NEC 079.88
chorionic plate 658.8
Clostridium (haemolyticum) (novyi)
NEC 041.84
perfringens 041.83
complicating pregnancy, childbirth, or
puerperium NEC 647.9
coronavirus 079.89
SARS-associated 079.82
corpus luteum *(see also* Salpingo-oophoritis)
614.2
cyst—*see* Cyst
Ducrey's bacillus (any site) 099.0
due to or resulting from
device, implant, or graft (any) (presence of)—*see* Complications
injection, inoculation, infusion, transfusion, or vaccination (prophylactic) (therapeutic) 999.3
injury NEC—*see* Wound, open, by site,
complicated
surgery 998.59
Enterobacter aerogenes NEC 041.85
enterococcus NEC 041.04
enterostomy 569.61
enterovirus NEC 079.89
episiotomy 674.3
Epstein-Barr virus 075
Escherichia coli NEC 041.4
generalized 038.42
ethmoidal (chronic) (sinus) *(see also*
Sinusitis, ethmoidal) 473.2
Eubacterium 041.84

Infection, infected, infective *(continued)*
fallopian tube *(see also* Salpingo-oophoritis) 614.2
fungus NEC
fingernail or toenail 110.1
perianal (area) 110.3
Fusobacterium 041.84
Gardnerella vaginalis 041.89
gastric *(see also* Gastritis) 535.5
generalized NEC *(see also* Septicemia)
038.9
genital organ or tract 614.9
with or following
abortion—*see* Abortion, by type,
with sepsis
following abortion 639.0
ectopic or molar pregnancy *(see also*
categories 630–633.9) 639.0
complicating pregnancy 646.6
puerperal, postpartum, childbirth 670.8
major 670.0
minor or localized 646.6
genitourinary tract NEC 599.0
gonococcal NEC *(see also* Gonococcus)
098.0
gram-negative bacilli NEC 041.85
anaerobic 041.84
Helicobactor pylori 041.86
Hemophilus influenzae NEC 041.5
generalized 038.41
Herpes zoster 053.9
human immunodeficiency virus (HIV) V08
with symptoms, symptomatic 042
human immunodeficiency virus type
2 (HIV 2) 079.53
human T-cell lymphotrophic virus
type I (HTLV-I) 079.51
human T-cell lymphotrophic virus
type II (HTLV-II) 079.52
human herpesvirus 6 058.81
herpesvirus 7 058.82
herpesvirus 8 058.89
herpesvirus NEC 058.89
human papillomavirus 079.4
hydronephrosis 591
inguinal glands 683
due to soft chancre 099.0
intrauterine *(see also* Endometritis) 615.9
complicating delivery 646.6
kidney (cortex) (hematogenous)
with or following
abortion—*see* Abortion, by type,
with urinary tract infection

Infection, infected, infective *(continued)*
    following abortion 639.8
    with or following
      ectopic or molar pregnancy *(see also*
        categories 630–633.9)
        639.8
      complicating pregnancy or puerperium
        646.6
    pyelonephritis (acute) 590.1
    Klebsiella pneumoniae NEC 041.3
    labia (majora) (minora) *(see also* Vulvitis)
      616.10
    lymph gland (axillary) (cervical)
      (inguinal) 683
    mima polymorpha NEC 041.85
    mixed flora NEC 041.89
    Monilia *(see also* Candidiasis) 112.9
    Mycoplasma NEC 041.81
    nipple—*see* Infection, breast
    obstetrical surgical wound 674.3
    Oidium albicans *(see also* Candidiasis)
      112.9
    operation wound 998.59
    ovary *(see also* Salpingo-oophoritis)
      614.2
    parainfluenza virus 079.89
    paraurethral ducts 597.89
    pelvic *(see also* Disease, pelvis, inflamma-
      tory) 614.9
    Peptococcus or peptostreptococcus
      041.84
    perirectal 569.49
    peritoneal *(see also* Peritonitis) 567.9
    periurethral 597.89
    pleuropneumonia-like organisms NEC
      (PPLO) 041.81
    pneumococcal NEC 041.2
      generalized (purulent) 038.2
    Pneumococcus NEC 041.2
    posttraumatic NEC 958.3
    Proprionibacterium 041.84
    Proteus (mirabilis) (morganii) (vulgaris)
      NEC 041.6
    Pseudomonas NEC 041.7
      pneumonia 482.1
    puerperal, postpartum (major) 670
      minor 646.6
    purulent—*see* Abscess
    putrid, generalized—*see* Septicemia
    pyemic—*see* Septicemia
    rectum (sphincter) 569.49
    respiratory
      influenzal (acute) (upper) 487.1

Infection, infected, infective *(continued)*
    respiratory *(continued)*
      rhinovirus 460
      upper (acute) (infectious) NEC
        465.9
        with flu, grippe, or influenza
          487.1
        multiple sites NEC 465.8
        streptococcal 034.0
        viral NEC 465.9
    Saccharomyces *(see also* Candidiasis)
      112.9
    septic, generalized or speticemic—*see*
      Septicemia
    seroma 998.51
    Serratia (marcescens) 041.85
      generalized 038.44
    sinus *(see also* Sinusitis) 473.9
    Skene's duct or gland *(see also* Urethritis)
      597.89
    skin (local) (staphylococcal) (streptococ-
      cal) NEC
      abscess—*see* Abscess, by site
      cellulitis—*see* Cellulitis, by site
    sphenoidal (chronic) (sinus) *(see also*
      Sinusitis, sphenoidal) 473.3
    staphylococcal NEC 041.10
      aureus 041.11
        methicillin
          resistant (MRSA) 041.12
          susceptible (MSSA) 041.11
      generalized (purulent) 038.10
        aureus 038.11
        specified organism NEC 038.19
      pneumonia 482.40
        aureus 482.41
        methicillin
          resistant (MRSA) 482.42
          susceptivle (MSSA) 482.41
        specified type NEC 482.49
      septicemia 038.10
        aureus 038.11
        methicillin
          resistant (MRSA) 038.12
          susceptible (MSSA) 038.11
        specified organism NEC 038.19
      specified NEC 041.19
    steatoma 706.2
    streptococcal NEC 041.00
      generalized (purulent) 038.0
      group
        A 041.01
        B 041.02

Infection, infected, infective *(continued)*
streptococcal *(continued)*
C 041.03
D (enterococcus) 041.04
G 041.05
pneumonia—*see* Pneumonia, streptococcal
septicemia 038.0
sore throat 034.0
specified NEC 041.09
Trichomonas 131.9
bladder 131.09
cervix 131.09
specified site NEC 131.8
urethra 131.02
urogenitalis 131.00
vagina 131.01
vulva 131.01
tubal or tubo-ovarian (*see also* Salpingo-
oophoritis) 614.2
tuberculosis NEC (*see also* Tuberculosis)
011.9
urethra (*see also* Urethritis) 597.80
urinary (tract) NEC 599.0
with or following
abortion—*see* Abortion, by type,
with urinary tract infection
following abortion 639.8
ectopic or molar pregnancy (*see also*
categories 630–633.9) 639.8
candidal 112.2
complicating pregnancy, childbirth, or
puerperium 646.6
asymptomatic 646.5
diplococcal (acute) 098.0
chronic 098.2
due to Trichomonas (vaginalis) 131.00
gonococcal (acute) 098.0
chronic or duration of 2 months or
over 098.2
trichomonal 131.00
tuberculous (*see also* Tuberculosis)
016.3
uterus, uterine (*see also* Endometritis)
615.9
utriculus masculinus NEC 597.89
vagina (granulation tissue) (wall) (*see also*
Vaginitis) 616.10
varicella 052.9
varicose veins—*see* Varicose, veins
verumontanum 597.89
vesical (*see also* Cystitis) 595.9
virus, viral (*see also* Infection, retrovirus)

Infection, infected, infective *(continued)*
079.99
adenovirus, in diseases classified elsewhere—*see* category 079
in diseases classified elsewhere—*see*
category 079
salivary gland disease specified type
NEC 079.89
in diseases classified elsewhere—*see*
category 079
unspecified nature or site 079.99
warts 078.10
specified NEC 078.19
vulva (*see also* Vulvitis) 616.10
yeast (*see also* Candidiasis) 112.9
Infertility
female (associated with) (due to) 628.9
adhesions, peritubal 614.6 (628.2)
anomaly (congenital)
cervical mucus 628.4
cervix 628.4
fallopian tube 628.2
uterus 628.3
vagina 628.4
anovulation 628.0
endometritis, tuberculous (*see also*
Tuberculosis) 016.7 (628.3)
nonimplantation 628.3
ovarian failure 256.39 (628.0)
pituitary–hypothalamus NEC 253.8
(628.1)
anterior pituitary NEC 253.4 (628.1)
hyperfunction NEC 253.1 (628.1)
panhypopituitarism 253.2 (628.1)
specified NEC 628.8
Stein-Leventhal syndrome 256.4
(628.0)
tubal (block) (occlusion) (stenosis)
628.2
male (due to) 606.9
absolute 606.0
azoospermia 606.0
drug therapy 606.8
extratesticular cause NEC 606.8
germinal cell
aplasia 606.0
desquamation 606.1
infection 606.8
obstruction, afferent ducts 606.8
oligospermia 606.1
radiation 606.8
spermatogenic arrest (complete) 606.0
incomplete 606.1

Infertility *(continued)*
systemic disease 606.8
previous, requiring supervision of pregnancy V23.0
Infestation
complicating pregnancy, childbirth, or puerperium 647.9
Epidermophyton—*see* Dermatophytosis
Monilia (albicans) (*see also* Candidiasis) 112.9
vagina 112.1
vulva 112.1
pubic louse 132.2
Trichomonas 131.9
bladder 131.09
cervix 131.09
specified site NEC 131.8
urethra 131.02
urogenital 131.00
vagina 131.01
vulva 131.01
Infiltrate, infiltration
calcium salt (muscle) 275.49
chemotherapy, vesicant 999.81
liver 573.8
skin, lymphocytic (benign) 709.8
vesicant agent NEC 999.82
Inflammation, inflamed, inflammatory
(with exudation)
accessory sinus (chronic) (*see also* Sinusitis) 473.9
amnion—*see* Amnionitis
anus 569.49
appendix (*see also* Appendicitis) 541
areola 611.0
puerperal, postpartum 675.0
Bartholin's gland 616.8
bladder (*see also* Cystitis) 595.9
breast 611.0
postpartum 675.2
broad ligament (*see also* Disease, pelvis, inflammatory) 614.4
acute 614.3
catarrhal 460
vagina 616.10
cervix (uteri) (*see also* Cervicitis) 616.0
cicatrix (tissue)—*see* Cicatrix
Douglas' cul-de-sac or pouch (chronic) (*see also* Disease, pelvis, inflammatory) 614.4
acute 614.3
due to (presence of) any device, implant, or graft classifiable to

Inflammation, inflamed, inflammatory *(continued)*
996.3–996.5—*see* Complications
follicular, pharynx 472.1
genital organ (diffuse) (internal) 614.9
with or following
abortion—*see* Abortion, by type, with sepsis
following abortion 639.0
ectopic or molar pregnancy (*see also* categories 630–633.9) 639.0
complicating pregnancy, childbirth, or puerperium 646.6
labium (majus) (minus) (*see also* Vulvitis) 616.10
mammary glad 611.0
puerperal, postpartum 675.2
nasal sinus (chronic) (*see also* Sinusitis) 473.9
nerve NEC 729.2
nipple 611.0
postpartum 675.0
ovary (*see also* Salpingo-oophoritis) 614.2
parametrium (chronic) (*see also* Disease, pelvis, inflammatory) 614.4
acute 614.3
pelvis (*see also* Disease, pelvis, inflammatory) 614.9
peritoneum (*see also* Peritonitis) 567.9
periuterine (*see also* Disease, pelvis, inflammatory) 614.9
rectum 569.49
respiratory, upper (*see also* Infection, respiratory, upper) 465.9
retroperitoneal (*see also* Peritonitis) 567.9
Skene's duct or gland (*see also* Urethritis) 597.89
tubal or tubo-ovarian (*see also* Salpingo-oophoritis) 614.2
uterine ligament (*see also* Disease, pelvis, inflammatory) 614.4
acute 614.3
uterus (catarrhal) (*see also* Endometritis) 615.9
vagina (*see also* Vaginitis) 616.10
vein (*see also* Phlebitis) thrombotic
leg or lower extremity 451.2
deep (vessels) NEC 451.19
superficial (vessels) 451.0
vulva (*see also* Vulvitis) 616.10
Influenza, influenzal 487.1
abdominal 487.8

Influenza, influenzal *(continued)*
Asian 487.1
avian 488.0
bronchial 487.1
bronchopneumonia 487.0
catarrhal 487.1
cold (any type) 487.1
epidemic 487.1
hemoptysis 487.1
laryngitis 487.1
novel (2009) H1N1 488.1
novel A/H1N1 488.1
pharyngitis 487.1
pneumonia (any form) 487.0
respiratory (upper) 487.1
sinusitis 487.1
stomach 487.8
swine 488.1
vaccination, prophylactic (against) V04.81
Inhalation
pneumonia—*see* Pneumonia, aspiration
stomach contents or secretions, in labor
and delivery 668.0
Inhibition, inhibited
orgasm 302.73
sexual
desire 302.71
excitement 302.72
Inhibitor, systemic lupus erythematosus
(presence of) 286.5
Injury (for internal organs, see Injury,
internal by site)
with or following
abortion—*see* Abortion, by type, with,
damage to pelvic organs
following abortion 639.2
ectopic or molar pregnancy (*see also*
categories 630–633.9) 639.2
abdomen, abdominal (viscera) (*see also*
Injury, internal, abdomen)
muscle or wall 959.12
anus 959.19
back 959.19
blood vessel NEC
abdomen
multiple 902.87
specified NEC 902.89
due to accidental puncture or laceration
during procedure 998.2
ovarian 902.89
artery 902.81
vein 902.82
pelvis
multiple 902.87

Injury *(continued)*
specified NEC 902.89
uterine 902.59
artery 902.55
vein 902.56
breast 959.19
buttock 959.19
clitoris 959.14
coccyx 959.19
complicating delivery 665.6
extremity (lower) (upper) NEC 959.8
genital organ(s) external 959.14
hymen 959.14
instrumental (during surgery) 998.2
nonsurgical—*see* Injury, by site
obstetrical 665.9
bladder 665.5
cervix 665.3
high vaginal 665.4
perineal NEC 664.9
urethra 665.5
uterus 665.5
internal
abdomen 866.00
appendix 863.85
with open wound into cavity 863.95
bladder (sphincter) 867.0
obstetrical trauma 665.5
open wound into cavity 867.1
broad ligament 867.6
with open wound into cavity 867.7
cervix (uteri) 867.4
obstetrical trauma 665.3
open wound into cavity 867.5
colon
with rectum 863.46
with open wound into cavity 863.56
multiple sites 863.46
with open wound into cavity 863.56
specified site NEC 863.49
with open wound into cavity
863.59
complicating delivery 665.9
fallopian tube 867.6
with open wound into cavity 867.7
genital organ NEC 867.6
with open wound into cavity 867.7
intrauterine (*see also* Injury, internal,
uterus) 867.4
with open wound into cavity 867.5
mesosalpinx 867.6
with open wound into cavity 867.7
ovary 867.6
with open wound into cavity 867.7

Injury *(continued)*

internal *(continued)*
   pelvis, pelvic (organs) (viscera) 867.8
      with
         fracture—*see* Fracture, pelvis
         open wound into cavity 867.9
         specified site NEC 867.6
            with open wound into cavity
               867.7
   rectum 863.45
      with
         colon 863.46
            with open wound into cavity
               863.56
         open wound into cavity 863.55
   round ligament 867.6
      with open wound into cavity 867.7
   ureter 867.2
      with open wound into cavity 867.3
   urethra (sphincter) 867.0
      obstetrical trauma 665.5
      open wound into cavity 867.1
   uterus 867.4
      obstetrical trauma NEC 665.5
      open wound into cavity 867.5
  labium (majus) (minus) 959.14
  multiple (sites not classifiable to the same
      four-digit category in 959.1)
      959.8
  pelvic (floor) 959.19
      complicating delivery 664.1
      obstetrical trauma 665.5
  perineum 959.14
  periurethral tissue
      complicating delivery 665.5
  pubic region 959.19
  pudenda 959.14
  rectovaginal septum 959.14
  sacrum 959.19
  soft tissue (of external sites) (severe)—*see*
      Wound, open, by site
  specified site NEC 959.8
  superficial
      anus (and other part[s] of trunk) 911
      breast (and other part[s] of trunk) 911
      clitoris (and other part[s] of trunk) 911
      labium (majus) (minus) (and other
         part[s] of trunk) 911
      multiple sites (not classifiable to the
         same three-digit category)
         919
      perineum (and other part[s] of trunk)
         911

Injury *(continued)*
  superficial *(continued)*
    skin NEC 919
    subcutaneous NEC 919
      vagina (and other part[s] of trunk) 911
      vulva (and other part[s] of trunk) 911
    supraclavicular fossa 959.19
    surgical complication (external or internal
        site) 998.2
    symphysis pubis 959.19
      complicating delivery 665.6
    trunk 959.19
    ultraviolet rays NEC 990
    vagina 959.14
    vulva 959.14

Insemination, artificial V26.1
Insertion
  cord (umbilical) lateral or velamentous
      663.8
  intrauterine contraceptive device V25.1
  placenta, vicious—*see* Placenta, previa
  subdermal implantable contraceptive V25.5
Insomnia—*see* Sleep, Sleeplessness
Instability
  urethral 599.83
  vasomotor 780.2
Insufficiency, insufficient
  anus 569.49
  arterial, peripheral 443.9
  arteriovenous 459.9
  cardiac (*see also* Insufficiency, myocardial)
      complicating surgery 997.1
      postoperative 997.1
  cardiovascular (*see also* Disease, cardiovas-
      cular) 429.2
  circulatory NEC 459.9
  gonadotropic hormone secretion 253.4
  myocardial, myocardium (with arterio-
      sclerosis)
    hypertensive (*see also* Hypertension,
        heart) 402.91
      benign 402.11
      malignant 402.01
    postoperative 997.1
  organic 799.89
  ovary 256.39
    postablative 256.2
  peripheral vascular (arterial) 443.9
  placental—*see* Placenta, insufficiency
  platelets 287.5
  prenatal care in current pregnancy V23.7
  renal 593.9
    due to procedure 997.5

Insufficiency, insufficient *(continued)*
respiratory 786.09
urethral sphincter 599.84
vascular 459.9
peripheral 443.9
renal *(see also* Hypertension, kidney)
403.90
weight gain during pregnancy 646.8
Insufflation, fallopian
fertility testing V26.21
following sterilization reversal V26.22
Intoxication
acid 276.2
alcohol (acute) 305.0
with alcoholism 303.0
hangover effects 305.0
hallucinogenic (acute) 305.3
potassium (K) 276.7
septic
with of following
abortion—*see* Abortion, by type,
with sepsis
following abortion 639.0
ectopic or molar pregnancy *(see also*
categories 630–633.9) 639.0
during labor 659.3
generalized—*see* Septicemia
puerperal, postpartum, childbirth 670.2
serum (prophylactic) (therapeutic) 999.5
uremic—*see* Uremia
water 276.6
Intrauterine contraceptive device—*see*
Contraception
Inversion *(see also* Anomaly)
cervix 622.8
nipple 611.79
congenital 757.6
puerperal, postpartum 676.3
sleep rhythm 780.55
uterus (postinfectional) (postpartal, old)
(chronic) 621.7
complicating delivery 665.2
vagina—*see* Prolapse, vagina
Involution, involutional *(see also* condition)
breast, cystic or fibrocystic 610.1
ovary, senile 620.3
paraphrenia (climacteric) (menopause)
297.2
Irritability (nervous) 799.2
bowel (syndrome) 564.1
bronchial *(see also* Bronchitis) 490
colon 564.1
urethra 599.84

Irritation
anus 569.49
cervix *(see also* Cervicitis) 616.0
intestine 564.9
perineum 709.9
peritoneum *(see also* Peritonitis) 567.9
vagina 623.9
Ischomenia 626.8
Ischuria 788.5
Isoimmunization NEC *(see also*
Incompatibility) 656.2
Itch *(see also* Pruritus) 698.9
dhobie 110.3
genital organs 698.1
perianal 698.0
winter 698.8

J
Jaundice (yellow)
catarrhal (acute) 070.1
with hepatic coma 070.0
febrile (acute) 070.1
with hepatic coma 070.0
from injection, inoculation, infusion,
or transfusion (blood)
(other substance) (onset
within 8 months after administration)—*see* Hepatitis,
viral
hepatocellular 573.8
homologous (serum)—*see* Hepatitis, viral
infectious (acute) (subacute) 070.1
with hepatic coma 070.0

K
Keloid, cheloid (kelis) 701.4
Keloma 701.4
Keratoma, senile 702.0
Keratosis
actinic 702.0
genital (external) 629.8
nigricans 701.2
seborrheic 702.19
inflamed 702.11
senilis 702.0
solar 702.0
vagina 623.1
Ketoacidosis 276.2
diabetic 250.1
Ketonuria 791.6
Kink, kinking
appendix 543.9
organ or site, congenital NEC—*see*

Kink, kinking *(continued)*
    Anomaly, specified type
    NEC, by site
  vein(s) (caval) (peripheral) 459.2
Knot, umbilical cord (true) 663.2
Kraurosis
  ani 569.49
  vagina 623.8
  vulva 624.09

L

Labiated hymen 752.49
Labile
  blood pressure 796.2
  vasomotor system 443.9
Labor—*see* Delivery, labor
Laceration (*see also* Wound, open, by site)
  with or following
    abortion—*see* Abortion, by type, with
      damage to pelvic organs
      following abortion 639.2
    ectopic pregnancy (*see also* categories
      633.0–633.9) 639.2
    molar pregnancy (*see also* categories
      630–632) 639.2
  accidental, complicating surgery 998.2
  anus (sphincter) 879.6
    complicated 879.7
    complicating delivery—*see* Delivery,
      laceration
    nontraumatic, nonpuerperal 565.0
  bladder (urinary)
    obstetrical trauma 665.5
  blood vessel—*see* Injury, blood vessel, by
    site
  bowel
    obstetrical trauma 665.5
  broad ligament
    nontraumatic 620.6
    obstetrical trauma 665.6
    syndrome (nontraumatic) 620.6
  causing eversion of cervix uteri (old)
    622.0
  central, complicating delivery 664.4
  cervix (uteri)
    nonpuerperal, nontraumatic 622.3
    obstetrical trauma (current) 665.3
    old (postpartal) 622.3
    traumatic—*see* Injury, internal, cervix
  internal organ (abdomen) (pelvis)
    NEC—*see* Injury, internal, by
      site
  labia, complicating delivery 664.0

Laceration *(continued)*
  pelvic
    floor (muscles)
      complicating delivery 664.1
      nonpuerperal 618.7
      old (postpartal) 618.7
    organ NEC
      complicating delivery 665.5
      obstetrical trauma 665.5
  perineum, perineal (old) (postpartal)
    618.7
    complicating delivery—*see* Delivery,
      complicated by trauma
    muscles, complicating delivery
      664.1
    nonpuerperal, current injury 879.6
      complicated 879.7
    secondary (postpartal) 674.2
  peritoneum
    obstetrical trauma 665.5
  rectovaginal (septum)
    complicating delivery 665.4
      with perineum 664.2
        involving anal or rectal mucosa
        664.3
    nonpuerperal 623.4
    old (postpartal) 623.4
  spinal cord (meninges)—*see* Injury,
    spinal, by site
  urethra or periurethral
    nonpuerperal, nontraumatic 599.84
    obstetrical trauma 665.5
  uterus
    nonpuerperal, nontraumatic 621.8
    obstetrical trauma NEC 665.5
    old (postpartal) 621.8
  vagina
    complicating delivery—*see* Delivery,
      complicated by
    nonpuerperal, nontraumatic 623.4
    old (postpartal) 623.4
  vulva
    complicating delivery 664.0
    nonpuerperal, nontraumatic 624.4
    old (postpartal) 624.4
Lack of
  appetite (*see also* Anorexia) 783.0
  development—*see* Hypoplasia
  energy 780.79
  medical attention 799.89
  ovulation 628.0
  physical exercise V69.0
  prenatal care in current pregnancy V23.7

Lactation, lactating (breast) (puerperal) (postpartum)
  defective 676.4
  disorder 676.9
    specified type NEC 676.8
  excessive 676.6
  failed 676.4
  mastitis NEC 675.2
  mother (care and/or examination) V24.1
  nonpuerperal 611.6
  suppressed 676.5
Lacticemia, excessive 276.2
Laparoscopic procedure converted to open procedure V64.41
Laryngitis
  with influenza 487.1
  chronic 476.1
Laryngopharyngitis (acute) 465.0
  septic 034.0
Late effect(s) (of) (*see also* condition)
  foreign body in orifice (injury classifiable to 937–939) 908.5
  injury
    blood vessel, abdomen and pelvis (injury classifiable to 902) 908.4
    internal organ NEC, abdomen (injury classifiable to 863–864) 908.1
  pregnancy complication(s) 677
  radiation (conditions classifiable to 990) 909.2
  surgical and medical care 909.3
Lateroversion, uterus, uterine (cervix) (postinfectional) (postpartal, old) 621.6
  congenital 752.3
  in pregnancy or childbirth 654.4
Laxative habit (*see also* Abuse, drugs, non-dependent) 305.9
Leakage
  amniotic fluid 658.1
    with delayed delivery 658.2
  blood (microscopic), fetal, into maternal circulation
    affecting management of pregnancy or puerperium 656.0
  device, implant, or graft—*see* Complications
  spinal fluid at lumbar puncture site 997.09
  urine, continuous 788.37
Leiomyoma (*see also* Neoplasm, connective tissue, benign)
  uterus (cervix) (corpus) 218.9

Leiomyoma *(continued)*
  in pregnancy or childbirth 654.1
    causing obstructed labor 660.2
  interstitial 218.1
  intramural 218.1
  submucous 218.0
  subperitoneal or subserous 218.2
Leiomyomatosis (intravascular)—*see* Neoplasm, connective tissue, uncertain behavior
Leiomyosarcoma (*see also* Neoplasm, connective tissue, malignant)
Lentigo (congenital) 709.09
  Maligna (*see also* Neoplasm, skin, in situ)
    melanoma—*see* Melanoma
Lesion
  anorectal 569.49
  calcified—*see* Calcification
  congenital—*see* Anomaly
  cystic—*see* Cyst
  degenerative—*see* Degeneration
  inflammatory—*see* Inflammation
  nonallopathic, in region (of)
    abdomen 739.9
    hip or pelvic 739.5
  obstructive—*see* Obstruction
  organ or site NEC—*see* Disease, by site
  perirectal 569.49
  peritoneum (granulomatous) 568.89
  pigmented (skin) 709.00
  polypoid—*see* Polyp
  sinus (accessory) (nasal) (*see also* Sinusitis) 473.9
  skin 709.9
  syphilitic—*see* Syphilis
  ulcerated or ulcerative—*see* Ulcer
  uterus NEC 621.9
  vagina 623.8
  vascular 459.9
    umbilical cord 663.6
  warty—*see* Verruca
Lethargy 780.79
Leukodermia 709.09
Leukoplakia
  anus 569.49
  cervix (uteri) 622.2
  rectum 569.49
  urethra (postinfectional) 599.84
  uterus 621.8
  vagina 623.1
  vulva 624.09
Leukorrhea (vagina) 623.5
  due to Trichomonas (vaginalis) 131.00

Leydig cell—*see* Carcinoma, Tumor
Leydig–Sertoli cell tumor—*see* Carcinoma,
    Tumor
LGSIL (low grade squamous intraepithelial
    lesion)
  anus 796.73
  cervix 795.03
  vagina 795.13
Lice (infestation) (crab) (pediculus pubis)
    132.2
Lichen
  albus or atrophicus 701.0
  myxedematous 701.8
  planus (acute) (chronicus) (hypertrophic)
    (verrucous) 701.0
  sclerosus (et atrophicus) 701.0
  urticatus 698.2
Light-for-dates, affecting management of
    pregnancy 656.5
Linitis (gastric) 535.4
Lipoadenoma—*see* Neoplasm, by site,
    benign
Lipofibroma—*see* Lipoma, by site
Lipogranuloma, sclerosing 709.8
Lipoma, lipofibroma
  breast (skin) 214.1
  intra-abdominal 214.3
  peritoneum 214.3
  retroperitoneum 214.3
  skin 214.1
  subcutaneous tissue 214.1
Lipuria 791.1
**Listeriosis, suspected fetal damage affect-
    ing management of preg-
    nancy 655.4**
Listlessness 780.79
**Lithopedion affecting management of
    pregnancy 656.8**
Lithuria 791.9
Livedo 782.61
Locked twins 660.5
Long-term (current) drug use
    V58.69
  antibiotics V58.62
  anticoagulants V58.61
  anti-inflammatories, non-steroidal
    (NSAID) V58.64
  antiplatelets/antithrombotics V58.63
  aspirin V58.66
  insulin V58.67
  methadone V58.69
  steroids V58.65
  tamoxifen V07.51

Loss
  appetite 783.0
    nonorganic origin (psychogenic) 307.59
  consciousness, transient 780.2
  control, sphincter, rectum 787.6
  elasticity, skin 782.8
  fluid (acute) (with) 276.5
    hypernatremia 276.0
    hyponatremia 276.1
  hair 704.00
  height 781.91
  organ or part—*see* Absence, by site,
    acquired
  weight (cause unknown) 783.21
Low
  back syndrome 724.2
  basal metabolic rate (BMR) 794.7
  bladder compliance 596.52
  blood pressure (*see also* Hypotension)
    458.9
    reading (incidental) (nonspecific) 796.3
  implantation or insertion, placenta—*see*
    Placenta, previa
  risk, human papillomavirus (HPV) DNA
    test positive
    anal 796.79
    cervical 795.09
    vaginal 795.19
Lumbago, Lumbalgia 724.2
Lump (*see also* Mass)
  abdominal or pelvic 789.3
  breast 611.72
Lump *(continued)*
  skin 782.2
  umbilicus 789.3
Lupus 710.0
  discoid (local) 695.4
  disseminated 710.0
  erythematodes or erythematosus (dis-
    coid) (local) 695.4
    disseminated 710.0
    systemic 710.0
    inhibitor (presence of) 286.5
  hydralazine, correct substance properly
    administered 695.4
  nontuberculous, not disseminated 695.4
Luteoma 220
Lymphadenitis
  with or following
    abortion—*see* Abortion, by type, with
      sepsis
      following abortion 639.0
    ectopic pregnancy (*see also* categories

Lymphadenitis *(continued)*
       633.0–633.9) 639.0
    molar pregnancy (*see also* categories
       630–632) 639.0
    breast, puerperal, postpartum 675.2
    chancroidal (congenital) 099.0
    gonorrheal 098.89
    purulent, septic or streptococcal 683
    syphilitic (early) (secondary) 091.4
    venereal 099.1
Lymphadenopathy (general) 785.6
Lymphadenosis 785.6
    acute 075
Lymphangitis
    with or following
       abortion—*see* Abortion, by type, with
          sepsis
          following abortion 639.0
       abscess—*see* Abscess, by site
       cellulitis—*see* Abscess, by site
       ectopic pregnancy (*see also* categories
          633.0–633.9) 639.0
       molar pregnancy (*see also* categories
          630–632) 639.0
    acute (with abscess or cellulitis)
       specified site—*see* Abscess, by site
    breast, puerperal, postpartum 675.2
    chancroidal 099.0
    puerperal, postpartum, childbirth 670.8
Lymphedema (*see also* Elephantiasis), surgi-
       cal, postmastectomy (syn-
       drome) 457.0
Lymphoblastosis, acute benign 075
Lymphogranuloma (malignant) 201.9
    venereal (any site) 099.1
       with stricture of rectum 099.1
Lymphoma
    benign—*see* Neoplasm, by site, benign
    compound 200.8
    histiocytic (diffuse) 200.0
    immunoblastic (type) 200.8
    large cell 200.7
    lymphocytic (cell type) (diffuse) 200.1
       with plasmacytoid differentiation,
          diffuse 200.8
       intermediate or poor differentiation
          (diffuse) 200.1
       well differentiated (diffuse) 200.1
    lymphosarcoma type 200.1
    mixed cell type (diffuse) 200.8
    nodular, histiocytic 200.0
    small cell and large cell, mixed (diffuse)
       200.8

Lymphomatosis, granulomatous 099.1
Lymphopathia, venereum 099.1

M
Macromastia (*see also* Hypertrophy, breast)
       611.1
Macules and papules 709.8
Maintenance
    chemotherapy or other drug regimen or
          treatment V58.1
    radiotherapy V58.0
Mal lie—*see* Presentation, fetal
Malabsorption, folate, congenital 281.2
Malacoplakia, urethra 599.84
Malaise 780.79
Male type pelvis
    with disproportion (fetopelvic) 653.2
       causing obstructed labor 660.1
Malfunction (*see also* Dysfunction)
    catheter device—*see* Complications,
          mechanical, catheter
    colostomy 569.62
    cystostomy 997.5
    device, implant, or graft NEC—*see*
          Complications
Malignancy—*see* Neoplasm, by site,
          malignant
Malingerer, malingering V65.2
Malnutrition (calorie)
    complicating pregnancy 648.9
    lack of care, or neglect (child) (infant)
          995.52
       adult 995.84
Malposition
    cervix—*see* Malposition, uterus
    congenital
       genitalia, genital organ(s) or tract,
          external 752.49
       ovary 752.0
       ureter 753.4
       uterus 752.3
    device, implant, or graft—*see*
          Complications
    fetus NEC—*see* Presentation, fetal
    pelvic organs or tissues
       in pregnancy or childbirth 654.4
          causing obstructed labor 660.2
    placenta—*see* Placenta, previa
    uterus (acquired) (postinfectional) (post-
          partal, old) 621.6
       anteflexion or anteversion (*see also*
          Anteversion, uterus) 621.6
       congenital 752.3

Malposition *(continued)*
in pregnancy or childbirth 654.4
causing obstructed labor 660.2
inversion 621.6
lateral (flexion) (version) *(see also*
Lateroversion, uterus)* 621.6
retroflexion or retroversion *(see also*
Retroversion, uterus)* 621.6
Malposture 729.90
Malpresentation, fetus—*see* Presentation,
fetal
Mammographic
calcification 793.89
calculus 793.89
microcalcification 793.81
Mammoplasia 611.1
Mania (monopolar)
puerperal (after delivery) 296.0
single episode 296.0
Marital conflict V61.10
Mark
port wine, raspberry or strawberry
757.32
stretch 701.3
tattoo 709.09
Masculinovoblastoma 220
Mass
abdominal 789.3
anus 787.99
breast 611.72
cystic—*see* Cyst
lymph node 785.6
malignant—*see* Neoplasm, by site,
malignant
pelvis, pelvic 789.3
perineum 625.8
rectum 787.99
skin 782.2
specified organ NEC—*see* Disease of
specified organ or site
superficial (localized) 782.2
umbilicus 789.3
uterus 625.8
vagina 625.8
vulva 625.8
Mastalgia 611.71
Mastitis (acute) (diffuse) (interstitial)
(lobular) (nonpuerperal)
(parenchymatous) (simple)
(subacute) 611.0
chronic (cystic) (fibrocystic) 610.1
cystic or fibrocystic 610.1
infective 611.0

Mastitis *(continued)*
lactational 675.2
lymphangitis 611.0
periductal 610.4
plasma cell 610.4
puerperal, postpartum, 675.2
purulent 675.1
stagnation 676.2
retromammary 611.0
puerperal, postpartum 675.1
submammary 611.0
puerperal, postpartum 675.1
Mastoplasia 611.1
Maternity—*see* Delivery
Measles 055.9
complication 055.8
vaccination, prophylactic (against) V04.2
Meatitis, urethral *(see also* Urethritis)* 597.89
Meatus, meatal—*see* condition
Meconium
in liquor noted during delivery 656.8
obstruction in mucoviscidosis 277.01
passage of 792.3
noted during delivery—omit code
Melancholia
menopausal (climacteric) 296.2
recurrent episode 296.3
single episode 296.2
puerperal 296.2
Melanoderma, melanodermia 709.09
Melanoma (malignant) 172.9
abdominal wall 172.5
breast 172.5
buttock 172.5
genital organ (external) NEC 184.4
gluteal region 172.5
labium
majus 184.1
minus 184.2
metastatic
of or from specified site—*see*
Melanoma, by site
site not of skin—*see* Neoplasm, by site,
malignant, secondary
unspecified site 172.9
nodular—*see* Melanoma, by site
perianal skin or perineum 172.5
skin NEC 172.8
trunk NEC 172.5
vagina vault 184.0
vulva 184.4
Melanosis 709.09
precancerous *(see also* Neoplasm, sk

Melanosis *(continued)*
    in situ)
    malignant melanoma in—*see* Melanoma
Melanuria 791.9
Melasma 709.09
Melena 578.1
   due to ulcer—*see* Ulcer, by site, with
      hemorrhage
Menarche, precocious 259.1
Meningismus (infectional) (pneumococcal)
    influenzal NEC 487.8
Meningitis
   actinomyocotic 039.8 (320.7)
   candidal carrier (suspected) of V02.59
   due to other bacterial diseases classified
      elsewhere 320.7
   H. influenza 320.0
   pneumococcal 320.1
   staphylococcal 320.3
   sterile 997.09
   streptococcal (acute) 320.2
Meningococcus, meningococcal
   carrier (suspected) of V02.59
Menolipsis 626.0
Menometrorrhagia 626.2
Menopause, menopausal (symptoms)
    (syndrome) 627.2
   arthritis (any site) NEC 716.3
   artificial 627.4
   bleeding 627.0
   crisis 627.2
Menopause, menopausal *(continued)*
   depression (single episode) 296.2
     recurrent episode 296.3
   postsurgical 627.4
   premature 256.31
    postirradiation 256.2
    postsurgical 256.2
   psychoneurosis 627.2
   toxic polyarthritis NEC 716.39
Menorrhagia (primary) 626.2
   menopausal 627.0
   postmenopausal 627.1
   premenopausal 627.0
   puberty (menses retained) 626.3
Menstrual (*see also* Menstruation)
   extraction or regulation V25.3
   molimen 625.4
   period, normal V65.5
Menstruation
   absent 626.0
   anovulatory 628.0
   delayed 626.8
   difficult 625.3

Menstruation *(continued)*
   disorder 626.9
    specified NEC 626.8
   during pregnancy 640.8
   excessive 626.2
   frequent 626.2
   infrequent 626.1
   irregular 626.4
   latent 626.8
   membranous 626.8
   painful (primary) (secondary) 625.3
   passage of clots 626.2
   precocious 626.8
   protracted 626.8
   retained 626.8
   retrograde 626.8
   scanty 626.1
   suppressed 626.8
   vicarious (nasal) 625.8
Metaplasia
   breast 611.89
   cervix—omit code
   endometrium (squamous) 621.8
   squamous cell
    amnion 658.8
    cervix—*see* condition
    uterus 621.8
Metastasis, metastatic
   abscess—*see* Abscess
   calcification 275.40
   cancer, neoplasm, or disease
    from specified site—*see* Neoplasm, by
      site, malignant
    to specified site—*see* Neoplasm, by site,
      secondary
   deposits (in)—*see* Neoplasm, by site,
     secondary
   pneumonia 038.8 (484.8)
Metritis (catarrhal) (septic) (suppurative)
    (see also Endometritis) 615.9
   puerperal, postpartum, childbirth 670.1
   septic 670.2
Metropathia hemorrhagica 626.8
Metroperitonitis (*see also* Peritonitis,
    pelvic) 614.5
Metrorrhagia 626.6
   arising during pregnancy—*see*
      Hemorrhage, pregnancy
   postpartum NEC 666.2
   primary 626.6
Metrovaginitis (*see also* Endometritis)
    615.9
   gonococcal (acute) 098.16
    chronic or duration of 2 months or
      over 098.36

Micromastia 611.82
Microthelia 757.6
Microthromboembolism—*see* Embolism
Micturition
    disorder NEC 788.69
    frequency 788.41
    nocturnal 788.43
    painful 788.1
    psychogenic 306.53
Miescher's disease (granulomatosis disciformis) 709.3
Migraine (idiopathic) 346.9
    with aura (acute-onset) (without headache) (prolonged) (typical) 346.0
    without aura 346.1
        chronic 346.7
        transformed 346.7
    abdominal (syndrome) 346.2
    allergic (histamine) 346.2
    atypical 346.8
    basilar 346.0
    classic(al) 346.0
    hemiplegic 346.3
        familial 346.3
        sporadic 346.3
    lower-half 339.00
    menstrual 346.4
    menstrually related 346.4
    pure menstrual 346.4
    specified form NEC 346.8
    variant 346.2
Milium (*see also* Cyst, sebaceous) 706.2
    colloid 709.3
Milk
    excess secretion 676.6
    fever 672
    retention 676.2
Milk-leg (deep vessels) 671.4
    complicating pregnancy 671.3
    nonpuerperal 451.19
    postpartum 671.4
Misadventure (prophylactic) (therapeutic)—*see* Complications 999.9
Miscarriage—*see* Abortion, spontaneous
Missed
    abortion 632
    delivery (at or near term) 656.4
    labor (at or near term) 656.4
Misshapen reconstructed breast 612.0
Mittelschmerz 625.2
Mola destruens 236.1
Molar pregnancy 631
    hydatidiform—*see* Hydatidiform
Mole (pigmented) (*see also* Neoplasm, skin, benign)

Mole *(continued)*
    blood 631
    cancerous—*see* Melanoma
    carneous 631
    destructive 236.1
    ectopic—*see* Pregnancy, ectopic
    fleshy 631
    hemorrhagic 631
    hydatid, hydatidiform—*see* Hydatidiform mole
    melanoma—*see* Melanoma
    nonpigmented—*see* Neoplasm, skin, benign
    pregnancy NEC 631
    skin—*see* Neoplasm, skin, benign
    tubal—*see* Pregnancy, tubal
Molimen, molimina (menstrual) 625.4
Molluscum (contagiosum) (epitheliale) 078.0
    fibrosum—*see* Lipoma, by site
    pendulum—*see* Lipoma, by site
Moniliasis (*see also* Candidiasis)
    vulvovaginitis 112.1
Mononucleosis, infectious 075
Mood swings 296.99
Morning sickness 643.0
Mucinosis (cutaneous) (papular) 701.8
Mucocele
    appendix 543.9
    uterus 621.8
Mucocutaneous lymph node syndrome 446.1
Mucositis (cervix) (vagina) (vulva) **616.81**
Mucoviscidosis 277.00
    with meconium obstruction 277.01
Mucus in stool 792.1
Müllerian anomaly—*see* Anomaly, Müllerian
Müllerian mixed tumor—*see* Neoplasm, by site, malignant
Multiparity V61.5
    affecting management of
        labor and delivery 659.4
        pregnancy V23.7
    requiring contraceptive management (*see also* Contraception) V25.9
Mumps 072.9
    with or without complication 072.8
    vaccination, prophylactic (against) V04.6
Murmur (cardiac) (heart) (nonorganic) (organic) 785.2
    benign—omit code
    cardiorespiratory 785.2
    functional—omit code
    presystolic, mitral—*see* Insufficiency, mitral
    undiagnosed 785.2
Mycosis (vagina) (vaginitis) 112.1
Myofascitis (acute) 729.1
    low back 724.2

Myofibrositis (*see also* Myositis) 729.1
Myoma (*see also* Neoplasm, connective
      tissue, benign)
  cervix (stump) (uterus) (*see also*
      Leiomyoma) 218.9
  malignant—*see* Neoplasm, connective
      tissue, malignant
  uterus (cervix) (corpus) (*see also*
      Leiomyoma) 218.9
    in pregnancy or childbirth 654.1
      causing obstructed labor 660.2
Myosarcoma—*see* Neoplasm, connective
      tissue, malignant
Myosis, stromal (endolymphatic) 236.0
Myositis 729.1
  multiple—*see* Polymyositis
Myxedema (*see also* Hypothyroidism)
  cutis, papular 701.8
  postpartum 674.8

N
Nägele's pelvis 738.6
  with disproportion (fetopelvic) 653.0
    causing obstructed labor 660.1
Narcosis, carbon dioxide (respiratory)
    786.09
Nasopharyngitis (acute) (infective) (suba-
    cute) 460
  septic or streptococcal 034.0
  suppurative (chronic) 472.2
  ulcerative (chronic) 472.2
Nausea (*see also* Vomiting) 787.02
  with vomiting 787.01
  gravidarum—*see* Hyperemesis, gravidarum
Near-syncope 780.2
Necrosis, necrotic
  arteritis 446.0
  breast (aseptic) (fat) (segmental) 611.3
  fat, fatty (generalized)

Necrosis, necrotic *(continued)*
  omentum 567.8
  peritoneum 567.8
  skin (subcutaneous) 709.3
  kidney (bilateral)
    complicating
      abortion 639.3
      ectopic or molar pregnancy 639.3
      pregnancy 646.2
    following labor and delivery 669.3
    traumatic 958.5
  liver (acute) (congenital) (subacute)
    with or following
      abortion—*see* Abortion, by type,
        with specified complication
        NEC
      following abortion 639.8
      ectopic pregnancy (*see also*
        categories 630–633.9) 639.8
      molar pregnancy (*see also* categories
        630–632) 639.8
    complicating pregnancy 646.7
    puerperal, postpartum 674.8
    toxic 573.3
  lymphatic gland 683
  mammary gland 611.3
  ovary (*see also* Salpingo-oophoritis) 614.2
  perineum 624.8
  placenta (*see also* Placenta, abnormal) 656.7
  skin or subcutaneous tissue 709.8
    due to burn—*see* Burn, by site
  subcutaneous fat 709.3
  tubular (acute) (anoxic) (toxic) due to a
    procedure 997.5
  vagina 623.8
  vulva 624.8
Neglect (adult) 995.84

Neoplasm Table

The terms used in this table are defined as follows:

■ Malignant neoplasms are cancerous and capable of dissemination and/or local infiltration.

■ Primary neoplasms are the original site of the neoplasm.

■ Secondary neoplasms are a second cancerous neoplasm appearing at a body site other than the original one.

■ Carcinoma in situ is cancerous but confined or "noninvasive" in nature.

■ Benign neoplasms are noncancerous.

■ Uncertain behavior means the tissue has neoplastic characteristics, but the pathologist cannot yet determine its behavior. Further testing is required.

■ Unspecified behavior means the nature of the neoplasm is undetermined pending laboratory results.

| | Malignant | | | | | |
	Primary	Secondary	Ca in situ	Benign	Uncertain Behavior	Unspecified
abdomen, abdominal wall	173.5	198.2	232.5	216.5	238.2	239.2
connective tissue	171.5	198.89	—	215.5	238.1	239.2
adipose tissue (*see also* Neoplasm, connective tissue)	171.9	198.89	—	215.9	238.1	239.2
adnexa (uterine)	183.9	198.82	233.39	221.8	236.3	239.5
anorectum, anorectal (junction)	154.8	197.5	230.7	211.4	235.2	—
anus, anal	154.3	197.5	230.6	211.4	235.5	—
canal	154.2	197.5	230.5	211.4	235.5	—
contiguous sites with rectosigmoid junction or rectum	154.8	—	—	—	—	—
areola	174.0	198.81	233.0	217	238.3	239.3
Bartholin's gland	184.1	198.82	233.32	221.2	236.3	239.5
bile or biliary tract	156.9	197.8	230.8	211.5	235.3	239.0
intrahepatic duct	155.1	197.8	230.8	211.5	235.3	239.0
intralobular, continguous sites	155.1	197.8	230.8	211.5	235.3	239.0
bowel—*see* Neoplasm, intestine						
breast (connective tissue) (glandular tissue) (soft parts)	174.9	198.81	233.0	217	238.3	239.3

(continued)

Neoplasm Table *(continued)*

	Malignant					
	Primary	Secondary	Ca in situ	Benign	Uncertain Behavior	Unspecified
breast *(continued)*						
areola	174.0	198.81	233.0	217	238.3	239.3
axillary tail	174.6	198.81	233.0	217	238.3	239.3
central portion	174.1	198.81	233.0	217	238.3	239.3
contiguous sites	174.8	—	—	—	—	—
ectopic sites	174.8	198.81	233.0	217	238.3	239.3
inner	174.8	198.81	233.0	217	238.3	239.3
lower	174.8	198.81	233.0	217	238.3	239.3
lower-inner quadrant	174.3	198.81	233.0	217	238.3	239.3
lower-outer quadrant	174.5	198.81	233.0	217	238.3	239.3
mastectomy site (skin)	173.5	198.2	—	—	—	—
specified as breast tissue	174.8	198.81	—	—	—	—
midline	174.8	198.81	233.0	217	238.3	239.3
nipple	174.0	198.81	233.0	217	238.3	239.3
outer	174.8	198.81	233.0	217	238.3	239.3
skin	173.5	198.2	232.5	216.5	238.2	239.2
tail (axillary)	174.6	198.81	233.0	217	238.3	239.3
upper	174.8	198.81	233.0	217	238.3	239.3
upper-inner quadrant	174.2	198.81	233.0	217	238.3	239.3
upper-outer quadrant	174.4	198.81	233.0	217	238.3	239.3
cavity, peritoneal	158.9	197.6	—	211.8	235.4	—
cervix (cervical) (uteri) (uterus)	180.9	198.82	233.1	219.0	236.0	239.5
canal	180.0	198.82	233.1	219.0	236.0	239.5
contiguous sites	180.8	—	—	—	—	—
endocervix (canal) (gland)	180.0	198.82	233.1	219.0	236.0	239.5
exocervix	180.1	198.82	233.1	219.0	236.0	239.5
external os	180.1	198.82	233.1	219.0	236.0	239.5
internal os	180.0	198.82	233.1	219.0	236.0	239.5
nabothian gland	180.0	198.82	233.1	219.0	236.0	239.5
squamocolumnar junction	180.8	198.82	233.1	219.0	236.0	239.5
stump	180.8	198.82	233.1	219.0	236.0	239.5
clitoris	184.3	198.82	233.32	221.2	236.3	239.5
colon *(see also* Neoplasm, intestine, large and rectum)	154.0	197.5	230.4	211.4	235.2	—
connective tissue NEC	171.9	198.89	—	215.9	238.1	239.2
abdomen	171.5	198.89	—	215.5	238.1	239.2
abdominal wall	171.5	198.89	—	215.5	238.1	239.2
breast *(see also* Neoplasm, breast)	174.9	198.81	233.0	217	238.3	239.3
chest (wall)	171.4	198.89	—	215.4	238.1	239.2
pararectal	171.6	198.89	—	215.6	238.1	239.2
paravaginal	171.6	198.89	—	215.6	238.1	239.2

(continued)

Neoplasm Table *(continued)*

	Malignant					
	Primary	Secondary	Ca in situ	Benign	Uncertain Behavior	Unspecified
connective tissue NEC *(continued)*						
pelvis (floor)	171.6	198.89	—	215.6	238.1	239.2
pelvo-abdominal	—	198.89	—	215.8	238.1	239.2
perineum	171.6	198.89	—	215.6	238.1	239.2
perirectal (tissue)	171.6	198.89	—	215.6	238.1	239.2
periurethral (tissue)	171.6	198.89	—	215.6	238.1	239.2
presacral	171.6	198.89	—	215.6	238.1	239.2
rectovaginal septum or wall	171.6	198.89	—	215.6	238.1	239.2
rectovesical (tissue)	171.6	198.89	—	215.6	238.1	239.2
thoracic (duct) (wall)	171.4	198.89	—	215.4	238.1	239.2
umbilicus	171.5	198.89	—	215.5	238.1	239.2
cul-de-sac (Douglas')	158.8	197.6	—	211.8	235.4	—
digestive organs	159.9	197.8	230.9	211.9	235.5	239.0
contiguous sites with peritoneum	159.8	—	—	—	—	—
disseminated	199.0	199.0	234.9	229.9	238.9	199.0
duodenojejunal junction	152.8	197.4	230.7	211.2	235.2	239.0
endometrium (gland) (stroma)	182.0	198.82	233.2	219.1	236.0	239.5
esophagus	150.9	197.8	230.1	211.0	235.5	239.0
contiguous sites	150.8	—	—	—	—	—
specified part NEC	150.8	197.8	230.1	211.0	235.5	239.0
fallopian tube (accessory)	183.2	198.82	233.39	221.0	236.3	239.5
fetal membrane	181	198.82	233.2	219.8	236.1	239.5
follicle, nabothian	180.0	198.82	233.1	219.0	236.0	239.5
Gartner's duct	184.0	198.82	233.31	221.1	236.3	239.5
generalized	199.0	199.0	234.9	229.9	238.9	199.0
genitourinary tract	184.9	198.82	233.39	221.9	236.3	239.5
gland, glandular (lymphatic) (system)—*see* Neoplasm, lymph gland						
hymen	184.0	198.82	233.31	221.1	236.3	239.5
intestine, intestinal						
large (colon)	153.9	197.5	230.3	211.3	235.2	—
appendix	153.5	197.5	230.3	211.3	235.2	—
and rectum	154.0	197.5	230.4	211.4	235.2	—
small	152.9	197.4	230.7	211.2	235.2	239.0
contiguous sites	152.8	—	—	—	—	—
labia, labium (skin)	184.4	198.82	233.32	221.2	236.3	239.5
majora	184.1	198.82	233.32	221.2	236.3	239.5
minora	184.2	198.82	233.32	221.2	236.3	239.5
ligament						
broad	183.3	198.82	233.39	221.0	236.3	239.5

(continued)

Neoplasm Table *(continued)*

	Malignant					
	Primary	Secondary	Ca in situ	Benign	Uncertain Behavior	Unspecified
ligament *(continued)*						
broad	183.3	198.82	233.39	221.0	236.3	239.5
Mackenrodt's	183.8	198.82	233.39	221.8	236.3	239.5
round	183.5	198.82	—	221.0	236.3	239.5
uterine	183.4	198.82	—	221.0	236.3	239.5
utero-ovarian	183.8	198.82	233.39	221.8	236.3	239.5
uterosacral	183.4	198.82	—	221.0	236.3	239.5
liver, primary	155.0	—	—	—	—	—
mesosalpinx	183.3	198.82	233.3	221.0	236.3	239.5
mesovarium	183.3	198.82	233.39	221.0	236.3	239.5
mons pubis	184.4	198.82	233.39	221.2	236.3	239.5
Müllerian duct	184.8	198.82	233.39	221.8	236.3	239.5
multiple sites NEC	199.0	199.0	234.9	229.9	238.9	199.0
nabothian gland (follicle)	180.0	198.82	233.1	219.0	236.0	239.5
omentum	158.8	197.6	—	211.8	235.4	—
ovary	183.0	198.6	233.39	220	236.2	239.5
parametrium	183.4	198.82	—	221.0	236.3	239.5
paravaginal	195.3	198.89	—	229.8	238.8	239.89
paroophoron	183.3	198.82	233.3	221.0	236.3	239.5
parovarium	183.3	198.82	233.39	221.0	236.3	239.5
pelvirectal junction	154.0	197.5	230.4	211.4	235.2	—
pelvic floor	195.3	198.89	234.8	229.8	238.8	239.89
perianal (skin)	173.5	198.2	232.5	216.5	238.2	239.2
perineum	195.3	198.89	234.8	229.8	238.8	239.89
perirectal (tissue)	195.3	198.89	—	229.8	238.8	239.89
peritoneum, peritoneal (cavity)	158.9	197.6	—	211.8	235.4	—
contiguous sites	158.8	—	—	—	—	—
with digestive organs	159.8	—	—	—	—	—
periurethral tissue	195.3	198.89	—	229.8	238.8	239.89
placenta	181	198.82	233.2	219.8	236.1	239.5
pudenda, pudendum	184.4	198.82	233.32	221.2	236.3	239.5
rectouterine pouch	154.0	197.5	230.4	211.4	235.2	—
rectum (ampulla)	154.1	197.5	230.4	211.4	235.2	—
and colon	154.0	197.5	230.4	211.4	235.2	—
contiguous sites with anus or rectosigmoid junction	154.8	—	—	—	—	—
retroperitoneal/ retroperitoneum	158.0	197.6	—	211.8	235.4	—
contiguous sites	158.8	—	—	—	—	—
rectovaginal septum or wall	195.3	198.89	234.8	229.8	238.8	239.89
rectovesical septum	195.3	198.89	234.8	229.8	238.8	239.89

(continued)

Neoplasm Table *(continued)*

	Malignant					
	Primary	Secondary	Ca in situ	Benign	Uncertain Behavior	Unspecified
scar NEC *(see also* Neoplasm, skin)	173.9	198.2	232.9	216.9	238.2	239.2
septum						
urethrovaginal	184.9	198.82	233.39	221.9	236.3	239.5
vesicovaginal	184.9	198.82	233.39	221.9	236.3	239.5
skin NEC	173.9	198.2	232.9	216.9	238.2	239.2
abdominal wall	173.5	198.2	232.5	216.5	238.2	239.2
anus	173.5	198.2	232.5	216.5	238.2	239.2
breast	173.5	198.2	232.5	216.5	238.2	239.2
perineum	173.5	198.2	232.5	216.5	238.2	239.2
specified sites NEC	173.8	198.2	232.8	216.8	232.8	239.2
submammary fold	173.5	198.2	232.5	216.5	238.2	239.2
trunk	173.5	198.2	232.5	216.5	238.2	239.2
stomach	151.9	197.8	230.2	211.1	235.2	239.0
contiguous sites	151.4	197.8	230.2	211.1	235.2	239.0
wall NEC	151.9	197.8	230.2	211.1	235.2	239.0
tubo-ovarian	183.8	198.82	233.39	221.8	236.3	239.5
umbilicus, umbilical	173.5	198.2	232.5	216.5	238.2	239.2
unknown site or unspecified	199.1	199.1	234.9	229.9	238.9	239.9
urethrovaginal (septum)	184.9	198.82	233.39	221.9	236.3	239.5
utero-ovarian	183.8	198.82	233.39	221.8	236.3	239.5
ligament	183.3	198.82	—	221.0	236.3	239.5
uterus *(see also* Neoplasm, cervix)	179	198.82	233.2	219.9	236.0	239.5
adnexa NEC	183.9	198.82	233.3	221.8	236.3	239.5
contiguous sites	183.8	—	—	—	—	—
body	182.0	198.82	233.2	219.1	236.0	239.5
contiguous sites	182.8	—	—	—	—	—
cornu	182.0	198.82	233.2	219.1	236.0	239.5
corpus	182.0	198.82	233.2	219.1	236.0	239.5
endometrium	182.0	198.82	233.2	219.1	236.0	239.5
fundus	182.0	198.82	233.2	219.1	236.0	239.5
isthmus	182.1	198.82	233.2	219.1	236.0	239.5
ligament	183.4	198.82	—	221.0	236.3	239.5
broad	183.3	198.82	233.3	221.0	236.3	239.5
round	183.5	198.82	—	221.0	236.3	239.5
lower segment	182.1	198.82	233.2	219.1	236.0	239.5
myometrium	182.0	198.82	233.2	219.1	236.0	239.5
squamocolumnar junction	180.8	198.82	233.1	219.0	236.0	239.5
vagina, vaginal (fornix) (vault) (wall)	184.0	198.82	233.3	221.1	236.3	239.5
vaginovesical	184.9	198.82	233.39	221.9	236.3	239.5
vesicocervical tissue	184.9	198.82	233.39	221.9	236.3	239.5

(continued)

Neoplasm Table *(continued)*

| | Malignant | | | | | |
	Primary	Secondary	Ca in situ	Benign	Uncertain Behavior	Unspecified
vesicovaginal	184.9	198.82	233.39	221.9	236.3	239.5
septum	184.9	198.82	233.39	221.9	236.3	239.5
vestibular gland, greater	184.1	198.82	233.32	221.2	236.3	239.5
vulva	184.4	198.82	233.32	221.2	236.3	239.5
vulvovaginal gland	184.4	198.82	233.32	221.2	236.3	239.5
wolffian (body) (duct)	184.8	198.82	233.39	221.8	236.3	239.5

Nephritis, polycystic 753.12
Nerves or nervous (*see also* condition) 799.2
Neuritis
  arising during pregnancy 646.4
  lumbosacral 724.4
  sciatic 724.3
Neuropathy, entrapment, median nerve
      354.0
Neurosis, neurotic
  anxiety (state) 300.00
    generalized 300.02
    panic type 300.01
  bladder 306.53
  compulsive, compulsion 300.3
  depressive (reaction) (type) 300.4
  genitourinary 306.50
  menopause, unspecified type 627.2
  obsessive or obsessive-compulsive
      300.3
  posttraumatic (acute) (situational)
      308.3
  sexual 302.70
Nevus (*see also* Neoplasm, skin, benign)
  anemic, anemicus 709.09
  avasculosus 709.09
  blue, malignant—*see* Melanoma
  flammeus 757.32
  magnocellular, specified site—*see*
      Neoplasm, by site, benign
Nevus *continued*)
  malignant—*see* Melanoma
  pigmented, giant—*see* Neoplasm, skin,
      uncertain behavior
  port wine 757.32
  sanguineous 757.32
  strawberry 757.32
  vascular 757.32
Night sweats 780.8
Nisbet's chancre 099.0
Nocturnal (*see also* condition)
  dyspnea (paroxysmal) 786.09
  enuresis 788.36
  frequency (micturition) 788.43
Nodal rhythm disorder 427.89
Nodule(s), nodular
  arthritic—*see* Arthritis, nodosa
  breast 793.89
  cutaneous 782.2
  inflammatory—*see* Inflammation
  rheumatic 729.89
  skin NEC 782.2
  solitary, lung, emphysematous 492.8
  subcutaneous 782.2

Nonclosure—*see* Imperfect, closure
Noncompliance with medical treatment
      V15.81
  renal dialysis V45.12
Nonhealing wound, surgical 998.83
Nosebleed 784.7
Noxious substances transmitted through
      placenta or breast milk
  diethylstilbestrol (DES) 760.76
  suspected, affecting management of preg-
      nancy 655.5

O

Obesity (constitutional) (exogenous) (famil-
      ial) (nutritional) (simple)
      278.00
  due to hyperalimentation 278.00
  morbid 278.01
  of pregnancy 649.1
  severe 278.01
Obliteration
  appendix (lumen) 543.9
  endometrium 621.8
  fallopian tube 628.2
  lymphatic vessel, postmastectomy 457.0
  organ or site, congenital NEC—*see*
      Atresia
  placental blood vessels—*see* Placenta,
      abnormal
  urethra 599.84
  vein 459.9
Observation (for)
  criminal assault V71.6
  injuries (accidental) V71.4
  malignant neoplasm, suspected V71.1
  postpartum
    immediately after delivery V24.0
    routine follow-up V24.2
  pregnancy
    high-risk V23.9
      specified problem NEC V23.89
    normal (without complication) V22.1
      with nonobstetric complication V22.2
      first V22.0
  rape or seduction, alleged V71.5
    injury during V71.5
  suspected (undiagnosed) (unproven)
    child or wife battering victim V71.6
    condition NEC V71.89
      maternal and fetal
        amniotic cavity and membrane
            problem V89.01
        cervical shortening V89.05

Observation (for) *(continued)*
    fetal anomaly V89.03
    fetal growth problem V89.04
    oligohydramnios V89.01
    other specified problem NEC
        V89.09
    placental problem V89.02
    polyhydramnios V89.01
  hydatidiform mole V71.89
  malignant neoplasm V71.1
Obsessive, obsessive-complusive 300.3
Obstetrical trauma NEC (complicating
        delivery) 665.9
  with or following
    abortion—*see* Abortion, by type, with
        damage to pelvic organs
    following abortion 639.2
    ectopic pregnancy (*see also* categories
        633.0–633.9) 639.2
    molar pregnancy (*see also* categories
        630–632) 639.2
Obstruction, obstructed, obstructive
  airway
    with
      asthma NEC (*see also* Asthma) 493.9
      bronchiectasis 494.0
      bronchitis (*see also* Bronchitis, with
        obstruction) 491.20
      emphysema NEC 492.8
      chronic (with) 496
      asthma NEC (*see also* Asthma) 493.2
      bronchiectasis 494.0
      bronchitis (*see also* Bronchitis,
        chronic obstructive) 491.20
      emphysema NEC 492.8
    asthma (chronic) (with obstructive pul-
        monary disease) 493.2
  circulatory 459.9
  device, implant, or graft—*see*
      Complications
  due to foreign body accidentally left in
      operation wound 998.4
  fallopian tube (bilateral) 628.2
  foreign body—*see* Foreign body
  labor (by)—*see* Delivery, complicated by
  rectum 569.49
  respiratory, chronic 496
  thrombotic—*see* Thrombosis
  ureter, due to calculus 592.1
  ureteropelvic junction, congenital 753.21
  ureterovesical junction, congenital 753.22
  urethra 599.6
    congenital 753.6

Obstruction, obstructed, obstructive
    (continued)
  urinary (moderate) 599.6
    organ or tract (lower) 599.6
  uterus 621.8
  vagina 623.2
  vein, venous 459.2
    caval (inferior) (superior) 459.2
    thrombotic—*see* Thrombosis
    vessel NEC 459.9
Occlusion (*see also* Closure)
  anus 569.49
  breast (duct) 611.89
  cervical canal, cervix (uteri) (*see also*
      Stricture, cervix) 622.4
  fallopian tube 628.2
    congenital 752.19
  hymen 623.3
    congenital 752.42
  organ or site, congenital NEC—*see* Atresia
  urethra (*see also* Stricture, urethra) 598.9
    congenital 753.6
  uterus 621.8
Oligohydramnios 658.0
  due to premature rupture of membranes
      658.1
Oligospermia 606.1
Oliguria 788.5
  with or complicating
    abortion—*see* Abortion, by type, with
      renal failure
    following abortion 639.3
    ectopic pregnancy (*see also* categories
      633.0–633.9) 639.3
    molar pregnancy (*see also* categories
      630–632) 639.3
    pregnancy 646.2
      with hypertension—*see* Toxemia, of
        pregnancy
  due to a procedure 997.5
  following labor and delivery 669.3
  specified due to a procedure 997.5
Omentum (*see also* Peritonitis) 567.9
Oophoritis—*see* Salpingo-oophoritis
Open, opening—*see* Imperfect, closure
Orthopnea 786.02
Osteoarthritis or osteoarthropathy—*see*
      Osteoarthrosis
Osteoarthrosis (degenerative) (hyper-
      trophic) (rheumatoid) 715.9
  generalized 715.09
  primary or idiopathic 715.1
  polyarticular 715.09
Osteopenia 733.90

Osteoporosis (generalized) 733.00
  disuse 733.03
  drug-induced 733.09
  idiopathic 733.02
  postmenopausal 733.01
  screening V82.81
  senile 733.01
  specified type NEC 733.09
Osteosis cutis 709.3
Outcome of delivery
  multiple birth (more than two) V27.9
    all liveborn V27.5
    all stillborn V27.7
    some liveborn V27.6
    unspecified V27.9
  single V27.9
    liveborn V27.0
    stillborn V27.1
  twins V27.9
    both liveborn V27.2
    both stillborn V27.4
    one liveborn, one stillborn V27.3
Ovaritis (cystic) (*see also* Salpingo-oophoritis)
    614.2
Overdevelopment (*see also* Hypertrophy)
  breast 611.1
Overeating 783.6
  nonorganic origin 307.51
Overload
  fluid 276.6
  potassium (K) 276.7
  sodium (Na) 276.0
Ovulation (cycle)
  failure or lack of 628.0
  pain 625.2
Ovum, blighted, dropsical or pathologic
    631
OX syndrome 758.6

P
Pachyderma, pachydermia, pachyder-
    matitis 701.8
Paget's disease (osteitis deformans)
  with infiltrating duct carcinoma of the
    breast—*see* Neoplasm, breast,
    malignant
  extramammary (*see also* Neoplasm, skin,
    malignant)
    anus, skin 173.5
  malignant
    breast (mammary) (nipple) 174.0
    specified site NEC—*see* Neoplasm,
      skin, malignant
    unspecified site 174.0
Paget-Schroetter syndrome (intermittent
    venous claudication) 453.8

Pain(s)
  abdominal 789.0
  acute 338.1
    due to
      postoperative 338.18
      trauma 338.11
  adnexa (uteri) 625.9
  anginoid (*see also* Pain, precordial) 786.51
  anus 569.42
  arm 729.5
  axillary 729.5
  back (postural) 724.5
    low 724.2
  breast 611.71
  broad ligament 625.9
  cecum, colon 789.0
  chest (centra) 786.50
    midsternal or substernal 786.51
    wall 786.52
  chronic 338.2
    due to
      pain syndrome 338.4
      postoperative 338.28
      trauma 338.21
  coronary—*see* Angina
  costochondral 786.52
  diaphragm 786.52
  due to (presence of) any device, implant,
    or graft classifiable to 996.3–
    996.5—*see* Complications
  extremity (lower) (upper) 729.5
  flank 789.0
  gas (intestinal) 787.3
  head (*see also* Headache) 784.0
  intermenstrual 625.2
  kidney 788.0
  labor, false or spurious 644.1
  lumbar region 724.2
  menstrual 625.3
  neoplasm related (acute) (chronic) 338.3
  ovary 625.9
  ovulation 625.2
  pelvic 625.9
  perineum 625.9
  postoperative—*see* Pain, by site
  premenstrual 625.4
  rectum 569.42
  respiration 786.52
  rheumatic NEC 729.0
    muscular 729.1
  round ligament (stretch) 625.9
  sciatic 724.3
  skin 782.0
  umbilicus 789.05
  urinary (organ) (system) 788.0

Pain(s) *(continued)*
  uterus 625.9
  vagina 625.9
  vulva 625.9
Painful *(see also* Pain)
  coitus 625.0
    psychogenic 302.76
  menstruation 625.3
    psychogenic 306.52
  scar NEC 709.2
  urination 788.1
  wire sutures 998.89
Palliative care V66.7
Pallor 782.61
Palpable
  lymph nodes 785.6
  ovary 620.8
  uterus 625.8
Palpitation (heart) 785.1
Panarteritis 446.0
Pancytopenia (acquired)
  with malformations 284.09
  congenital 284.09
Panic (attack) (state) 300.01
  reaction to exceptional stress (transient)
    308.0
Papanicolaou smear
  anus 796.70
    with
      atypical squamous cells
        cannot exclude high grade squa-
          mous intraepithelial lesion
          (ASC-H) 796.72
        of undetermined significance
          (ASC-US) 796.71
      cytologic evidence of malignancy
        796.76
      high grade squamous intraepithelial
        lesion (HGSIL) 796.74
      low grade squamous intraepithelial
        lesion (LGSIL) 796.73
    glandular 796.70
    satisfactory but lacking transformation
      zone 796.77
    specified finding NEC 796.79
    unsatisfactory cytology 796.78
  cervix (screening test) V76.2
    with
      atypical squamous cells
        cannot exclude high grade squa-
          mous intraepithelial lesion
          (ASC-H) 795.02
        of undetermined significance

Papanicolaou smear *(continued)*
      (ASC-US) 795.01
    cytologic evidence of malignancy 795.06
      high grade squamous intraepithelial
        lesion (HGSIL) 795.04
      low grade squamous intraepithelial
        lesion (LGSIL) 795.03
    as part of gynecological examination
      V72.31
    for Medicare patient
      high risk V15.89
      not high risk V76.2, V72.31
    for suspected malignant neoplasm
      V76.2
    glandular 795.00
    high risk human papillomavirus (HPV)
      DNA test positive 795.05
    inadequate cytology sample 795.08
    low risk human papillomavirus (HPV)
      DNA test positive 795.09
  cervix *(continued)*
    with *(continued)*
      no disease found V71.1
      nonspecific abnormal finding795.00
      nonspecific finding NEC 795.09
      satisfactory but lacking transformation
        zone 795.07
    screening V76.2
      following hysterectomy for malig-
        nant condition V67.01
    specified finding NEC 795.19
    to confirm findings of recent normal
      smear following initial abnormal
      smear V72.32
    unsatisfactory cervical cytology
      795.08
    other specified site *(see also* Screening,
      malignant neoplasm)
    for Medicare patient
      high risk V15.89
      not high risk V76.49, V72.31
    nonspecific abnormal finding 796.9
  vagina V76.47
    with
      atypical squamous cells
        cannot exclude high grade squa-
          mous intraepithelial lesion
          (ASC-H) 795.12
        of undetermined significance
          (ASC-US) 795.11
      cytologic evidence of malignancy
        795.16
      high grade squamous intraepithelial

Papanicolaou smear *(continued)*|
　　lesion (HGSIL) 795.14
　　low grade squamous intraepithelial
　　　lesion (LGSIL) 795.13
　　abnormal NEC 795.19
　　for Medicare patient
　　　high risk V15.89
　　　not high risk V76.47, V72.31
　　glandular 795.10
　　high risk human papillomavirus (HPV)
　　　DNA test positive 795.15
　　inadequate cytology sample 795.18
　　low risk human papillomavirus (HPV)
　　　DNA test positive 795.19
　　screening V76.47
　　　following hysterectomy for malig-
　　　　nant condition V67.01
　　unsatisfactory cytology 795.18
Papillitis, anus or rectum 569.49
Papilloma (serous surface) (*see also*
　　　　Neoplasm, by site, benign)
　　borderline malignancy
　　specified site—*see* Neoplasm, by site,
　　　　uncertain behavior
　　unspecified site 236.2
　　specified site—*see* Neoplasm, by site,
　　　　benign
　　unspecified site 220
Papule 709.8
Paralysis, paralytic (complete) (incomplete)
　　anus (sphincter) 569.49
　　bladder (sphincter) 596.53
　　　neurogenic 596.54
　　　puerperal, postpartum, childbirth
　　　　665.5
　　Hyrtl's sphincter (rectum) 569.49
　　rectum (sphincter) 569.49
　　respiratory (muscle) (system) (tract)
　　　　786.09
　　uremic—*see* Uremia
Paramenia 626.9
Parametritis (chronic) (*see also* Disease,
　　　　pelvis, inflammatory) 614.4
　　acute 614.3
　　puerperal, postpartum, childbirth 670
Paraphrenia (climacteric) (menopausal)
　　　　297.2
Parorexia NEC 307.52
Parvovirus 079.83
Patent (*see also* Imperfect closure)
　　canal of Nuck 752.41
　　cervix (os) 622.5
　　　complicating pregnancy 654.5

Paternity testing V70.4
Pause, sinoatrial 427.81
Pectenitis, pectenosis 569.49
Pendulous
　　abdomen 701.9
　　　in pregnancy or childbirth 654.4
　　breast 611.8
Penetration, pregnant uterus by
　　　　instrument
　　with or following
　　　abortion—*see* Abortion, by type, with
　　　　damage to pelvic organs
　　　following abortion 639.2
　　　ectopic or molar pregnancy (*see also*
　　　　categories 630–633.9) 639.2
　　complication of delivery 665.1
Penta X syndrome 758.81
Perforation, perforative, perforated (non-
　　　　traumatic)
　　with or following
　　　abortion—*see* Abortion, by type, with
　　　　damage to pelvic organs
　　　following abortion 639.2
　　　ectopic or molar pregnancy (*see also*
　　　　categories 630–633.9) 639.2
　　appendix 540.0
　　　with peritoneal abscess 540.1
　　bladder (urinary)
　　　obstetrical trauma 665.5
　　bowel
　　　obstetrical trauma 665.5
　　broad ligament
　　　obstetrical trauma 665.6
　　by
　　　device, implant, or graft—*see*
　　　　Complications
　　　foreign body left accidentally in opera-
　　　　tion wound 998.4
　　　instrument (any) during a procedure,
　　　　accidental 998.2
　　cecum 540.0
　　　with peritoneal abscess 540.1
　　cervix (uteri) (*see also* Injury, internal,
　　　　cervix)
　　　obstetrical trauma 665.3
　　foreign body (external site)—*see* Wound,
　　　　open, by site, complicated
　　gastric (ulcer)—*see* Ulcer, stomach, with
　　　　perforation
　　intestine (with)
　　　obstetrical trauma 665.5
　　pelvic
　　　floor (with)

Perforation, perforative, perforated
(continued)
obstetrical trauma 664.1
organ (with)
obstetrical trauma 665.5
perineum—*see* Laceration, perineum
ectopic pregnancy (*see also* categories
630–632) 639.2
molar pregnancy (*see also* categories
630–632) 639.2
rectum 569.49
surgical (accidental) (by instrument)
(blood vessel) (nerve)
(organ) 998.2
traumatic
external—*see* Wound, open, by site
internal organ—*see* Injury, internal, by
site
urethra (with or following)
obstetrical trauma 665.5
uterus (*see also* Injury, internal, uterus
by intrauterine contraceptive device)
996.32
obstetrical trauma—*see* Injury, internal,
uterus, obstetrical trauma
vagina—*see* Laceration, vagina
viscus NEC 799.89
Periangiitis 446.0
Pericarditis (acute)
due to disease classified elsewhere
420.0
idiopathic 420.91
other specified 420.99
unspecified 420.90
Peripartum cardiomyopathy 674.5
Peritonitis (acute) (fibrinous) (localized)
(with adhesions) (with effu-
sion) 567.9
with or following
abortion—*see* Abortion, by type, with
sepsis
following abortion 639.0
abscess 567.2
appendicitis 540.0
with peritoneal abscess 540.1
ectopic pregnancy (*see also* categories
630–633.9) 639.0
molar pregnancy (*see also* categories
630–632) 639.0
aseptic 998.7
bacterial 567.2
chlamydial 099.56
chronic proliferative 567.8

Peritonitis *(continued)*
diffuse, disseminated NEC, generalized
(acute) 567.2
fibrinopurulent, fibrinous or fibropuru-
lent 567.2
gonococcal 098.86
pelvic (acute) 614.5
chronic NEC 614.7
with adhesions 614.6
pneumococcal 567.1
proliferative, chronic 567.8
puerperal, postpartum, childbirth 670
purulent or septic 567.2
staphylococcal or streptococcal 567.2
subdiaphragmatic 567.2
subphrenic 567.2
suppurative 567.2
talc 998.7
urine 567.8
Persistence, persistent (congenital)
communication—*see* Fistula, congenital
convolutions, fallopian tube 752.19
Gartner's duct 752.11
hymen (tag) in pregnancy or childbirth
654.8
causing obstructed labor 660.2
mesonephric duct, fallopian tube 752.11
organ or site NEC—*see* Anomaly, specified type NEC
ovarian rests in fallopian tube 752.19
pupillary membrane Rhesus (Rh) titer
999.7
Person (with)
affected by
family member
currently on deployment (military)
V61.01
returned from deployment (military)
(current or past conflict)
V61.02
currently deployed in theater or in support of military war, peacekeeping and humanitarian
operations V62.21
history of military war, peacekeeping and
humanitarian deployment
(current or past conflict)
V62.22
concern (normal) about sick person in
family V61.49
consulting on behalf of another V65.19
feared
complaint in whom no diagnosis was

Person (with) *(continued)*
   made V65.5
  condition not demonstrated V65.5
 feigning illness V65.2
 healthy, accompanying sick person V65.0
 "worried well" V65.5
Petechia, petechiae 782.7
Pheochromoblastoma, specified site—*see*
   Neoplasm, by site, malignant
Phlebitis (pyemic) (septic) (suppurative)
 complicating pregnancy or puerperium
   671.2
 deep (vessels) NEC 451.19
  femoral vein 451.11
 due to implanted device—*see*
   Complications
 during or resulting from a procedure 997.2
 following infusion, perfusion, or transfusion 999.2
 intracranial sinus (any) (venous)
  nonpyogenic in pregnancy or puerperium 671.5
 lower extremity 451.2
  deep (vessels) 451.19
   specified vessel NEC 451.19
  superficial (vessels) 451.0
   femoral vein 451.11
 pelvic
  with or following
   abortion—*see* Abortion, by type,
    with sepsis
    following abortion 639.0
    ectopic pregnancy (*see also* categories
     630–633.9) 639.0
    molar pregnancy (*see also* categories
     630–632) 639.0
  puerperal, postpartum 671.4
 postoperative 997.2
 pregnancy 671.9
  deep 671.3
  specified type NEC 671.5
  superficial 671.2
 puerperal, postpartum, childbirth 671.9
  deep 671.4
  lower extremities 671.2
  pelvis 671.4
  specified site NEC 671.5
  superficial 671.2
 ulcer, ulcerative
  lower extremity 451.2
   deep (vessels) 451.19
    femoral vein 451.11
   specified vessel NEC 451.19

Phlebitis, (continued)
 superficial (vessels) 451.0
 uterus (septic) (*see also* Endometritis)
  615.9
 varicose (leg) (lower extremity) (*see also*
  Varicose, vein) 454.1
Phlegmasia
 alba dolens (deep vessels) 451.19
  complicating pregnancy 671.3
  nonpuerperal 451.19
  postpartum, childbirth 671.4
 cerulea dolens 451.19
Phthiriasis (pubis) (any site) 132.2
Pica 307.52
Pick's tubular adenoma 220
Pigmentation (abnormal) 709.00
 anomalies NEC 709.00
  specified NEC 709.09
 metals 709.00
Placenta, placental
 ablatio, abruptio 641.2
 abnormal, abnormality 656.7
  with hemorrhage 641.8
 accessory lobe—*see* Placenta, abnormal
 accreta (without hemorrhage) 667.0
  with hemorrhage 666.0
 adherent (without hemorrhage) 667.0
  with hemorrhage 666.0
 apoplexy—*see* Placenta, separation
 battledore, bilobate or bipartita—*see*
  Placenta, abnormal
 carneous mole 631
 centralis—*see* Placenta, previa
 circumvallata—*see* Placenta, abnormal
 cyst (amniotic)—*see* Placenta, abnormal
 deficiency—*see* Placenta, insufficiency
 degeneration—*see* Placenta, insufficiency
 detachment (partial) (premature) (with
  hemorrhage) 641.2
 disease 656.7
 duplex—*see* Placenta, abnormal
 dysfunction—*see* Placenta, insufficiency
 fenestrata—*see* Placenta, abnormal
 fibrosis—*see* Placenta, abnormal
 fleshy mole 631
 hematoma—*see* Placenta, abnormal
 hemorrhage NEC—*see* Placenta, separation
 hormone disturbance or malfunction—*see*
  Placenta, abnormal
 hyperplasia—*see* Placenta, abnormal
 increta (without hemorrhage) 667.0
  with hemorrhage 666.0
 infarction 656.7

Placenta, placental *(continued)*
  insertion, vicious—*see* Placenta, previa
  insufficiency, affecting management of
      pregnancy 656.5
  lateral—*see* Placenta, previa
  low implantation or insertion—*see*
      Placenta, previa
  low-lying—*see* Placenta, previa
  malformation—*see* Placenta, abnormal
  malposition—*see* Placenta, previa
  marginalis, marginata—*see* Placenta, previa
  marginal sinus (hemorrhage) (rupture)
      641.2
  multilobed—*see* Placenta, abnormal
  multipartita—*see* Placenta, abnormal
  necrosis—*see* Placenta, abnormal
  percreta (without hemorrhage) 667.0
    with hemorrhage 666.0
  polyp 674.4
  previa (complete) (partial) (with hemor-
      rhage) 641.1
    before labor, without hemorrhage
      (with cesarean delivery)
      641.0
    during pregnancy (with or without
      hemorrhage) 641.0
  retention (with hemorrhage) 666.0
    fragments, complicating puerperium
      (delayed hemorrhage) 666.2
      without hemorrhage 667.1
    postpartum, puerperal 666.2
      without hemorrhage 667.0
  separation (normally implanted) (partial)
      (premature) (with hemor-
      rhage) 641.2
  septuplex—*see* Placenta, abnormal
  small—*see* Placenta, insufficiency
  softening (premature)—*see* Placenta,
      abnormal
  spuria—*see* Placenta, abnormal
  succenturiata—*see* Placenta, abnormal
  trapped (with hemorrhage) 666.0
    without hemorrhage 667.0
  trilobate—*see* Placenta, abnormal
  tripartita—*see* Placenta, abnormal
  triplex—*see* Placenta, abnormal
  varicose vessel—*see* Placenta, abnormal
  vicious insertion—*see* Placenta, previa
Placentitis complicating pregnancy 658.4
Platypelloid pelvis 738.6
  with disproportion (fetopelvic) 653.2
    causing obstructed labor 660.1
Pleuralgia 786.52

Pleurodynia 786.52
PMDD (premenstrual dysphoric disorder)
    625.4
PMS 625.4
Pneumatosis
  peritonei 568.89
  pulmonum 492.8
Pneumococcemia 038.2
Pneumococcus, pneumococcal—*see*
    condition
Pneumonia (acute) (primary) (purulent)
    486
  with influenza, flu, or grippe 487.0
  adenoviral 480.0
  anaerobes 482.81
  apex, apical—*see* Pneumonia, lobar
  aspiration, due to aspiration of micro-
      organisms
    bacterial 482.9
      specified type NEC 482.89
    specified organism NEC 483.8
      bacterial NEC 482.89
    viral 480.9
      specified type NEC 480.8
  atypical (disseminated) (focal) (primary)
      486
    with influenza 487.0
  bacterial 482.9
    specified type NEC 482.89
  Bacteroides (fragilis) (oralis) (melanino-
      genicus) 482.81
  basal, basic, basilar—*see* Pneumonia, lobar
  broncho-, bronchial (diffuse) (hemor-
      rhagic) (involving lobes)
      (lobar) (*see also* Pneumonia,
      due to) 485
    with influenza 487.0
    bacterial 482.9
      specified type NEC 482.89
  capillary 466.19
    with bronchospasm or obstruction
      466.19
  catarrhal—*see* Pneumonia, broncho-
  central—*see* Pneumonia, lobar
  Clostridium (haemolyticum) (novyi)
      NEC 482.81
  disseminated (focal)—*see* Pneumonia,
      broncho-
  due to
    Bacterium anitratum 482.83
    Chlamydia, chlamydial 483.1
    Diplococcus (pneumoniae) 481
    Eaton's agent 483.0

Pneumonia *(continued)*
   Escherichia coli (E. coli) 482.82
   Friedländer's bacillus 482.0
   Hemophilus influenzae (H. influenzae) 482.2
   Herellea 482.83
   Klebsiella pneumoniae 482.0
   Mycoplasma (pneumoniae) 483.0
   pleuropneumonia-like organism (PPLO) 483.0
   Pneumococcus 481
   Proteus 482.83
   pseudomonas 482.1
   embolic, embolism (*see* Embolism, pulmonary)
  Eubacterium 482.81
  fibrinous—*see* Pneumonia, lobar
  Fusobacterium (nucleatum) 482.81
  giant cell (*see also* Pneumonia, viral) 480.9
  gram-negative bacteria NEC 482.83
   anaerobic 482.81
  hypostatic (broncho-) (lobar) in varicella 052.1
  influenzal (broncho-) (lobar) (virus) 487.0
  interstitial
   with influenzal 487.0
   pseudomonas 482.1
  lobar (pneumococcal, any type) (*see also* Pneumonia, due to) 481
   with influenza 487.0
   bacterial 482.9
    specified type NEC 482.89
   specified organism NEC 483.8
    bacterial NEC 482.89
  metastatic NEC 038.8 (484.8)
  patchy—*see* Pneumonia, broncho
  Peptococcus 482.81
  Peptostreptococcus 482.81
  pneumococcal (broncho-) (lobar) 481
  postoperative 997.39
  primary atypical 486
  Proprionibacterium 482.81
  respiratory syncytial virus 480.1
  resulting from a procedure 997.3
  SARS-associated coronavirus 480.3
  Serratia (marcascens) 482.83
  Staphylococcal (bronch) (lobar) 482.40
   aureus 482.41
    methicillin
     resistant 482.42
     susceptible (MSSA) 482.41
  Streptococcus pneumoniae 481

Pneumonia *(continued)*
  traumatic (complication) (early) (secondary) 958.8
  TWAR agent 483.1
  varicella 052.1
  Veillonella 482.81
  viral, virus (broncho-) (interstitial) (lobar) 480.9
   with influenza, flu, or grippe 487.0
   adenoviral 480.0
   parainfluenza 480.2
   respiratory syncytial 480.1
   SARS-associated coronavirus 480.3
   specified type NEC 480.8
Pneumonitis (acute) (primary) (*see also* Pneumonia) 486
  postanesthetic
   obstetric 668.0
   overdose or wrong substance given 968.4
  postoperative 997.3
   obstetric 668.0
Poisoning
  contraceptives, oral 962.2
  gonadotropins 962.4
  ovarian hormones 962.2
  pituitary hormones 962.4
Pollakiuria 788.41
  psychogenic 306.53
Polyalgia 729.90
Polycystic (congenital) (disease)
  kidney 753.12
  ovary, ovaries 256.4
Polydipsia 783.5
Polyembryoma—*see* Neoplasm, by site, malignant
Polygalactia 676.6
Polyhydramnios (*see also* Hydramnios) 657
Polyp, polypus
  adenomatous—*see* Neoplasm, by site, benign
  anus, anal (canal) (nonadenomatous) 569.0
   adenomatous 211.4
  Bartholin's gland 624.6
  bladder 236.7
  broad ligament 620.8
  cervix (uteri) 622.7
   adenomatous 219.0
   in pregnancy or childbirth 654.6
    causing obstructed labor 660.2
   mucous 622.7
   nonneoplastic 622.7

Polyp, polypus *(continued)*
clitoris 624.6
colon *(see also* Polyp, adenomatous)
211.3
corpus uteri 621.0
endometrium 621.0
fallopian tube 620.8
labia 624.6
malignant—*see* Neoplasm, by site,
malignant
myometrium 621.0
neoplastic—*see* Neoplasm, by site, benign
paratubal 620.8
placenta, placental 674.4
rectosigmoid 211.4
rectum (nonadenomatous) 569.0
adenomatous 211.4
urethra 599.3
uterine ligament 620.8
uterus (body) (corpus) (mucous) 621.0
in pregnancy or childbirth 654.1
causing obstructed labor 660.2
vagina 623.7
vulva 624.6
Polyphagia 783.6
Polyserositis (peritoneal) 568.82
Polythelia 757.6
Polyuria 788.42
Positive
culture (nonspecific) 795.39
AIDS virus (HIV) V08
blood 790.7
stool 792.1
urine 791.9
serology
AIDS virus (HIV) V08
inconclusive 795.71
syphilis with signs or symptoms—*see*
Syphilis, by site and stage
false 795.6
skin test 795.7
tuberculin (without active tuberculosis)
795.5
Wassermann reaction, false 795.6
Postcaval ureter 753.4
Postmastectomy lymphedema (syndrome)
457.0
Postmenopausal
endometrium (atrophic) 627.8
suppurative *(see also* Endometritis) 615.9
hormone replacement therapy V07.4
status (age related) (natural) V49.81
Postpartum *(see also* Puerperal)

observation
immediately after delivery V24.0
routine follow-up V24.2
Postperfusion syndrome NEC 999.8
Post-term (pregnancy) 645.1
Postvasectomy sperm count V25.8
Precipitate labor 661.3
Preclimacteric bleeding (menorrhagia) 627.0
Precocious
adrenarche 259.1
menarche 259.1
menstruation 626.8
puberty NEC 259.1
sexual development NEC 259.1
Prediabetes, prediabetic 790.29
complicating pregnancy, childbirth, or
puerperium 648.8
Pre-eclampsia (mild) 642.4
with pre-existing hypertension 642.7
severe 642.5
**Pregnancy (complicated by) (management
affected by) NEC** 669.9
abnormal, abnormality of pelvic organs
or tissues *(see also* Pregnancy,
maternal conditions)
cervix 654.6
dysplasia 654.6
incompetent 654.5
malposition 654.4
tumor 654.6
cord (umbilical) 663.9
cystocele 654.4
ovary, tumor 654.4
pelvic organs or tissues NEC 654.9
adhesions, pelvic peritoneal 648.9
bony pelvis 653.0
contraction (general) 653.1
inlet 653.2
outlet 653.3
perineum 654.8
uterus 654.4
bicornis or bicornuate 654.0
congenital malformation 654.0
displacement NEC 654.4
double 654.0
herniation 654.4
incarceration 654.3
malposition 654.4
prolapse 654.4
retroversion 654.3
size (congenital) 654.0
spasms (abnormal) 646.8
torsion 654.4

Pregnancy *(continued)*
 tumor (body) (fibroid) 654.1
 urinary system, tumor 646.6
 vagina, tumor 654.7
 vulva (tumor) 654.8
 amnion, amniotic fluid
 amnionitis 658.4
 effusion 658.1
 delayed delivery following 658.2
 fluid embolism 673.1
 hydramnios 657.0
 hydrops amnii 657.0
 hydrorrhea 658.1
 nodosum 658.8
 oligohydramnios NEC 658.0
 polyhydramnios 657.0
 rupture of membranes—*see* Pregnancy,
 rupture
 bleeding (*see also* Pregnancy, hemorrhage)
 spotting 649.5
 dead ovum, retained 631
 delivery (*see also* Delivery)
 early onset (spontaneous) 644.2
 ectopic (ruptured) NEC 633.90
 with intrauterine pregnancy 633.91
 abdominal 633.00
 with intrauterine pregnancy 633.01
 broad ligament—*see* Pregnancy,
 ectopic, cornual
 cornual 633.80
 with intrauterine pregnancy 633.81
 ovarian 633.20
 with intrauterine pregnancy 633.21
 specified type NEC 633.80
 with intrauterine pregnancy 633.81
 tubal (with rupture) 633.10
 with intrauterine pregnancy
 633.11
 embolism (pulmonary)
 air 673.0
 amniotic fluid 673.1
 blood-clot 673.2
 cerebral 674.0
 pulmonary NEC 673.2
 pyemic 673.3
 septic 673.3
 examination, pregnancy (test)
 incidental finding V22.2
 negative result V72.41
 not confirmed V72.40
 positive result V72.42
 prenatal care only V22.1
 first pregnancy V22.0
 false 300.11

Pregnancy *(continued)*
 fetal conditions (suspected) 656.8 (*see
 also* Pregnancy, presentation)
 size and growth
 excessive growth 656.6
 growth retardation 656.5
 unusually large fetus 653.5
 uterine size-date discrepancy 649.6
 abnormality 655.9
 abdominal 655.8
 acid–base balance 656.8
 cardiovascular 655.8
 central nervous system 655.0
 chromosomal 655.1
 facial 655.8
 gastrointestinal 655.8
 genitourinary 655.8
 heart rate or rhythm 659.7
 limb 655.8
 specified NEC 655.8
 acidemia 656.3
 anencephaly 655.0
 aneuploidy 655.1
 conjoined twins 678.1
 damage (suspected) from
 drugs (obstetric, anesthesia or sedative) 655.5
 environmental toxins 655.8
 hereditary disease in family 655.2
 intrauterine contraceptive device 655.8
 maternal
 alcohol addiction 655.4
 disease NEC 655.4
 drug use 655.5
 listeriosis 655.4
 rubella 655.3
 toxoplasmosis 655.4
 viral infection 655.3
 radiation 655.6
 death (near term) 656.4
 early (before 22 completed weeks
 gestation) 632
 decreased fetal movements 655.7
 distress 656.8
 high risk conditions V23.9
 insufficient prenatal care V23.7
 specific problem NEC V23.89
 hydrocephalus 655.0
 meconium in liquor 656.8
 papyraceous 646.0
 postmaturity
 post-term 645.1
 prolonged 645.2
 spina bifida (with myelomeningocele)
 655.0

Pregnancy *(continued)*
fetal conditions (suspected) *(continued)*
hemorrhage 641.9
accidental 641.2
cerebrovascular 674.0
due to
afibrinogenemia or other coagulation defect 641.3
leiomyoma, uterine 641.8
placenta—*see* Pregnancy, placenta
early (before 22 completed weeks gestation) NEC 640.9
threatened abortion 640.0
unavoidable 641.1
fetal–maternal hemorrhage 656.0
hydatidiform mole (delivered) (undelivered) 630
hyperemesis—*see* Pregnancy, maternal conditions, vomiting
labor (*see also* Delivery)
false (pains) 644.1
onset of contractions before 37 weeks 644.0
maternal conditions (*see also* Pregnancy, fetal conditions, damage and Pregnancy, previous)
albuminuria 646.2
with
hypertension—*see* Hypertension, complicating pregnancy
amniotic fluid 658.4
chloasma (gravidarum) 646.8
convulsions (eclamptic) (uremic) 642.6
with pre-existing hypertension 642.7
current disease or condition (nonobstetric)
abnormal glucose tolerance 648.8
abscess or cellulitis, genitourinary tract 646.6
anemia 648.2
appendicitis 648.9
bacilluria or bacteriuria, asymptomatic 646.5
biliary problems 646.8
bone and joint disorders 648.7
cardiovascular disease 648.6
congenital 648.5
cerebrovascular disorder 674.0
coagulation defects 649.3
drug dependence 648.3
endometritis 670
gallbladder disease 646.8

Pregnancy *(continued)*
maternal conditions *(continued)*
current disease or condition *(continued)*
genital organ or tract 646.6
goiter 648.1
gonorrhea 647.1
hepatitis (acute) (malignant) (subacute) 646.7
viral 647.6
icterus gravis 646.7
infection 647.9
infective and parasitic diseases NEC 647.8
inflammation
genital organs 646.6
liver 646.7
nerves (peripheral) 646.4
urinary organs 646.6
injury NEC 648.9
malaria 647.4
mental disorders 648.4
nutritional deficiency 648.9
renal disease or failure NEC 646.2
with secondary hypertension 642.1
rubella 647.5
periodontal disease 648.9
prediabetes 648.8
pruritus (neurogenic) 646.8
smoking (cigarettes) 649.0
syphilis 647.0
thyroid dysfunction 648.1
tuberculosis 647.3
urinary organs (tract) infection 646.6
asymptomatic 646.5
venereal disease 647.2
death, maternal NEC 646.9
deciduitis 646.6
diabetes 648.0
gestational 648.8
pre-diabetes 648.8
drug abuse 648.4
eclampsia, eclamptic (coma) (convulsions) (delirium) (nephritis) (uremia) 642.6
with pre-existing hypertension 642.7
excessive weight gain NEC 646.1
fatigue 646.8
hypertension—*see* Hypertension, complicating pregnancy
hysteralgia 646.8
insufficient prenatal care V23.7

Pregnancy *(continued)*
  maternal conditions *(continued)*
    maternal age
      elderly
        multigravida V23.82
          complicating pregnancy 659.6
        primigravida V23.81
          complicating pregnancy 659.5
      young
        multigravida V23.84
          complicating pregnancy 659.8
        primigravida V23.83
          complicating pregnancy 659.8
    maternal weight
      insufficient weight gain 646.8
      maternal obesity syndrome 646.1
      obesity 649.1
    menstruation 640.8
    multiparity (grand) 659.4
    preclampsia (mild) 642.4
      severe 642.5
      superimposed on pre-existing hyper-
        tensive disease 642.7
    proteinuria (gestational) 646.2
      with hypertension—*see* Toxemia, of
        pregnancy
    septicemia 647.8
      postpartum 670.2
    thrombophlebitis or thrombosis
        (superficial) 671.2
      deep 671.3
      septic 670.3
    varicose, varicosity
      labia, perineum or vulva 671.1
      veins (legs) 671.0
    vomiting 643.9
      due to organic disease or other cause
        643.8
      early 643.0
        with metabolic disturbance 643.1
      late (after 22 completed weeks ges-
        tation) 643.2
  missed
    abortion 632
    delivery or labor (at or near term) 656.4
  molar—*see* Pregnancy, hydatidiform
  multiple gestation NEC 651.9
    five or more fetus(es) NEC 651.8
      fetal loss and retention of one or
        more fetus(es) 651.6
    following (elective) fetal reduction
      651.7
    malpresentation in 652.6

Pregnancy *(continued)*
  multiple gestation *(continued)*
    multiparity V23.3
      specified type NEC 651.8
        with fetal loss and retention of
          one or more fetus(es) 651.6
      quadruplet NEC 651.2
        with fetal loss and retention of
          one or more fetus(es) 651.5
      superfecundation or superfetation
        NEC 651.9
      triplet pregnancy 651.1
        with fetal loss and retention of
          one or more fetus(es)
          651.4
      twin pregnancy 651.0
        vanishing twin 651.33
        with fetal loss and retention of
          one fetus 651.3
  placenta, placental
    abnormality 656.7
    abruptio or ablatio 641.2
    disease 656.7
    infarct 656.7
    low implantation 641.1
      without hemorrhage 641.0
    marginal sinus (rupture) (hemorrhage)
      641.2
    placentitis 658.4
    premature separation 641.2
    previa 641.1
      without hemorrhage 641.0
    trauma 641.8
    varicose vessels 656.7
  presentation or position of fetus
    abnormal position causing obstructed
      labor 660.0
    acromion 652.8
    brow 652.4
    chin 652.4
    compound 652.8
    crossbirth 652.3
    face 652.4
    in multiple gestation 652.6
    mal lie 652.9
    mentum 652.4
    oblique 652.3
    prolapse (fetal)
      arm or hand 652.7
      extremity 652.8
      foot or leg 652.8
      umbilical cord 663.0
    shoulder presentation 652.8

Pregnancy *(continued)*
  transverse 652.3
  unstable lie 652.0
  previous
    abortion V23.2
      habitual 646.3
    cesarean delivery 654.2
    difficult delivery V23.49
    forceps delivery V23.49
    hemorrhage, antepartum or postpartum V23.49
    hydatidiform mole V23.1
    infertility V23.0
    in utero procedure during previous pregnancy V23.86
    malignancy NEC V23.89
    neonatal death or stillbirth V23.5
    nonobstetric condition V23.89
    poor obstetrical history V23.49
    premature delivery V23.41
    preterm labor V23.41
    surgery
      any site, causing obstructed labor 660.2
      bariatric 649.2
      cervix 654.6
      gynecologic NEC 654.9
      pelvic soft tissues NEC 654.9
      perineum or vulva 654.8
      uterus NEC 654.9
        from previous cesarean delivery 654.2
      vagina 654.7
    trophoblastic disease V23.1
    vesicular mole V23.1
  resulting from
    assisted reproductive technology V23.85
    in vitro fertilization V23.85
  Rh immunization, incompatibility or sensitization 656.1
    antibodies (maternal)
      anti-c, anti-d or anti-e 656.1
      blood group (ABO) 656.2
  rupture
    premature, membranes 658.1
      with delayed delivery 658.2
    marginal sinus (hemorrhage) 641.2
    uterus (before onset of labor) 665.0
  suspected conditions not found
    amniotic cavity and membrane problem V89.01
    cervical shortening V89.05

Pregnancy *(continued)*
  fetal anomaly V89.03
  fetal growth problem V89.04
  oligohydramnios V89.01
  other specified problem NEC V89.09
  placental problem V89.02
  polyhydramnios V89.01
  threatened
    abortion 640.0
    premature delivery 644.2
    premature labor 644.0
  trauma, obstetric NEC 665.9
Premature (*see also* condition)
  menopause 256.31
  puberty 259.1
  ventricular systole 427.69
Premenstrual syndrome 625.4
Premenstrual tension 625.4
Presentation, fetal—*see* Pregnancy, presentation
Problem (with)
  alcoholism in family V61.41
  communication V40.1
  diet, inappropriate V69.1
  exercise, lack of V69.0
  family V61.9
    specified circumstance NEC V61.8
  feeding (elderly) (infant) nonorganic 307.50
  high-risk sexual behavior V69.2
  life circumstance NEC V62.89
  lifestyle V69.9
    specified NEC V69.8
  marital V61.10
    divorce V61.03
    estrangement V61.09
    sexual function V41.7
  multiparity V61.5
  none (feared complaint unfounded) V65.5
  partner V61.10
  phase of life V62.89
  psychosocial V62.9
    specified type NEC V62.89
  self-damaging behavior V69.8
  sexual function V41.7
  sleep, lack of V69.4
  substance abuse in family V61.42
Procedure (surgical) not done NEC V64.3
  because of
    contraindication V64.1
    patient's decision V64.2
      for reasons of conscience or religion V62.6

Prolapse, prolapsed
anus, anal (canal) (sphincter) 569.1
bladder (acquired) (mucosa) (sphincter)
(*see also* Cystocele) 618.01
breast implant (prosthetic) 996.54
cervix, cervical (hypertrophied)
618.1
congenital 752.49
postpartal (old) 618.1
stump 618.84
fallopian tube 620.4
funis—*see* Prolapse, umbilical cord
genital 618.9
specified NEC 618.89
organ or site, congenital NEC—*see*
Malposition, congenital
ovary 620.4
pelvic (floor) 618.89
perineum 618.89
pregnancy related—*see* Pregnancy and
Delivery
rectum (mucosa) (sphincter) 569.1
urethra (acquired) (infected) (mucosa)
599.5
congenital 753.8
uterovaginal 618.4
complete 618.3
incomplete 618.2
specified NEC 618.89
uterus (first, second or third degree)
(complete) (without vaginal
wall prolapse) 618.1
with mention of vaginal wall prolapse—*see* Prolapse,
uterovaginal
congenital 752.3
postpartal (old) 618.1
vagina (anterior) (posterior) (vault) (wall)
(without uterine prolapse)
618.00
with uterine prolapse 618.4
complete 618.3
incomplete 618.2
posthysterectomy 618.5
paravaginal 618.02
specified NEC 618.09
Prolonged, prolongation
bleeding time (*see also* Defect, coagulation) 790.92
"idiopathic" (in von Willebrand's
disease) 286.4
coagulation time (*see also* Defect, coagulation) 790.92

Prolonged, prolongation *(continued)*
prothrombin time (*see also* Defect, coagulation) 790.92
Prophylactic
administration of
agents affecting estrogen receptors
and estrogen levels NEC
V07.59
anastrozole (arimidex) V07.52
antibiotics V07.39
antitoxin, any V07.2
aromatase inhibitors V07.52
estrogen receptor downregulators
V07.59
exemestane (Aromasin) V07.52
fulvestrant (Faslodex) V07.59
gonadotropin-releasing hormone
(GnRH) agonist V07.59
goserelin acetate (Zoladex) V07.59
letrozole (Femara) V07.52
leuprolide acetate (leuprorelin)
(Lupron) V07.59
megestrol acetate (Megace) V07.59
other prophylactic chemotherapy
raloxifene (Evista) V07.51
RhoGAM V07.2
selective estrogen receptor modulators (SERMs) V07.51
tamoxifen (Nolvadex) V07.51
toremifene (Fareston) V07.51
hormone replacement (postmenopausal)
V07.4
immunotherapy V07.2
measure, specified type NEC V07.8
sterilization V25.2
Protein sickness (prophylactic) (therapeutic)
999.5
Proteinuria (*see also* Albuminuria)
791.0
gestational 646.2
with hypertension—*see* Toxemia, of
pregnancy
Prurigo 698.2
Pruritus, pruritic 698.9
ani 698.0
conditions NEC 698.9
essential 698.9
genital organ(s) 698.1
gravidarum 646.8
hiemalis 698.8
perianal 698.0
senile, senilis 698.8
Trichomonas 131.9
vulva, vulvae 698.1

Pseudoacanthosis, nigricans 701.8
Pseudoerosion cervix, congenital 752.49
Pseudohermaphroditism 752.7
  with chromosomal anomaly—*see*
          Anomaly, chromosomal
  without adrenocortical disorder 752.7
Pseudomenstruation 626.8
Pseudomucinous
  cyst (ovary) 220
  peritoneum 568.89
Pseudotabes 799.89
Psychoneurosis, psychoneurotic—*see*
      Neurosis
Psoriasis 696.1
  arthritic, arthropathic 696.0
Ptosis (adiposa), breast 611.81
Puberty
  bleeding 626.3
  delayed 259.0
  precocious (constitutional) (cryptogenic)
      (idiopathic) NEC 259.1
    due to ovarian hyperfunction
      256.1
      estrogen 256.0
  premature 259.1
Puerperal
  bleeding—*see* Puerperal, hemorrhage
  embolism (pulmonary)
    air 673.0
    amniotic fluid 673.1
    blood-clot 673.2
    cardiac 674.8
    cerebral 674.0
    fat 673.8
    intracranial sinus (venous) 671.5
    pyemic 673.3
    septic 673.3
    spinal cord 671.5
  examination, routine V24.2
    immediately after delivery V24.0
    lactating mother V24.1
  hemorrhage 666.1
    brain 674.0
    delayed (after 24 hours) (uterine)
      666.2
    metrorrhagia 666.2
  injury, secondary perineal tear 674.2
  lactation (disorders) 676.9
    failure 676.4
    glactophoritis 675.2
    glactorrhea 676.6
    lactating mother, routine visit V24.1
    specified type NEC 676.8

Puerperal *(continued)*
maternal conditions
  abscess
    breast (areola) 675.1
    cervix (uteri) 670.8
    nabothian 646.6
    suprapelvic 670.8
    tubo-ovarian 670.8
    vaginorectal 646.6
    vulvovaginal gland 646.6
  blood (conditions) (defects)
    afibrinogenemia or other coagula-
      tion defect 666.3
    anemia 648.2
    Valsuani's (progressive pernicious
      anemia) 648.2
    dyscrasia 666.3
    thrombocytopenia 666.3
  breast and nipple NEC 676.3 (*see also*
      Puerperal, lactation)
    atrophy 676.3
    caked 676.2
    cracked nipple 676.1
    engorgement 676.2
    fissure, nipple 676.1
    fistula
      breast or mammary gland 675.1
      nipple 675.0
    induration (fibrous) 676.3
    infection or inflammation, breast
      675.2
      with nipple 675.9
        specified type NEC 675.8
      areola 675.1
    inversion, nipple 676.3
    lymphangitis 675.2
    thelitis 675.0
  cardiovascular system
    cardiomyopathy 674.5
    thrombosis, phlebitis—*see* Puerperal,
      infection and inflammation
  cerebrovascular NEC 674.0
    apoplexy 674.0
    hematoma, subdural 674.0
    hemiplegia, cerebral 674.0
    ischemia, cerebral 674.0
    monoplegia, cerebral 674.0
    occlusion, precerebral artery 674.0
    paralysis, cerebral 674.0
    paralytic stroke 674.0
  convulsions (eclamptic) (uremia) 642.6
    with pre-existing hypertension
      642.7

Puerperal *(continued)*
  maternal conditions *(continued)*
    death, sudden (maternal) (cause
        unknown) 674.9
    diabetes (mellitus) 648.0
      gestational 648.8
    drug dependence 648.3
    eclampsia 642.6
      with pre-existing hypertension 642.7
    fever 670.8
      meaning sepsis 670.2
      meaning pyrexia (of unknown ori-
          gin) 672
    gangrene, gas or uterus 670.8
    gonorrhea 647.1
    hemorrhoids 671.8
    hepatorenal syndrome 674.8
    hypertension—*see* Hypertension, com-
        plicating pregnancy
    infection or inflammation
      adnexitis 670.8
      Bartholin's gland 646.6
      breast—*see* Puerperium, breast
      broad ligament 670.8
      cervix, endocervix 646.6
      deciduitis (acute) 670.8
      endometritis 670.1
      endotrachelitis 646.6
      fallopian tube 670.8
      generalized 670.0
      genital tract (major) 670.0
        minor or localized 646.6
      hematosalpinx, infectional 670.8
      kidney (bacillus coli) 646.6
        nephritis or nephrosis 646.2
          with hypertension 642.1
      lymphangitis 670.8
      pelvic (inflammatory disease) 670.8
      peritoneum 670.8
      periuterine 670.8
      phlebitis 671.9
        deep 671.4
        intracranial sinus (venous) 671.5
        pelvic 671.4
        specified site NEC 671.5
        superficial 671.2
      pyemia 670.2
      sepsis, septicemia 670.2
      tetanus 670.8
      urinary (tract) NEC 646.6
        asymptomatic 646.5
      venous complication 671.9
      vulvitis 646.6

Puerperal *(continued)*
  maternal conditions *(continued)*
    infection or inflammation *(continued)*
      vulvovaginitis 646.6
    malnutrition 648.9
    mental disorder 648.4
    necrosis
      kidney, tubular 669.3
        renal cortex 669.3
      liver (acute) (subacute) 674.8
      ovary 670.8
    nonobstetrical condition 648.9
    prediabetes 648.8
    pre-eclampsia (mild) 642.4
      with pre-existing hypertension
          642.7
      severe 642.5
    renal disease NEC 646.2
      failure, acute 669.3
    rubella 647.5
    thyroid dysfunction 648.1
    toxemia—*see* Puerperal, eclampsia and
          Puerperal, pre-eclampsia
    tuberculosis 647.3
    tubo-ovarian disease 670.8
    urinary system, urine
      albuminuria (acute) (subacute)
          646.2
        pre-eclamptic 642.4
      anuria 669.3
      bacteriuria, asymptomatic 646.5
      cystitis 646.6
      cystopyelitis 646.6
      oligouria 669.3
      paralysis, bladder (sphincter)
          665.5
      uremia 669.3
    uterus, subinvolution 674.8
    varicose veins (legs) 671.0
      vulva or perineum 671.1
    polyp, placental 674.4
    retention of decidua, placenta or
          secundines (fragments)
          (with delayed hemorrhage)
          666.2
      without hemorrhage 667.1
    wound disruption
      cesarean 674.1
      episiotomy 674.2
      perineal laceration 674.2
Pulse
  alternating 427.89
  bigeminal or trigeminal 427.89

Pulse *(continued)*
feeble, rapid, due to shock following
injury 958.4
rapid 785.0
slow 427.89
Puncture (traumatic) (by) (*see also* Wound,
open, by site)
accidental, complicating surgery 998.2
device, implant, or graft—*see*
Complications
foreign body
internal organs (*see also* Injury, internal,
by site)
left accidentally in operation wound
998.4
instrument (any) during a procedure,
accidental 998.2
internal organs, abdomen, chest, or
pelvis—*see* Injury, internal,
by site
Purpura
annularis telangiectodes 709.1
fibrinolytic (*see also* Fibrinolysis)
286.6
fulminans, fulminous 286.6
hemorrhagic (*see also* Purpura, thrombocytopenic) 287.3
thrombocytopenic 287.3
idiopathic 287.3
pigmentaria, progressiva 709.09
posttransfusion 287.4
telangiectasia annularis 709.1
thrombocytopenic—*see*
Thrombocytopenia
thrombohemolytic—*see* Fibrinolysis
Werlhof's 287.3
Purpuric spots 782.7
absorption, general—*see* Septicemia
stool 792.1
Pus (in) *(continued)*
tube (rupture) (*see also* Salpingo-oophoritis) 614.2
urine 791.9
Pustular rash 782.1
Pyelitis (congenital) (uremic)
with or following
abortion—*see* Abortion, by type, with
specified complication NEC
following abortion 639.8
ectopic pregnancy (*see also* categories
633.0–633.9) 639.8
molar pregnancy (*see also* categories
630–632) 639.8

Pyelitis *(continued)*
complicating pregnancy, childbirth, or
puerperium 646.6
gonococcal 098.19
chronic or duration of 2 months or
over 098.39
Pyemia, pyemic (purulent) (*see also*
Septicemia) 038.9
abscess—*see* Abscess
Bacillus coli 038.42
embolism—*see* Embolism, pyemic
fever 038.9
infection 038.9
phlebitis—*see* Phlebitis
pneumococcal 038.2
postvaccinal 999.3
puerperal 670.2
specified organism NEC 038.8
staphylococcal 038.10
aureus 038.11
specified organism NEC 038.19
streptococcal 038.0
Pyrexia—*see* Fever
Pyuria (bacterial) 791.9

Q
Quadruplet pregnancy—*see* Pregnancy,
multiple gestation
Quintuplet pregnancy—*see* Pregnancy,
multiple gestation

R
Radiation effects or sickness (*see also*
Effect, adverse, radiation)
Radiotherapy session V58.0
Rales 786.7
Rape—*see* Injury, by site
alleged, observation or examination V71.5
Rapid
feeble pulse, due to shock, following
injury 958.4
heart (beat) 785.0
respiration 786.06
Rash 782.1
nettle 708.8
pustular 782.1
rose 782.1
serum (prophylactic) (therapeutic) 999.5
toxic 782.1
Reaction (*see also* Depression, depressive
reaction)
allergic (*see also* Allergy) 995.3
drug, medicinal substance, and biological—*see* Allergy, drug

Reaction *(continued)*
serum 999.5
anaphylactic—*see* Shock, anaphylactic
anesthesia—*see* Anesthesia, complication
drug NEC 995.2
    allergic—*see* Allergy, drug
    correct substance properly adminis-
        tered 995.2
    obstetric anesthetic or analgesic NEC
        668.9
foreign
    body in operative wound (inadvertently
        left) 998.4
        due to surgical material intentionally
            left—*see* Complications
    substance accidentally left during a
        procedure 998.7
hypoglycemic, due to insulin 251.0
incompatibility
    blood group (ABO) (infusion) (trans-
        fusion) 999.6
    Rh (factor) (infusion) (transfusion)
        999.7
inflammatory—*see* Infection
infusion—*see* Complications, infusion
paranoid (chronic) menopausal 297.2
psychoneurotic—*see* Neurosis
serum (prophylactic) (therapeutic)999.5
    immediate 999.4
situational, acute, to stress 308.3
stress, acute 308.9
    with predominant disturbance (of)
        consciousness 308.1
        emotions 308.0
        mixed 308.4
        psychomotor 308.2
        specified type NEC 308.3
surgical procedure—*see* Complications,
        surgical procedure
transfusion (blood) (lymphocytes)—*see*
        Complications, transfusion
tuberculin skin test, nonspecific (without
        active tuberculosis) 795.5
    positive (without active tuberculosis)
        795.5
vaccination (any)—*see* Complications,
        vaccination
Rectocele (without uterine prolapse) 618.04
with uterine prolapse 618.4
    complete 618.3
    incomplete 618.2
in pregnancy or childbirth 654.4
    causing obstructed labor 660.2
vagina, vaginal (outlet) 618.0

Redundant, redundancy
clitoris 624.2
labia 624.3
organ or site, congenital NEC—*see*
        Accessory
vagina 623.8
Refusal of treatment (because of) (due to)
patient's decision NEC V64.2
reason of conscience or religion V62.6
Relaxation
anus (sphincter) 569.49
cervix (*see also* Incompetency, cervix)
        622.5
inguinal rings—*see* Hernia, inguinal
pelvic floor 618.89
pelvis 618.89
perineum 618.89
rectum (sphincter) 569.49
urethra (sphincter) 599.84
uterus (outlet) 618.89
vagina (outlet) 618.89
Remnant, cervix, cervical stump
        (acquired) (postoperative)
        622.8
Respiration
asymmetrical 786.09
bronchial 786.09
Cheyne-Stokes (periodic respiration)
        786.04
decreased, due to shock following injury
        958.4
disorder of 786.00
    specified NEC 786.09
insufficiency 786.09
painful 786.52
periodic 786.09
poor 786.09
wheezing 786.07
Respiratory syncytial virus (RSV)
bronchiolitis 466.11
pneumonia 480.1
vaccination, prophylactic (against)
        V04.82
Retention, retained
bladder (*see also* Retention, urine) 788.20
    psychogenic 306.53
cyst—*see* Cyst
dead
    fetus—*see* Pregnancy
    ovum 631
decidua—*see* Delivery
fluid 276.6
foreign body, current trauma—*see*
        Foreign body, by site or type

Retention, retained *(continued)*
  menses 626.8
  milk (puerperal) 676.2
  smegma, clitoris 624.8
  urine NEC—*see* Urine
  water (in tissue) (*see also* Edema) 782.3
Retraction
  cervix—*see* Retroversion, uterus
  nipple 611.79
    congenital 757.6
    puerperal, postpartum 676.0
  ring, uterus (Bandl's) (pathological)
    661.4
  uterus (*see also* Retroversion, uterus)
    621.6
Retrocaval ureter 753.4
Retroperitonitis (*see also* Peritonitis) 567.9
Retroversion, retroverted
  cervix (*see also* Retroversion, uterus)
    621.6
  uterus, uterine (acquired) (acute) (post-
    partal, old) 621.6
    congenital 752.3
    in pregnancy or childbirth 654.3
      causing obstructed labor 660.2
Rhesus, Rh (factor)
  incompatibility, immunization, or
    sensitization
    affecting management of pregnancy
      656.1
  titer elevated 999.7
  transfusion reaction 999.7
Rheumatism, rheumatic (acute NEC)
    729.0
  arthritis, chronic 714.0
  articular (chronic) NEC (*see also*
    Arthritis) 716.9
  chronic NEC 729.0
  intercostal 729.0
  joint (chronic) NEC (*see also* Arthritis)
    716.9
  muscular or neuromuscular 729.0
  myositis 729.1
  neuralgic 729.0
  neuritis (acute) (chronic) 729.2
  polyarthritis
    acute or subacute—*see* Fever, rheumatic
    chronic 714.0
  polyarticular NEC (*see also* Arthritis)
    716.9
  sciatic 724.3
  subacute NEC 729.0
Rheumatoid—*see* condition

Rhinitis (chronic) (purulent) 472.0 (*see also*
    Fever, hay)
  acute 460
  granulomatous 472.0
  infective 460
  obstructive 472.0
  pneumococcal 460
Rhythm (cardiac)
  atrioventricular nodal 427.89
  disorder 427.9
    coronary sinus 427.89
    ectopic 427.89
    nodal 427.89
  escape 427.89
  idioventricular, accelerated 427.89
  nodal 427.89
  sleep, inversion 780.55
Rhytidosis facialis 701.8
Rigid, rigidity (*see also* condition)
  abdominal 789.4
  hymen (acquired) (congenital) 623.3
Ring(s)
  Bandl's, complicating delivery 661.4
  contraction, complicating delivery 661.4
  hymenal, tight (acquired) (congenital)
    623.3
  retraction, uterus, pathological 661.4
Ringworm
  perianal (area) 110.3
  specified site NEC 110.8
Rosacea (acne) 695.3
Rose
  cold, fever 477.0
  rash 782.1
Rubella (German measles) 056.9
  complicating pregnancy, childbirth, or
    puerperium 647.5
  contact or exposure to V01.4
  maternal with suspected fetal damage
    affecting management of
    pregnancy 655.3
  specified complications NEC 056.79
  vaccination, prophylactic (against) V04.3
Rubeola (measles) (*see also* Measles) 055.9
  complicated 055.8
Rupture, ruptured
  with or following
    abortion—*see* Abortion, by type, with
      damage to pelvic organs
    following abortion 639.2
    ectopic pregnancy (*see also* categories
      633.0–633.9) 639.2
    molar pregnancy (*see also* categories
      630–632) 639.2

Rupture, ruptured *(continued)*
　abdominal viscera NEC 799.89
　　obstetrical trauma 665.5
　abscess (spontaneous)—*see* Abscess, by
　　　site
　amnion—*see* Rupture, membranes
　anus (sphincter)—*see* Laceration, anus
　appendix (with peritonitis) 540.0
　　with peritoneal abscess 540.1
　bladder (sphincter)
　　obstetrical trauma 665.5
　　traumatic—*see* Injury, internal, bladder
　blood vessel (*see also* Hemorrhage) 459.0
　cecum (with peritonitis) 540.0
　　with peritoneal abscess 540.1
　cervix (uteri)
　　obstetrical trauma 665.3
　　traumatic—*see* Injury, internal, cervix
　colon, traumatic—*see* Injury, internal,
　　　colon
　corpus luteum (infected) (ovary) 620.1
　cyst—*see* Cyst
　fallopian tube 620.8
　　due to pregnancy—*see* Pregnancy,
　　　tubal
　　traumatic—*see* Injury, internal, fallopian
　　　tube
　graafian follicle (hematoma) 620.0
　hymen 623.8
　internal organ, traumatic—*see* Injury,
　　　internal, by site
　meaning hernia—*see* Hernia
　membranes (spontaneous)—*see* Pregnancy
　muscle (traumatic) with open wound—*see*
　　　Wound, open, by site
　operation wound (*see also* Dehiscence)
　　　998.32
　　internal 998.31
　ovary, ovarian 620.8
　　corpus luteum 620.1
　　follicle (graafian) 620.0
　pelvic
　　floor, complicating delivery 664.1
　　organ NEC—*see* Injury, pelvic, organs
　perineum 624.8
　　during delivery (*see also* Laceration,
　　　perineum, complicating
　　　delivery) 664.4
　pregnant uterus—*see* Rupture, uterus
　pyosalpinx (*see also* Salpingo-oophoritis)
　　　614.2
　rectum 569.49
　　traumatic—*see* Injury, internal, rectum

Rupture, ruptured *(continued)*
　traumatic
　　with open wound—*see* Wound, open,
　　　by site
　　external site—*see* Wound, open, by site
　　internal organ (abdomen, chest, or
　　　pelvis) (*see also* Injury, inter-
　　　nal, by site)
　　meaning hernia—*see* Hernia
　umbilical cord 663.8
　ureter (traumatic) (*see also* Injury, internal,
　　　ureter) 867.2
　urethra 599.84
　　obstetrical trauma 665.5
　　traumatic—*see* Injury, internal
　　　urethra
　uterosacral ligament 620.8
　uterus (traumatic)—*see* Injury, internal
　　　uterus
　　during labor 665.1
　　nonpuerperal, nontraumatic 621.8
　　nontraumatic 621.8
　　pregnant (during labor) 665.1
　　　before labor 665.0
　vagina 878.6
　　complicated 878.7
　　complicating delivery—*see* Laceration,
　　　vagina, complicating delivery
　varicose vein—*see* Varicose, vein
　vesical (urinary) traumatic—*see* Injury,
　　　internal, bladder
　vessel (blood) 459.0
　vulva 878.4
　　complicated 878.5
　　complicating delivery 664.0

S

Salpingitis (*see also* Salpingo-oophoritis)
　　　614.2
　follicularis 614.1
　gonococcal (chronic) 098.37
　　acute 098.17
　interstitial, chronic 614.1
　isthmica nodosa 614.1
　old—*see* Salpingo-oophoritis, chronic
　puerperal, postpartum, childbirth 670.8
　specific (chronic) 098.37
　　acute 098.17
　tuberculous (acute) (chronic) (*see also*
　　　Tuberculosis) 016.6
　venereal (chronic) 098.37
　　acute 098.17
Salpingocele 620.4

Salpingo-oophoritis 614.2
  acute 614.0
    with or following
      abortion—*see* Abortion, by type,
        with sepsis
        following abortion 639.0
      ectopic pregnancy (*see also* categories
        633.0–633.9) 639.0
      molar pregnancy (*see also* categories
        630–632) 639.0
      gonococcal 098.17
      puerperal, postpartum, childbirth 670.8
  chronic 614.1
    gonococcal 098.37
  complicating pregnancy 646.6
  old—*see* Salpingo-oophoritis, chronic
  puerperal 670.8
  subacute (*see also* Salpingo-oophoritis,
    acute) 614.0
  tuberculous (acute) (chronic) (*see also*
    Tuberculosis) 016.6
  venereal—*see* Salpingo-oophoritis, gono-
    coccal
Salpingoperitonitis (*see also* Salpingo-
    oophoritis) 614.2
Sampling
  chorionic villus V28.89
Sarcoma (*see also* Neoplasm, connective
    tissue, malignant)
  endometrial (stromal) 182.0
  isthmus 182.1
Scar, scarring (*see also* Cicatrix) 709.2
  adherent 709.2
  atrophic 709.2
  cervix, in pregnancy or childbirth 654.6
    causing obstructed labor 660.2
  hypertrophic 701.4
  keloid 701.4
  labia 624.4
  painful 709.2
  uterus 621.8
    in pregnancy or childbirth NEC
      654.9
      from previous cesarean delivery
        654.2
  vulva 624.4
Sciatica (infectional) 724.3
Scleredema (adultorum) (Buschke's)
    710.1
Sclerocystic ovary (syndrome) 256.4
Scleroderma, sclerodermia (generalized)
    (progressive) 710.1
Scleromyxedema 701.8

Sclerose en plaques 340
Sclerosis, sclerotic
  Alzheimer's 331.0
  cardiovascular (*see also* Disease, cardiovas-
    cular) 429.2
  corpus cavernosum (female) 624.8
  endometrium 621.8
  gastritis 535.4
  general (vascular)—*see* Arteriosclerosis
  ovary 620.8
  senile—*see* Arteriosclerosis
  systemic (progressive) 710.1
  vascular—*see* Arteriosclerosis
Scoliotic pelvis 738.6
  with disproportion (fetopelvic) 653.0
    causing obstructed labor 660.1
Screening (for)
  alcoholism V79.1
  anemia, deficiency NEC V78.1
    iron V78.0
  antenatal
    alphafetoprotein levels, raised V28.1
    based on amniocentesis V28.2
      chromosomal anomalies V28.0
      raised alphafetoprotein levels V28.1
    fetal growth retardation using ultra-
      sonics V28.4
    genomic V28.89
    gestational age V28.8
    isoimmunization V28.5
    malformations using ultrasonics V28.3
    proteomic risk V28.89
      pre-term labor V28.82
    specified condition NEC V28.8
    Streptococcus B V28.6
  arterial hypertension V81.1
  bacteriuria, asymptomatic V81.5
  cancer—*see* Screening, malignant neo-
    plasm
  cardiovascular diseases V81.0–V81.2
  cholesterol level V77.91
  chromosomal anomalies
    by amniocentesis, antenatal V28.0
    maternal, postnatal V82.4
  depression V79.0
  diabetes mellitus V77.1
  disease or disorder
    bacterial
      and spirochetal sexually transmitted
        diseases V74.5
      disease V74.9
        sexually transmitted V74.5
    blood, blood-forming organ V78.9
      specified type NEC V78.8

Screening *(continued)*
disease or disorder *(continued)*
chlamydial V73.98
specified NEC V73.88
genitourinary NEC V81.6
sexually transmitted (bacterial) (spirochetal) V74.5
sickle-cell (trait) V78.2
thyroid V77.0
viral V73.99
human papillomavirus V73.81
specified type NEC V73.89
fecal occult blood V76.41, V76.51
genetic
carrier
female V26.31
male V26.34
other
female V26.32
male V26.39
testing of male partner of habitual
aborter V26.35
gonorrhea V74.5
heart disease NEC V81.2
hypertensive V81.1
hemoglobinopathies NEC V78.3
hypercholesterolemia or hyperlipdemia
V77.91
hypertension V81.1
lipoid disorder NEC V77.91
malignant neoplasm (of)
breast V76.10
mammogram NEC V76.12
for high-risk patient V76.11
specified type NEC V76.19
cervix V76.2
as part of gynecological examination
V72.31
for Medicare patient
high risk V15.89
not high risk V76.2, V72.31
colon or colorectal V76.51
intestine V76.50
colon V76.51
small V76.52
ovary V76.46
rectum V76.41
skin V76.43
vagina V76.47
following hysterectomy for malignant condition V67.01
for Medicare patient
high risk V15.89
not high risk V76.2, V72.31

Screening *(continued)*
measles V73.2
nephropathy V81.1
obesity V77.8
osteoporosis V82.81
renal disease V81.1
rubella V73.3
syphilis V74.5
tuberculosis, pulmonary V74.1
Welcome to Medicare exam V70.0
Sebaceous
cyst (*see also* Cyst, sebaceous) 706.2
gland disease NEC 706.9
Sebocystomatosis 706.2
Seborrhea, seborrheic 706.3
adiposa 706.3
keratosis 702.19
inflamed 702.11
wart 702.19
inflamed 702.11
Secondary (*see also* condition)
neoplasm—*see* Neoplasm, by site, malignant, secondary
Secretion, urinary
excessive 788.42
suppression 788.5
Seizure—*see* Epilepsy
Self-mutilation 300.9
Senile (*see also* condition)
cervix (atrophic) 622.8
degenerative atrophy, skin 701.3
endometrium (atrophic) 621.8
fallopian tube (atrophic) 620.3
lung 492.8
ovary (atrophic) 620.3
vagina, vaginitis (atrophic) 627.3
wart 702.0
Separation
anxiety, abnormal 309.21
placenta (normally implanted)—*see*
Placenta, separation
symphysis pubis, obstetrical trauma 665.6
Sepsis (generalized) 995.91 (*see also*
Septicemia)
genital organ NEC 614.9
localized, in operation wound 998.59
nadir 038.9
resulting from infusion, injection, transfusion, or vaccination 999.39
severe 995.92
urinary 599.0
meaning sepsis 995.91
meaning urinary tract infection 599.0

Septic (*see also* condition)
  embolus—*see* Embolism
  shock (endotoxic) 785.52
  sore throat (milk-borne) 034.0
    streptococcal 034.0
  thrombus—*see* Thrombosis
  uterus (*see also* Endometritis) 615.9
Septicemia, septicemic (generalized) (sup-
        purative) 038.9 (*see also*
        Sepsis)
  with or following
    abortion—*see* Abortion, by type, with
        sepsis
      following abortion 639.0
    ectopic pregnancy (*see also* categories
        633.0–633.9) 639.0
    infusion, injection, transfusion, or
        vaccination 999.39
    molar pregnancy (*see also* categories
        630–632) 639.0
  Aerobacter aerogenes 038.49
  anaerobic 038.3
  Bacillus coli 038.42
  Bacteroides 038.3
  Clostridium 038.3
  complicating labor 659.3
  cryptogenic 038.9
  enteric gram-negative bacilli 038.40
  Enterobacter aerogenes 038.49
  Escherichia coli 038.42
  Friedländer's (bacillus) 038.49
  gangrenous 038.9
  gonococcal 098.89
  gram-negative (organism) 038.40
    anaerobic 038.3
  Hemophilus influenzae 038.41
  pneumococcal 038.2
  postoperative 998.59
  Proteus vulgaris 038.49
  Pseudomonas (aeruginosa) 038.43
  puerperal, postpartum 670
  Serratia 038.44
  specified organism NEC 038.8
  staphylococcal 038.10
    aureus 038.11
      methicillin
        resistant (MRSA) 038.12
        suspectible (MSSA) 038.11
    specified organism NEC 038.19
  streptococcal (anaerobic) 038.0
  Streptococcus pneumoniae 038.2
  viral 079.99
  Yersinia enterocolitica 038.49

Septum, septate (congenital) (*see also*
        Anomaly, specified type NEC)
  hymen 752.49
  uterus (*see also* Double, uterus) 752.2
  vagina 752.49
    in pregnancy or childbirth 654.7
      causing obstructed labor 660.2
Seroma (postoperative) (noninfected) 998.13
  infected 998.51
Serositis, multiple, peritoneal 568.82
Serum
  allergy, allergic reaction 999.5
    shock 999.4
  complication or reaction NEC 999.5
  disease NEC 999.5
  hepatitis 070.3
  intoxication 999.5
  jaundice (homologous)—*see* Hepatitis,
        viral, type B
  neuritis 999.5
  rash or reaction NEC 999.5
Sextuplet, pregnancy—*see* Pregnancy,
        multiple
Sexual
  anesthesia 302.72
  function, disorder of (psychogenic) 302.70
    specified type NEC 302.79
  immaturity 259.0
  precocity (constitutional) (cryptogenic)
        (idiopathic) NEC 259.1
Shingles (*see also* Herpes, zoster) 053.9
Shirodkar suture, in pregnancy 654.5
Shock 785.50
  with, following or complicating
    abortion—*see* Abortion, by type, with
        shock
      following abortion 639.5
    ectopic or molar pregnancy (*see also*
        categories 630–633.9)
        639.5
  injury (immediate) (delayed) 958.4
  labor and delivery 669.1
  anaphylactic 995.0
    correct medicinal substance properly
        administered 995.0
    immunization 999.4
    serum 999.4
  anesthetic
    correct substance properly adminis-
        tered 995.4
    overdose or wrong substance given
        968.4
  cardiogenic 785.51
  circulatory 785.59

Shock *(continued)*
culture 309.29
due to drug, correct substance properly
  administered 995.0
endotoxic 785.52
  due to surgical procedure 998.0
gram-negative 785.52
hematogenic 785.59
hemorrhagic due to
  disease 785.59
  surgery (intraoperative) (postoperative)
    998.0
  trauma 958.4
hypovolemic NEC 785.59
  surgical 998.0
  traumatic 958.4
insulin 251.0
kidney traumatic (following crushing)
  958.5
pleural (surgical) 998.0
  due to trauma 958.4
postoperative (nonobstetric) 998.0
psychic (*see also* Reaction, stress, acute)
  308.9
  past history (of) V15.49
septic 785.52
  with or following
    surgical procedure 998.0
    transfusion NEC 999.89
surgical 998.0
therapeutic misadventure NEC (*see also*
  Complications) 998.89
thyroxin 962.7
toxic 040.82
transfusion—*see* Complications, transfusion
traumatic (immediate) (delayed) 958.4
Short, shortening, shortness
breath 786.05
cervical, cervix 649.7
  gravid uterus 649.7
  non-gravid uterus 622.5
    acquired 622.5
    congenital 752.49
round ligament 629.8
umbilical cord 663.4
urethra 599.84
vagina 623.8
Shunt, arterial-venous (dialysis) V45.11
Shutdown, renal
complicating or following
  abortion 639.3
  ectopic or molar pregnancy 639.3
  labor and delivery 669.3

Sickle-cell
anemia or disease (*see also* Disease, sickle-
  cell) 282.60
hemoglobin
  C disease (without crisis) 282.63
    with crisis or vaso-occlusive pain
      282.64
  D disease (without crisis) 282.68
    with crisis 282.69
  E disease (without crisis) 282.68
    with crisis 282.69
  thalassemia (without crisis) 282.41
    with crisis or vaso-occlusive pain 282.42
trait 282.5
Sickness
morning 643.0
protein (*see also* Complications, vaccination) 999.5
serum NEC 999.5
Sinus (*see also* Fistula)
arrhythmia 427.89
bradycardia 427.89
  chronic 427.81
draining—*see* Fistula
marginal, rupture or bleeding 641.2
rectovaginal 619.1
skin, noninfected—*see* Ulcer, skin
tachycardia 427.89
tract (postinfectional)—*see* Fistula
Sinusitis 473.9
with influenza, flu, or grippe 487.1
acute 461.9
  ethmoidal 461.2
  frontal 461.1
  maxillary 461.0
  specified type NEC 461.8
  sphenoidal 461.3
specified site NEC 473.8
SIRS (systemic inflammatory response
  syndrome) 995.90
due to
  infectious process 995.91
    with organ dysfunction 995.92
  noninfectious process 995.93
    with organ dysfunction 995.94
Skenitis (*see also* Urethritis) 597.89
gonorrheal (acute) 098.0
  chronic or duration of 2 months or
    over 098.2
Sleep
disorder or disturbance 780.50
  with apnea—*see* Apnea, sleep
initiation or maintenance 780.52

Sleep *(continued)*
   rhythm inversion 780.55
   wakefulness—*see* Hypersomnia
Sleeplessness *(see also* Insomnia) 780.52
   menopausal 627.2
Sloughing (multiple) (skin)
   abscess—*see* Abscess, by site
   appendix 543.9
   rectum 569.49
Small, smallness
   introitus, vagina 623.3
   ovary 620.8
   pelvis
      with disproportion (fetopelvic)
         653.1
         causing obstructed labor 660.1
   placenta—*see* Placenta, insufficiency
   uterus 621.8
Smokers', smoking
   bronchitis or cough 491.0
   complicating pregnancy 649.0
   syndrome *(see also* Abuse, drugs, nonde-
      pendent) 305.1
   throat 472.1
Smothering spells 786.09
Sore
   pressure 707.0
   skin NEC 709.9
   soft 099.0
   throat 462
      with influenza, flu, or grippe 487.1
      acute 462
      chronic 472.1
      epidemic 034.0
      gangrenous 462
      malignant or purulent 462
      septic 034.0
      streptococcal (ulcerative) 034.0
      ulcerated 462
      viral NEC 462
Sounds, friction, pleural or chest
      786.7
Spasm, spastic *(see also* condition), intes-
      tinal 564.9
Sperm counts
   fertility testing V26.21
   following sterilization reversal V26.22
   postvasectomy V25.8
Spitting blood *(see also* Hemoptysis)
      786.3
Split, splitting
   heart sounds 427.89
   urinary stream 788.61

Spots, spotting
   atrophic (skin) 701.3
   intermenstrual
      irregular 626.6
      regular 626.5
   of pregnancy 649.5
   purpuric 782.7
Sputum, abnormal (amount) (color)
      (excessive) (odor) (purulent)
      786.4
   bloody 786.3
Squamous *(see also* condition)
   epithelium in
      cervical canal (congenital) 752.49
      uterine mucosa (congenital) 752.3
   metaplasia, cervix—*see* condition
Starvation (inanition) (due to lack of
      food), voluntary NEC 307.1
Stasis
   dermatitis or eczema *(see also* Varix, with
      stasis dermatitis) 454.1
   ulcer, with varicose veins 454.0
   urine NEC *(see also* Retention, urine)
      788.20
State
   agitated, acute reaction to stress 308.2
   anxiety or apprehension (neurotic) *(see
      also* Anxiety) 300.00
      specified type NEC 300.09
   clouded (epileptic) (paroxysmal) 345.9
   depressive NEC 311
      neurotic 300.4
   menopausal 627.2
      artificial 627.4
      following induced menopause 627.4
   panic 300.01
Status (post)
   absence of organ, acquired (postsurgi-
      cal)—*see* Absence, by site,
      acquired
   asthmaticus *(see also* Asthma) 493.9
   bariatric surgery V45.86
      complicating pregnancy, childbirth, or
         puerperium 649.2
   breast
      correction V43.82
      implant removal V45.83
      reconstruction V43.82
   chemotherapy V66.2
      current V58.69
   circumcision, female—*see* Status, female
      genital muilation
   colostomy V44.3

Status (post) *(continued)*
  contraceptive device V45.59
    intrauterine V45.51
    subdermal V45.52
  cystostomy V44.50
  delinquent immunization V15.83
  dialysis V45.11
  drug therapy or regimen V67.59
    high-risk medication NEC V67.51
    estrogen receptor
      positive V86.0
      negative V86.1
  female genital mutilation 629.20
    type 1 (clitorectomy) 629.21
    type II (excision labia minora) 629.22
    type III (infibulation) 629.23
    type IV (other) 629.29
  gastrostomy V44.1
  hysterectomy V88.01
    partial with remaining cervical stump
      V88.02
    total V88.01
  ileostomy V44.2
  malignant neoplasm, ablated or excised—
      see History, malignant
      neoplasm
  organ replacement or transplant, by artifi-
      cial or mechanical device or
      prosthesis
    breast V43.82
    heart V43.2
    joint V43.6
  postmenopausal (age related) (natural)
      V49.81
  postpartum NEC V24.2
    care immediately following delivery V24.0
    routine follow-up V24.2
  sterilization, tubal ligation V26.51
  tracheostomy V44.0
  tubal ligation V26.51
  underimmunization V15.83
  vagina, artificial V44.7
Stenosis (cicatricial)
  anus, anal (canal) (sphincter) 569.2
  cardiovascular (*see also* Disease, cardiovas-
      cular) 429.2
  cervix, cervical (canal) 622.4
    congenital 752.49
    in pregnancy or childbirth 654.6
      causing obstructed labor 660.2
    due to (presence of) any device, implant,
      or graft—*see* Complications

Stenosis *(continued)*
  fallopian tube 628.2
    gonococcal (chronic) 098.37
    acute 098.17
    tuberculous (*see also* Tuberculosis)
      016.6
  hymen 623.3
  organ or site, congenital NEC—*see*
      Atresia
  rectum (sphincter) 569.2
    gonococcal 098.7
    inflammatory 099.1
  ureter, tuberculous (*see also* Tuberculosis)
      016.2
  urethra 598.9
    gonococcal 098.2 (598.01)
    gonorrheal 098.2 (598.01)
    infective 598.00
    late effect of injury 598.1
    postcatheterization 598.2
    postobstetric 598.1
    postoperative 598.2
    specified cause NEC 598.8
    traumatic 598.1
    valvular, congenital 753.6
  urinary meatus 598.9
    congenital 753.6
  uterus, uterine 621.5
    os (external) (internal)—*see* Stenosis,
      cervix
  vagina (outlet) 623.2
    congenital 752.49
    in pregnancy or childbirth 654.7
      causing obstructed labor 660.2
  vulva (acquired) 624.8
Sterilization, admission for V25.2
Stitch, burst (in external operation wound)
      998.32
  internal 998.31
Stoma malfunction (cystostomy)
      (ureterostomy) 997.5
Strangulation, strangulated
  appendix 543.9
  hemorrhoids 455.8
    external 455.5
    internal 455.2
  hernia (*see also* Hernia, by site)
  organ or site, congenital NEC—*see*
      Atresia
  ovary 620.8
    due to hernia 620.4
  umbilical cord—*see* Compression, umbili-
      cal cord

Streak, ovarian 752.0
Stress reaction (gross) (*see also* Reaction,
    stress, acute) 308.9
Stricture—*see* Stenosis
Stroke
    heart—*see* Disease, heart
    postoperative 997.02
Stromatosis, endometrial 236.0
Struma (*see also* Goiter) 240.9
    ovarii 220
        and carcinoid 236.2
        malignant 183.0
Stump—*see* Amputation, cervix
Subinvolution (uterus) 621.1
    breast (postlactational) (postpartum) 611.8
    chronic 621.1
    puerperal, postpartum 674.8
Subseptus uterus 752.3
Substance abuse in family V61.42
Succenturiata placenta—*see* Placenta,
    abnormal
Sugar
    blood
        high 790.29
        low 251.2
    in urine 791.5
Suicide, suicidal (attempted) (at risk for)
    (tendencies) 300.9
Superinvolution uterus 621.8
Supernumerary (congenital)—*see* Accessory
Suppression
    lactation 676.5
    menstruation 626.8
    ovarian secretion 256.39
    urine 788.5
Suppuration, suppurative (*see also* condi-
    tion)
    bladder (*see also* Cystitis) 595.89
    breast 611.0
        puerperal, postpartum 675.1
    fallopian tube (*see also* Salpingo-oophoritis)
        614.2
    pelvis (*see also* Disease, pelvis, inflamma-
        tory) 614.4
        acute 614.3
    uterus (*see also* Endometritis) 615.9
    vagina 616.10
    wound—*see* Wound, open, by site, com-
        plicated
Surgery
    cosmetic NEC V50.1
        breast reconstruction following mas-
            tectomy V51.0

Surgery *(continued)*
    elective (plastic)
        breast
            augmentation or reduction V50.1
            reconstruction following mastec-
                tomy V51.0
        circumcision, ritual or routine (in
            absence of medical indica-
            tion) V50.2
        ear piercing V50.3
    not done because of
        contraindication V64.1
        patient's decision V64.2
        specified reason NEC V64.3
    vagina 654.7
Survey
    fetal anatomic V28.81
Susceptibility, genetic (to)
    neoplasm, malignant, of
        breast V84.01
        endometrium V84.04
        other V84.09
        ovary V84.02
    other disease V84.8
Swelling, swollen
    abdominal (not referable to specific
        organ) 789.3
    anus 787.99
    breast 611.72
    cervical gland 785.6
    genital organ 625.8
    glands 785.6
    inflammatory—*see* Inflammation
    liver 573.8
    lymph nodes 785.6
    pelvis 789.3
    perineum 625.8
    rectum 787.99
    skin 782.2
    umbilicus 789.3
    uterus 625.8
    vagina 625.8
    vulva 625.8
Symptoms, specified (general) NEC
    breast NEC 611.79
    chest NEC 786.9
    development NEC 783.9
    digestive system or gastrointestinal tract
        NEC 787.99
    emotional state NEC 799.29
    genital organs NEC 625.9
    menopausal 627.2
    metabolism NEC 783.9

Symptoms, specified *(continued)*
   musculoskeletal, limbs NEC 729.89
   nutrition or metabolism NEC 783.9
   pelvis 625.9
   peritoneum NEC 789.9
   respiratory system NEC 786.9
   skin, integument NEC or subcutaneous
      tissue NEC 782.9
   urinary system NEC 788.99
Syncope (near) (pre-) 780.2
   complicating delivery 669.2
Syndrome (*see also* Disease)
   acid pulmonary aspiration 997.3
      obstetric (Mendelson's) 668.0
   acquired immune deficiency 042
   acute abdominal 789.0
   Ahumada-de Castillo or Argonz-Del
      Castillo (non-puerperal
      galactorrhea and amenor-
      rhea) 253.1
   Allen-Masters 620.6
   Alzheimer's 331.0
   angina (*see also* Angina) 413.9
   anterior
      chest wall 786.52
      compartment (tibial) 958.8
   anticardiolipin antibody 795.79
   anxiety (*see also* Anxiety) 300.00
   Asherman's 621.5
   autosomal (*see also* Abnormal, autosomes
      NEC)
      deletion 758.39
   battered
      adult (spouse) 995.81
      baby or child 995.54
   bilateral polycystic ovarian 256.4
   bladder neck (*see also* Incontinence,
      urine) 788.30
   blue bloater 491.20
      with
         acute bronchitis 491.22
         exacerbation (acute) 491.21
   Bonnevie-Ullrich 758.6
   broad ligament laceration 620.6
   Burnett's (milk-alkali) 275.42
   Bywaters' 958.5
   carpal tunnel 354.0
   Charcot's (intermittent claudication) 443.9
   Chiari-Frommel 676.6
   compression 958.5
   congestion-fibrosis (pelvic) 625.5
   dead fetus 641.3
   defibrination (*see also* Fibrinolysis) 286.6

Syndrome *(continued)*
   DIC (diffuse or disseminated intravascu-
      lar coagulopathy) (*see also*
      Fibrinolysis) 286.6
   dystocia, dystrophia 654.9
   fatigue, chronic 780.71
   Fitz-Hugh and Curtis 098.86
      due to
         Chlamydia trachomatis 099.56
         Neisseria gonorrhoeae (gonococcal
            peritonitis) 098.86
   Frommel–Chiari 676.6
   functional bowel 564.9
   genito-anorectal 099.1
   HELLP 642.5
   hyperactive bowel 564.9
   irritable bowel 564.1
   IVC (intravascular coagulopathy) (*see also*
      Fibrinolysis) 286.6
   Klinefelter's 758.7
   Li-Fraumeni V84.01
   Likoff's (angina in menopausal women)
      413.9
   low back 724.2
   Luetscher's (dehydration) 276.5
   Masters-Allen 620.6
   Mendelson's (resulting from a procedure)
      997.39
      during labor 668.0
      obstetric 668.0
   menopause 627.2
      postartificial 627.4
   menstruation 625.4
   migraine 346.0
   milk alkali (milk drinkers') 275.42
   mitral click (-murmur) 785.2
   mucocutaneous lymph node (MCLS)
      446.1
   ovarian remnant 620.8
   pelvic congestion (-fibrosis) 625.5
   postimmunization—*see* Complications,
      vaccination
   postmastectomy lymphedema 457.0
   postpartum panhypopituitary 253.2
   postperfusion NEC 999.89
   postphlebitic (asymptomatic) (with)
      459.10
      complication NEC 459.19
      inflammation 459.12
         and ulcer 459.13
      ulcer 495.11
         with inflammation 459.13
   postviral (asthenia) NEC 780.79
   potassium intoxication 276.7

Syndrome *(continued)*
  premenstrual (tension) 625.4
  pterygolymphangiectasia 758.6
  Raynaud's 443.0
  Rokitansky-Kuster-Hauser (congenital
      absence, vagina) 752.49
  sclerocystic ovary 256.4
  Secretan's (posttraumatic edema) 782.3
  sex chromosome mosaic 758.81
  sick
    cell 276.1
    sinus 427.81
  smokers' 305.1
  Stein's or Stein-Leventhal (polycystic
      ovary) 256.4
  sympathetic, pelvic 625.5
  systemic inflammatory response (SIRS)
      (due to) 995.90
    infectious process 995.91
      with organ dysfunction 995.92
    non-infectious process 995.93
      with organ dysfunction 995.94
  tachycardia-bradycardia 427.81
  Taylor's 625.5
  toxic shock 040.82
  Turner-Varny 758.6
  universal joint, cervix 620.6
  urethral 597.81
  vanishing twin 651.33
  Von Schroetter's (intermittent venous
      claudication) 453.8
  water retention 276.6
Synechia
  intrauterine (traumatic) 621.5
  vulvae, congenital 752.49
Syphilis, syphilitic (acquired)
  chancre (multiple) 091.0
    extragenital 091.2
    Rollet's 091.2
  congenital 090.0
  contact V01.6
  early NEC 091.0
    relapse (treated, untreated) 091.7
    skin 091.3
    symptomatic NEC 091.89
      extragenital chancre 091.2
      primary, except extragenital chancre
        091.0
      secondary (*see also* Syphilis, second-
        ary) 091.3
        relapse (treated, untreated) 091.7
      ulcer 091.3
  exposure to V01.6

Syphilis, syphilitic *(continued)*
  primary NEC 091.2
    anus 091.1
    and secondary (*see also* Syphilis, second-
        ary) 091.9
    extragenital chancre NEC 091.2
    genital 091.0
    specified site NEC 091.2
  secondary (and primary) 091.9
    anus 091.3
    mucous membranes 091.3
    skin 091.3
    specified form NEC 091.89
    vulva 091.3
  seronegative, with signs or symptoms—
        see Syphilis, by site and stage
  seropositive, with signs or symptoms—*see*
        Syphilis, by site or stage
  vagina 091.0
  vulva 091.0
    secondary 091.3

T
Tachycardia 785.0
  atrial, auricular or nodal 427.89
  paroxysmal 427.2
    with sinus bradycardia 427.81
    essential 427.2
    junctional 427.0
    ventricular (atrioventricular) (supraven-
        tricular) 427.1
  postoperative 997.1
Tachypnea 786.06
Tag (hypertrophied skin) (infected)
      701.9
  anus or rectum 455.9
  hemorrhoidal 455.9
  hymen 623.8
  perineal 624.8
  skin 701.9
    anus or rectum 455.9
  urethra, urethral 599.84
  vulva 624.8
Tear, torn (traumatic) (*see also* Wound,
      open, by site)
  with or following
    abortion—*see* Abortion, by type, with
        damage to pelvic organs
      following abortion 639.2
    ectopic or molar pregnancy (*see also*
        categories 630–633.9)
        639.2

Tear, torn *(continued)*
anus, anal (sphincter), nontraumatic,
       nonpuerperal (healed) (old)
       565.0
  complicating delivery (healed) (old)
       654.8
  not associated with third-degree lacera-
       tion 664.6
    with mucosa 664.3
bladder, obstetrical trauma 665.5
bowel, obstetrical trauma 665.5
broad ligament, obstetrical trauma 665.6
cervix
  obstetrical trauma (current) 665.3
  old 622.3
internal organ (abdomen, chest, or
       pelvis)—*see* Injury, internal,
       by site
pelvic
  floor, complicating delivery 664.1
  organ NEC, obstetrical trauma 665.5
perineum (*see also* Laceration, perineum)
  obstetrical trauma 665.5
periurethral tissue, obstetrical trauma
    665.5
rectovaginal septum—*see* Laceration,
    rectovaginal septum
umbilical cord, complicating delivery 663.8
urethra, obstetrical trauma 665.5
uterus—*see* Injury, internal, uterus
vagina—*see* Laceration, vagina
vulva, complicating delivery 664.0
Tenderness
abdominal (generalized) (localized) 789.6
rebound 789.6
skin 782.0
Teratoblastoma (malignant)—*see*
    Neoplasm, by site, malignant
Teratocarcinoma (*see also* Neoplasm, by
    site, malignant)
Teratoma (solid) (*see also* Neoplasm, by
    site, uncertain behavior)
benign—*see* Neoplasm, by site, benign
combined with choriocarcinoma—*see*
    Neoplasm, by site, malignant
cystic (adult)—*see* Neoplasm, by site,
    benign
differentiated type—*see* Neoplasm, by
    site, benign
immature—*see* Neoplasm, by site,
    malignant
malignant—*see* Neoplasm, by site,
    malignant

Teratoma *(continued)*
mature—*see* Neoplasm, by site, benign
ovary 220
  embryonal, immature, or malignant
    183.0
Terminal care V66.7
Test(s)
AIDS (virus human immunodeficiency
    virus) (HIV) V72.69
basal metabolic rate V72.69
blood
  alcohol V70.4
  drug V70.4
  for therapeutic drug monitoring V58.83
  for routine general physical examination
    V72.62
  prior to treatment or procedure V72.63
  typing V72.86
  Rh typing V72.86
fertility V26.21
genetic—*see* Screening
laboratory V72.60
  for medicolegal reason V70.4
  ordered as part of a routine general
    medical examination V72.62
  pre-operative V72.63
  pre-procedural V72.63
  specified NEC V72.69
nuchal translucency V28.89
paternity V70.4
pregnancy
  negative result V72.41
  positive result V72.42
  unconfirmed V72.40
preoperative V72.84
  specified NEC V72.83
procreative management NEC V26.29
Rh typing V72.86
specified type NEC V72.85
Tuberculin V74.1
Wassermann, false positive 795.6
Tetanus, tetanic (cephalic) (convulsions)
with or following
  abortion—*see* Abortion, by type, with
    sepsis
    following abortion 639.0
  ectopic or molar pregnancy (*see also*
    categories 630–633.9)
    639.0
  inoculation V03.7
    reaction (due to serum)—*see*
      Complications, vaccination
  puerperal, postpartum, childbirth 670.8

Thalassemia—*see* Sickle-cell
Thecoma 220
  malignant 183.0
Therapy
  chemotherapy V58.1
  postmenopausal hormone replacement
      V07.4
  radiation V58.0
Thermography (abnormal) 793.9
  breast 793.89
Thickened endometrium 793.5
Thickening
  breast 611.79
  hymen 623.3
  skin 782.8
Thirst, excessive 783.5
Threatened
  abortion or miscarriage 640.0
    with subsequent abortion (*see also*
      Abortion, spontaneous) 634.9
  labor 644.1
    premature 644.0
  miscarriage 640.0
  premature
    delivery 644.2
    labor 644.0
      before 22 completed weeks gestation
      640.0
Thrombocytopenia, thrombocytopenic
    287.5
  essential, hereditary or primary 287.3
  fetal 678.0
  puerperal, postpartum 666.3
  purpura 287.3
  secondary 287.4
  sex-linked 287.3
Thromboembolism—*see* Embolism
Thrombopenia (*see also* Thrombo-
    cytopenia) 287.5
Thrombophlebitis
  antepartum (superficial) 671.2
    deep 671.3
  cerebral (sinus) (vein), nonpyogenic, in
    pregnancy or puerperium
    671.5
  due to implanted device—*see*
    Complications, due to (pres-
    ence of) any device, implant,
    or graft
  during or resulting from a procedure
    NEC 997.2
  following infusion, perfusion, or transfu-
    sion 999.2

Thrombophlebitis *(continued)*
  leg or lower extremity 451.2
    deep (vessels) 451.19
    superficial (vessels) 451.0
  pelvic
    with or following
      abortion—*see* Abortion, by type,
        with sepsis
      following abortion 639.0
      ectopic or molar pregnancy (*see also*
        categories 630–633.9) 639.0
    puerperal 671.4
  postoperative 997.2 (*see also* Puerperal)
Thrombosis, thrombotic
  due to (presence of) any device, implant,
    or graft classifiable to
    996.3–996.5—*see*
    Complications, due to (pres-
    ence of) any device, implant,
    or graft
  femoral (vein) 453.8
    deep 453.41
    with inflammation or phlebitis 451.11
  inflammation, vein—*see*
    Thrombophlebitis
  leg or lower extremity
    with inflammation or phlebitis—*see*
      Thrombophlebitis
    deep (vessels) 453.40
      distal 453.42
    superficial (vessels) 453.8
  pampiniform plexus 620.8
  pregnancy 671.2
    deep (vein) 671.3
    superficial (vein) 671.2
  resulting from presence of shunt or other
    internal prosthetic device—
    see Complications
  specified site NEC 453.8
  umbilical cord (vessels) 663.6
  vein
    deep 453.8
    lower extremity—*see* Thrombosis,
      lower extremity
Thyromegaly 240.9
Tight, tightness
  chest 786.59
  hymen 623.3
  introitus (acquired) (congenital) 623.3
  urethral sphincter 598.9
Tipping pelvis 738.6
  with disproportion (fetopelvic) 653.0
    causing obstructed labor 660.1

Tiredness 780.79

Tobacco abuse (affecting health) NEC (*see also* Abuse, drugs, nondependent) 305.1

complicating pregnancy 649.0

Torsion

cervix—*see* Malposition, uterus 621.6

fallopian tube 620.5

hydatid of Morgagni 620.5

Torsion *(continued)*

organ or site, congenital NEC—*see* Anomaly, specified type NEC

ovary (pedicle) 620.5

congenital 752.0

umbilical cord—*see* Compression, umbilical cord

uterus (*see also* Malposition, uterus) 621.6

Tortuous

fallopian tube 752.19

organ or site, congenital NEC—*see* Distortion

urethra 599.84

vein—*see* Varicose, vein

Toxemia 799.89

with abortion—*see* Abortion, by type, with toxemia

bacterial—*see* Septicemia

eclamptic 642.6

with pre-existing hypertension 642.7

fatigue 799.89

of pregnancy—*see* Pregnancy and Puerperal

septic (*see also* Septicemia) 038.9

staphylococcal 038.10

aureus 038.11

specified organism NEC 038.19

stasis 799.89

Toxic shock syndrome 040.82

Transfusion, blood

fetal twin to twin 678.0

incompatible 999.6

reaction or complication—*see* Complications, transfusion

without reported diagnosis V58.2

Translocation (*see also* Anomaly, chromosomes)

autosomes NEC 758.5

balanced autosomal in normal individual 758.4

Down's syndrome 758.0

Transplants, ovarian, endometrial 617.1

Trapped placenta (with hemorrhage) 666.0

without hemorrhage 667.0

Trauma, traumatism (*see also* Injury, by site)

causing hemorrhage of pregnancy or delivery 641.8

complicating or following

abortion—*see* Abortion, by type, with damage to pelvic organs

following abortion 639.2

ectopic or molar pregnancy (*see also* categories 630–633.9) 639.2

during delivery NEC 665.9

previous major, affecting management of pregnancy, childbirth, or puerperium V23.89

psychic (current) (*see also* Reaction, adjustment)

previous (history) V15.49

Trichomoniasis 131.9

bladder 131.09

cervix 131.09

specified site NEC 131.8

urethra 131.02

urogenitalis 131.00

vagina 131.01

vulva 131.01

vulvovaginal 131.01

Trigeminy 427.89

postoperative 997.1

Trigonitis (bladder) (chronic) (pseudomembranous) 595.3

tuberculous (*see also* Tuberculosis) 016.1

Triplet pregnancy—*see* Pregnancy, multiple

Trophoneurosis, disseminated 710.1

Tuberculosis, tubercular, tuberculous 011.9

bladder 016.1

broad ligament 016.7

bronchiectasis 011.5

bronchopneumonia 011.6

cervix 016.7

complex, primary 010.0

complicating pregnancy, childbirth, or puerperium 647.3

contact V01.1

converter (tuberculin skin test) (without disease) 795.5

cyst, ovary 016.6

cystitis 016.1

endometrium 016.7

fallopian tube 016.6

genitourinary NEC 016.9

ovary or oviducts (acute) (chronic) 016.6

Tuberculosis, tubercular, tuberculous
(continued)
pelvic organ 016.7
placenta 016.7
primary, complex 010.0
pulmonary 011.9
ureter 016.2
urethra, urethral 016.3
urinary organ or tract 016.3
uterus 016.7
vaccination, prophylactic (against) V03.2
vagina 016.7
vulva 016.7 (616.51)
Tuboplasty, after previous sterilization
V26.0
Tumor (*see also* Neoplasm, by site, unspecified nature)
any site, causing obstructed labor 660.2
basal cell—*see* Neoplasm, skin, uncertain behavior
benign—*see* Neoplasm, by site, benign
Brenner 220
borderline malignancy 236.2
malignant 183.0
proliferating 236.2
carcinoid—*see* Carcinoid
cervix, in pregnancy or childbirth 654.6
dermoid—*see* Neoplasm, by site, benign
endodermal sinus, specified site—*see*
Neoplasm, by site, malignant
unspecified site 183.0
epithelial
benign—*see* Neoplasm, by site, benign
malignant—*see* Neoplasm, by site, malignant
fatty—*see* Lipoma
fetal, causing disproportion 653.7
fibroid—*see* Leiomyoma
gonadal stromal—*see* Neoplasm, by site, uncertain behavior
granulosa cell (theca cell) 236.2
malignant 183.0
hilar cell 220
Krukenberg's 198.6
Leydig cell
benign, specified site—*see* Neoplasm, by site, benign
unspecified site 220
malignant, specified site—*see*
Neoplasm, by site, malignant
unspecified site 183.0
specified site—*see* Neoplasm, by site, uncertain behavior

Tumor *(continued)*
unspecified site 236.2
lipid (lipoid) cell, ovary 220
markers elevated carcinogen embryonic antigen (CEA) 795.81
elevated cancer antigen 125 (CA125) 795.82
Müllerian, mixed—*see* Neoplasm, by site, malignant
ovarian stromal 236.2
ovary, in pregnancy or childbirth 654.4
papillary—*see* Papilloma
pelvic, in pregnancy or childbirth 654.9
Sertoli cell with lipid storage or Sertoli-Leydig cell
specified site—*see* Neoplasm, by site, benign
unspecified site 220
theca (teca-lutein) cell 220
theca cell-granulosa cell 236.2
uterus, in pregnancy or childbirth 654.1
vagina, in pregnancy or childbirth 654.7
vulva, in pregnancy or childbirth 654.8
yolk sac, specified site—*see* Neoplasm, by site, malignant
unspecified site 183.0
Twin pregnancy—*see* Pregnancy, multiple
Twist, twisted
organ or site, congenital NEC—*see* Anomaly, specified type NEC
ovarian pedicle 620.5
umbilical cord—*see* Compression, umbilical cord

U
Ulcer, ulcerated, ulcerating, ulceration, ulcerative
anorectal 569.41
anus (sphincter) (solitary) 569.41
aphthous, genital organ(s) 616.50
bladder (solitary) (sphincter)
submucosal (*see also* Cystitis) 595.1
tuberculous (*see also* Tuberculosis) 016.1
breast 611.0
cancerous—*see* Neoplasm, by site, malignant
cervix (uteri) (trophic) 622.0
with mention of cervicitis 616.0
chancroidal 099.0
chronic (cause unknown)—*see* Ulcer, skin

Ulcer, ulcerated, ulcerating, ulceration,
ulcerative *(continued)*
cystitis (interstitial) 595.1
decubitus (unspecified site) *(see also*
Ulcer, pressure) 707.00
duodenum (peptic) (with) 532.9
acute (with) 532.3
hemorrhage alone 532.0
hemorrhage and perforation 532.2
perforation alone 532.1
chronic (with) 532.7
hemorrhage alone 532.4
hemorrhage and perforation 532.5
perforation alone 532.6
genital organ 629.8
granuloma of pudenda 099.2
hemorrhoids 455.8
external 455.5
internal 455.2
labium (majus) (minus) 616.50
Lipschütz's 616.50
malignant—*see* Neoplasm, by site,
malignant
peptic (site unspecified) 533.9
acute (with) 533.3
hemorrhage alone 533.0
hemorrhage and perforation 533.2
perforation alone 533.1
chronic (with) 533.7
hemorrhage alone 533.4
hemorrhage and perforation 533.6
perforation alone 533.5
pressure 707.00
rectum (sphincter) (solitary) 569.41
skin (chronic) (nonhealing) (perforating)
(pyogenic) 707.9
decubitus *(see also* Ulcer, pressure)
707.00
varicose—*see* Ulcer, varicose
solitary, anus or rectum (sphincter) 69.41
stasis (leg) (venous) 454.0
inflamed or infected 454.2
stercoral, stercoraceous anus or rectum
569.41
submucosal, bladder 595.1
unspecified site NEC—*see* Ulcer, skin
urethra (meatus) *(see also* Urethritis)
597.89
uterus 621.8
cervix 622.0
with mention of cervicitis 616.0
vagina 616.89
varicose—*see* Varicose

Ulcer, ulcerated, ulcerating, ulceration,
ulcerative *(continued)*
vulva (acute) (infectional) 616.50
herpetic 054.12
tuberculous 016.7 (616.51)
vulvobuccal, recurring 616.50
X-ray—*see* Ulcer, by site
Underweight 783.22
**Unicornis, unicorporeus or uniformis
uterus** 752.3
Unilateral *(see also* condition)
development, breast 611.89
organ or site, congenital NEC—*see*
Agenesis
vagina 752.49
Universal joint, cervix 620.6
Unsatisfactory
cytology smear
anal 796.78
cervical 795.08
vaginal 795.18
Unstable lie—*see* Pregnancy, presentation
Uremia, uremic
with or complicating
abortion—*see* Abortion, by type, with
renal failure
complicating abortion 639.3
ectopic or molar pregnancy *(see also*
categories 630–633.9)
639.3
hypertension *(see also* Hypertension,
kidney) 403.91
labor and delivery 669.3
extrarenal hypertensive (chronic) *(see also*
Hypertension, kidney)
403.91
Ureterostomy status with complication
997.5
Urethralgia 788.99
Urethritis (acute) (chronic) (recurrent)
(subacute) 597.80
diplococcal (acute) 098.0
chronic or duration of 2 months or
over 098.2
due to Trichomonas (vaginalis) 131.02
gonococcal (acute) 098.0
chronic or duration of 2 months or
over 098.2
nongonococcal (sexually transmitted)
099.40
Chlamydia trachomatis 099.41
Reiter's 099.3
specified organism NEC 099.49

Urethritis *(continued)*
  nonspecific (sexually transmitted) *(see also* Urethritis, nongonococcal) 099.40
  not sexually transmitted 597.80
  tuberculous *(see also* Tuberculosis) 016.3
Urethrocele 618.03
  with uterine prolapse 618.4
    complete 618.3
    incomplete 618.2
Urethrorrhagia 599.84
Urethrorrhea 788.7
Urethrostomy status with complication 997.5
Urethrotrigonitis 595.3
Uricosuria 791.9
Urine, urinary, urination *(see also* condition)
  abnormality NEC 788.69
  blood in *(see also* Hematuria) 599.70
  discharge, excessive 788.42
  enuresis 788.30
  frequency 788.41
  hesitancy 788.64
  incontinence 788.30
    active 788.30
      stress 625.6
        and urge 788.33
      mixed (stress and urge) 788.33
    neurogenic 788.39
    overflow 788.38
  intermittent stream 788.61
  nocturnal 788.43
  painful 788.1
  psychogenic 306.53
  pus in 791.9
  retention or stasis NEC 788.20
    bladder, incomplete emptying 788.21
    psychogenic 306.53
    specified NEC 788.29
  secretion
    deficient 788.5
    excessive 788.42
    frequency 788.41
  straining on urination 788.65
  stream
    intermittent, splitting 788.61
    slowing, weak 788.62
  urgency 788.63
Urinoma NEC 599.9
  urethra 599.84
Uroarthritis, infectious 099.3

Urodialysis 788.5
Urticaria 708.9
  allergic 708.0
  cholinergic 708.5
  chronic 708.8
  cold, familial 708.2
  dermatographic 708.3
  factitial 708.3
  giant 995.1
  idiopathic 708.1
  nonallergic 708.1
  papulosa (Hebra) 698.2
  recurrent periodic 708.8
  serum 999.5
  specified type NEC 708.8
  thermal (cold) (heat) 708.2
  vibratory 708.4
Uterine size-date discrepancy 649.6
Uteromegaly 621.2

V
Vaccination
  complication or reaction—*see* Complications, vaccination
  delayed V64.00
  not done (contraindicated) V64.0
    because of patient's decision V64.2
    guardian or parent refusal V64.05
  prophylactic (against) V05.9
    chicken pox, varicella V05.4
    common cold V04.7
    disease (single) NEC V05.9
      bacterial NEC V03.9
        specified type NEC V03.89
      combination, specified type NEC V06.8
      specified type NEC V05.8
    hepatitis, viral V05.3
    influenza V04.81
      with *Streptococcus pneumoniae* (pneumococcus) V06.6
      Hemophilus influenzae, type B (Hib) V03.81
    measles-mumps-rubella (MMR) V06.4
    measles (alone) V04.2
    mumps (alone) V04.6
    poliomyelitis V04.0
    respiratory syncytial virus (RSV) V04.82
    rubella (alone) V04.3
    Streptococcus pneumoniae (pneumococcus) V03.82
      with influenza V06.6

Vaccination *(continued)*
prophylactic *(continued)*
tetanus toxoid (alone) V03.7
tuberculosis (BCG) V03.2
viral
disease NEC V04.89
hepatitis V05.3
Vaginal—*see* condition
Vaginismus (reflex) 625.1
functional or psychogenic 306.51
Vaginitis (acute) (chronic) 616.10
with or following
abortion—*see* Abortion, by type, with
sepsis
following abortion 639.0
ectopic or molar pregnancy (*see also*
categories 630–633.9)
639.0
adhesive, congenital 752.49
atrophic, postmenopausal 627.3
bacterial 616.10
blennorrhagic (acute) 098.0
chronic or duration of 2 months or
over 098.2
candidal 112.1
chlamydial 099.53
complicating pregnancy or puerperium
646.6
congenital (adhesive) 752.49
due to
C. albicans 112.1
Trichomonas (vaginalis) 131.01
gonococcal (acute) 098.0
chronic or duration of 2 months or
over 098.2
granuloma 099.2
Monilia 112.1
mycotic 112.1
postirradiation 616.10
postmenopausal atrophic 627.3
senile (atrophic) 627.3
trichomonal 131.01
tuberculous (*see also* Tuberculosis) 016.7
venereal NEC 099.8
VAIN I (vaginal intraepithelial neoplasia I)
623.0
VAIN II (vaginal intraepithelial neoplasia
II) 623.0
VAIN III (vaginal intraepithelial neoplasia
III) 233.31
Valve, valvular (formation) (*see also*
condition)
cervix, internal os 752.49
congenital NEC—*see* Atresia

Valve, valvular *(continued)*
ureter 753.29
pelvic junction 753.21
vesical orifice 753.22
urethra 753.6
Varicella (with) 052.9
complication 052.8
specified NEC 052.7
exposure to V01.71
pneumonia 052.1
vaccination and inoculation (against)
(prophylactic) V05.4
Varicocele
ovary 456.5
perineum 456.6
Varicose, varix (lower extremity) (ruptured) (with) 454.9
anus—*see* Hemorrhoids
bladder 456.5
broad ligament 456.5
edema 454.8
inflamed or infected 454.1
with ulcer 454.2
in pregnancy or puerperium 671.0
perineum 671.1
vulva 671.1
labia (majora) 456.6
ovary 456.5
pain 454.8
pelvis 456.5
perineum 456.6
in pregnancy or puerperium
671.1
placenta—*see* Placenta, abnormal
rectum—*see* Hemorrhoids
stasis dermatitis 454.1
with ulcer 454.2
swelling 454.8
ulcerated 454.0
inflamed or infected 454.2
uterine ligament 456.5
vulva 456.6
in pregnancy, childbirth, or puerperium
671.1
Vasodilation 443.9
Vasoplasty, after previous sterilization
V26.0
Venereal—*see* Disease, venereal
Verruca (filiformis) 078.10
acuminata (any site) 078.11
plana (juvenilis) plantaris 078.19
seborrheica 702.19
inflamed 702.11

Verruca *(continued)*
  senilis 702.0
  venereal 078.19
  viral NEC 078.10
Version—*see* Delivery
Vesicle, cutaneous or skin 709.8
Vestibulitis, vulvar 616.10
VIN I (vulvar intraepithelial neoplasia I)
    624.01
VIN II (vulvar intraepithelial neoplasia II)
    624.02
VIN III (vulvar intraepithelial neoplasia III)
    233.32
Viremia 790.8
Vitiligo 709.01
  vulva 624.8
Voluntary starvation 307.1
Volvulus, fallopian tube, or oviduct
    620.5
Vomiting 787.03
  with nausea 787.01
    allergic 535.4
    bilious (cause unknown) 787.04
    blood (*see also* Hematemesis) 578.0
    of or complicating pregnancy—*see*
        Pregnancy
    physiological 787.03
    psychogenic 307.54
    uremic—*see* Uremia
Vulvismus 625.1
Vulvitis (acute) (chronic) 616.10
  with or following
    abortion—*see* Abortion, by type, with
        sepsis
      following abortion 639.0
    ectopic or molar pregnancy (*see also*
        categories 630–633.9) 639.0
  adhesive, congenital 752.49
  blennorrhagic (acute) 098.0
    chronic or duration of 2 months or
        over 098.2
  chlamydial 099.53
  complicating pregnancy or puerperium
      646.6
  due to Ducrey's bacillus 099.0
  gonococcal (acute) 098.0
    chronic or duration of 2 months or
        over 098.2
  herpetic 054.11
  leukoplakic 624.09
  monilial 112.1
  puerperal, postpartum, childbirth 646.6
  trichomonal 131.01

Vulvodynia 625.70
  specified NEC 625.79
Vulvovaginitis (*see also* Vulvitis) 616.10
  chlamydial 099.53
  gonococcal (acute) 098.0
    chronic or duration of 2 months or
        over 098.2
  herpetic 054.11
  monilial 112.1
  trichomonal *(Trichomonas vaginalis)*
      131.01

W
Wart (common) (infectious) (viral) 078.10
  common 078.19
  external genital organs (venereal) 078.11
  flat 078.19
  genital 078.11
  juvenile 078.19
  moist 078.10
  plantar 078.12
  seborrheic 702.19
    inflamed 702.11
  senile 702.0
  specified NEC 078.19
  syphilitic 091.3
  venereal 078.11
Wasting pelvic muscle 618.83
Water intoxication, loading or poisoning
    276.6
Weak, weakness (generalized) 780.79
  pelvic fundus
    pubocervical tissue 618.81
    rectovaginal tissue 618.82
  urinary stream 788.62
Weight
  gain (abnormal) (excessive) 783.1
    during pregnancy 646.1
      insufficient 646.8
  loss (cause unknown) 783.21
Welcome to Medicare exam V70.0
Wheal 709.8
Wheezing 786.07
"Worried well" V65.5
Wound, open (laceration) (with initial hem-
        orrhage, not internal) 879.8
  abdomen wall (anterior) 879.2
    complicated 879.3
    lateral 879.4
      complicated 879.5
  anus 879.6
  bladder—*see* Injury, internal, bladder
  blood vessel—*see* Injury, blood vessel, by
      site

Wound, open *(continued)*
 breast 879.0
  complicated 879.1
 buttock 877.0
  complicated 877.1
 clitoris 878.8
  complicated 878.9
 fallopian tube—*see* Injury, internal, fallopian tube
 genital organs (external) NEC 878.8
  complicated 878.9
  internal—*see* Injury, internal, by
    site
 hymen 878.6
  complicated 878.7
 labium (majus) (minus) 878.4
  complicated 878.5
 multiple, unspecified site(s) 879.8
 nonhealing surgical 998.83
 pelvic floor or region 879.6
  complicated 879.7
 perineum 879.6
  complicated 879.7
 pubic region 879.2
  complicated 879.3
 pudenda 878.8
  complicated 878.9
 rectovaginal septum 878.8
  complicated 878.9
 skin NEC 879.8
 subcutaneous NEC 879.8
 surgical, nonhealing 998.83
 trunk (multiple) NEC 879.6
  complicated 879.7
  specified site NEC 879.6
   complicated 879.7
 umbilical region 879.2
  complicated 879.3
 urinary organs (internal)—*see* Injury,
    internal
 vagina 878.6
  complicated 878.7
 vulva 878.4
  complicated 878.5

X
Xanthofibroma—*see* Neoplasm, connective
    tissue, benign
Xanthosis 709.09
 surgical 998.81
Xerosis, cutis or skin 706.8
XO syndrome 758.6
XXX syndrome 758.81

XXXXY syndrome 758.81
XXY syndrome 758.82
XYY syndrome 758.81

Y
Yawning 786.09
Yeast infection (*see also* Candidiasis) 112.9

3

TABULAR LIST

Volume 1, Diseases: Tabular List contains more than 14,000 codes. This volume contains the numeric listing of categories and subcategories used to describe classifications of diseases, conditions, illnesses, and injuries. Some codes are further divided in sub-subcategories.

For example, the chapter "Diseases of the Genitourinary System" (codes 580–629) contains five sections, including "Disorders of Breast" (codes 610–611) and "Inflammatory Disease of Female Pelvic Organs" (codes 614–616). The section "Disorders of Breast" is divided into two categories, "Benign mammary dysplasias" (610) and "Other disorders of breast" (611). Category 610 is further divided into seven subcategories (610.1–610.9), including "Fibroadenosis of breast" (610.2).

TABULAR LIST (VOLUME 1) CONVENTIONS

Volume 1 conventions relate to coding multiple diagnoses, inclusion and exclusion statements, the abbreviation NOS (not otherwise specified), variable and fixed code descriptions, V codes, and E codes.

MULTIPLE DIAGNOSES

ICD-9-CM conventions sometimes indicate that two diagnoses are required to completely describe a patient's condition. The code identifying the underlying etiology is reported first, followed by the code for the manifestation. The following phrases listed under a code number in ICD-9-CM indicate both that two codes are necessary and the order in which the codes must be reported.

"Code first" means that another code is listed first. The exact wording varies: the wording may be "Code first underlying cause," "Code first underlying disease," or "Code, if applicable, any causal condition first." For example, under code 628.1 (Infertility, female, of pituitary-hypothalamic origin), is the statement:

Code first underlying cause, as:
    adiposogenital dystrophy (253.8)
    anterior pituitary disorder (253.0–253.4)

Therefore, a code for the underlying cause of the infertility (253.0–253.4 or 253.8) is listed first on the claim form followed by code 628.1.

"Use additional code" means that two codes are required, but this code is listed first. For example, a note under code 660.0 (Obstruction caused by malposition of fetus at onset of labor) states:

Use additional code from 652.0–652.9 to identify condition

Therefore, code 660.0 is listed first on the claim form followed by a code to identify the specific fetal malposition, such as breech or transverse presentation (652.0–652.9).

INCLUDES AND EXCLUDES NOTES AND INCLUSION TERMS

These notes provide additional information to assist the user in determining if a code is appropriate in a specific case. "Includes" notes appear under a code or code category to further define or give examples of the conditions reported using this code. The terms may be synonyms or, in the case of "other specified" codes, a list of various conditions assigned to that code. The inclusion terms are not necessarily exhaustive. It is not necessary for the documentation in the patient's medical record to use one of the inclusion terms in order for that code to be reported. For example, code 620.1 lists two inclusion terms:

> 620.1   Corpus luteum cyst or hematoma
> corpus luteum hemorrhage
> rupture and lutein cyst

The documentation may or may not use one of the inclusion terms.

For example, a note following code category 628 (infertility, female) states:

> Includes: primary and secondary sterility

The 628 code series is further divided into subcategories 628.0–628.9. This "includes" note applies to all the codes listed in the category. The documentation may or may not indicate that the patient has primary or secondary sterility.

"Excludes" notes appear under a code or code category to indicate that the conditions listed are not to be reported using this code, but are reported using a different one. If the documentation indicates the condition in the exclusion term, then this code is not reported. For example, a note following code 625.6 states:

> 625.6   Stress incontinence, female
> Excludes: mixed incontinence (788.33)
> Stress incontinence, male (788.32)

If the documentation indicates that the patient has either mixed or male stress incontinence, then code 625.6 is not reported. It would not be appropriate to report both 625.6 and 788.33 or 788.32.

For example, a note following code category 620 (noninflammatory disorders of ovary, fallopian tube, and broad ligament) states:

> Excludes: hydrosalpinx (614.1)

The 620 code series is further divided into subcategories 620.0–620.9. This note applies to all the codes listed in the category. Therefore, a hydrosalpinx is not reported as a noninflammatory disorder (620 series), but as chronic salpingitis (614.1). However, if the documentation indicates that the patient has both a hydrosalpinx (614.1) and a hematoma of the broad ligament (620.7), it would be appropriate to report both codes.

NOT OTHERWISE SPECIFIED

The abbreviation NOS (not otherwise specified) means that there is insufficient documentation in the patient record to choose between several ICD-9-CM codes. For example, a diagnosis of inflammatory disease of the ovary would be reported using 614.9 (unspecified inflammatory disease of female pelvic organs and tissues) which has an inclusion note "pelvic infection or inflammation, female NOS." It would be preferable, however, for the physician to provide enough documentation to enable the coder to select a more specific code from category 614, which includes codes indicating disease of specific organs and the chronic or acute nature of the condition.

NOT ELSEWHERE CLASSIFIED

The abbreviation NEC (not elsewhere classified) means that there is sufficient documentation in the patient record to describe the condition but ICD-9-CM does not include a specific code for it. For example, an ultrasound performed to determine gestational age is reported using code V28.8 (screening, antenatal, specified condition NEC) because there is no specific code for antenatal screening for gestational age.

VARIABLE AND FIXED CODE DESCRIPTIONS

Code descriptions may have either variable or fixed code descriptions. For fixed code descriptions, the complete code number with all required digits is listed next to the description for that code. For variable code descriptions, the fourth or fifth digit must be selected from a digit list found at the beginning of the code category. An example of a fixed description is code 995.83 (Adult sexual abuse). An example of a varied description is code 250.6 (Diabetes with neurological manifestations). The user must select a fifth digit (0–3) from a digit list under the code category heading 250 (Diabetes mellitus) to indicate the type of diabetes and whether it is controlled or uncontrolled.

Most codes in the obstetric chapter of ICD-9-CM (codes 630–677) have variable descriptions and use a digit list. These digit lists are described in Chapter 11.

INFECTIOUS AND PARASITIC DISEASES (001–139)

Categories for "late effects" of infectious and parasitic diseases are to be found at 137–139.

Includes: diseases generally recognized as communicable or transmissible as well as a few diseases of unknown but possibly infectious origin

Excludes: acute respiratory infections (460–466)
certain localized infections
influenza (487.0–487.8, 488)

TUBERCULOSIS

Includes: infection by *Mycobacterium tuberculosis* (human) (bovine)
The following fifth-digit subclassification is for use with category 016:

0   unspecified
1   bacteriological or histological examination not done
2   bacteriological or histological examination unknown (at present)
3   tubercle bacilli found (in sputum) by microscopy
4   tubercle bacilli not found (in sputum) by microscopy, but found by bacterial culture
5   tubercle bacilli not found by bacteriological examination, but tuberculosis confirmed histologically
6   tubercle bacilli not found by bacteriological or histological examination, but tuberculosis confirmed by other methods (inoculation of animals)

010   Primary tuberculous infection
     010.0   Primary tuberculous infection

011   Pulmonary tuberculosis
     011.5   Tuberculous bronchiectasis
     011.6   Tuberculous pneumonia (any form)
     011.9   Pulmonary tuberculous, unspecfiied

016   Tuberculosis of genitourinary system
     Requires fifth digit. See beginning of section 010–018 for definitions.
     016.0   Kidney
             Renal tuberculosis
             Use additional code to identify manifestation
     016.1   Bladder
     016.2   Ureter
     016.3   Other urinary organs
     016.6   Tuberculous oophoritis and salpingitis
     016.7   Other female genital organs
             Tuberculous:
                 cervicitis
                 endometritis
     016.9   Genitourinary tuberculosis, unspecified

OTHER BACTERIAL DISEASES

Excludes: bacterial venereal diseases (098.0–099.8)

034 Streptococcal sore throat

    034.0 Streptococcal sore throat

        Septic:

            angina

            sore throat

        Streptococcal:

            angina

            laryngitis

            pharyngitis

            tonsillitis

038 Septicemia

Use additional code for systemic inflammatory response syndrome (SIRS) (995.91–995.92)

    038.0 Streptococcal septicemia

    038.1 Staphylococcal septicemia

        038.10 Staphylococcal septicemia, unspecified

        038.11 Methicillin susceptible *Staphylococcus aureus* septicemia

            MSSA septicemia

            Staphylococcus aureus septicemia NOS

        038.12 Methicillin resistant Staphylococcus aureus septicemia

        038.19 Other staphylococcal septicemia

    038.2 Pneumococcal septicemia (*Streptococcus pneumoniae* septicemia)

    038.3 Septicemia due to anaerobes

        Septicemia due to bacteroides

        Excludes: that due to anaerobic streptococci (038.0)

    038.4 Septicemia due to other gram-negative organisms

        038.40 Gram-negative organism, unspecified

            Gram-negative septicemia NOS

        038.41 *Hemophilus influenzae (H. influenzae)*

        038.42 *Escherichia coli (E. coli)*

        038.43 Pseudomonas

        038.44 Serratia

        038.49 Other

    038.8 Other specified septicemias

        Excludes: septicemia (due to) gonococcal (098.89)

    038.9 Unspecified septicemia

        Septicemia NOS

        Excludes: bacteremia NOS (790.7)

TABULAR LIST: INFECTIOUS AND PARASITIC DISEASES (001–139)

040 Other bacterial diseases
Excludes: bacteremia NOS (790.7)
bacterial infection NOS (041.9)
040.8 Other specified bacterial diseases
040.82 Toxic shock syndrome
Use additional code to identify the organism
040.89 Other

041 Bacterial infection in conditions classified elsewhere and of unspecified site
Codes in this category are used as an additional code to identify the bacterial agent in diseases classified elsewhere. Codes in this category also are used to classify bacterial infections of unspecified nature or site.
Excludes: septicemia (038.0–038.9)
041.0 Streptococcus
041.00 Streptococcus, unspecified
041.01 Group A
041.02 Group B
041.03 Group C
041.04 Group D (Enterococcus)
041.05 Group G
041.09 Other Streptococcus
041.1 Staphylococcus
041.10 Staphylococcus, unspecified
041.11 Methicillin susceptible Staphylococcus aureus (MSSA)
Staphylococcus aureus NOS
041.12 Methicillin resistant Staphylococcus aureus
Methicillin-resistant Staphylococcus aureus (MRSA)
041.19 Other Staphylococcus
041.2 Pneumococcus
041.3 Klebsiella pneumoniae
041.4 *Escherichia coli (E.coli)*
041.5 *Hemophilus influenzae (H. influenzae)*
041.6 Proteus (mirabilis) (morganii)
041.7 Pseudomonas
041.8 Other specified bacterial infections
041.81 Mycoplasma
Eaton's agent
Pleuropneumonia-like organisms (PPLO)
041.82 *Bacteroides fragilis*
041.83 *Clostridium perfringens*
041.84 Other anaerobes
Gram-negative anaerobes

041.85 Other gram-negative organisms
Aerobacter aerogenes
Gram-negative bacteria NOS
Mima polymorpha
Serratia
Excludes: gram-negative anaerobes (041.84)
041.86 *Helicobacter pylori [H. pylori]*
041.89 Other specified bacteria
041.9 Bacterial infection, unspecified

HUMAN IMMUNODEFICIENCY VIRUS (HIV) INFECTION

042 Human immunodeficiency virus (HIV) disease, symptomatic
Acquired immune deficiency syndrome (AIDS)
AIDS-like syndrome
AIDS-related complex
ARC
Use additional code(s) to identify all manifestations of HIV
Use additional code to identify HIV-2 infection (079.53)
Excludes: asymptomatic HIV infection status (V08)
exposure to HIV virus (V01.79)
nonspecific serologic evidence of HIV (795.71)

VIRAL DISEASES GENERALLY ACCOMPANIED BY EXANTHEM

052 Chickenpox
052.0 Postvaricella encephalitis
Postchickenpox encephalitis
052.1 Varicella (hemorrhagic) pneumonitis
052.7 With other specified complications
052.8 With unspecified complication
052.9 Varicella without mention of complication
Chickenpox NOS
Varicella NOS

053 Herpes zoster
Includes: shingles
zona
053.7 With other specified complications
053.71 Otitis externa due to herpes zoster
053.79 Other
053.8 With unspecified complication
053.9 Herpes zoster without mention of complication
Herpes zoster NOS

054 Herpes simplex
054.0 Eczema herpeticum
Kaposi's varicelliform eruption
054.1 Genital herpes
054.10 Genital herpes, unspecified
Herpes progenitalis
054.11 Herpetic vulvovaginitis
054.12 Herpetic ulceration of vulva
054.19 Other

055 Measles
Includes: morbilli
Rubeola
055.8 With unspecified complication
055.9 Measles without mention of complication

056 Rubella
Includes: German measles
056.7 With other specified complications
056.79 Other
056.8 With unspecified complications
056.9 Rubella without mention of complication

058 Other human herpesvirus
Excludes: congenital herpes (771.2)
cytomegalovirus (078.5)
Epstein-Barr virus (075)
herpes simplex (054.0–054.9)
herpes zoster (053.0–053.9)
human herpesvirus (1–3) (NOS) (054.0–054.9)
human herpesvirus 4 (075)
human herpesvirus 5 (078.5)
varicella (052.0–052.9)
varicella-zoster virus (052.0–053.9)
058.8 Other human herpesvirus infections
058.81 Human herpesvirus 6 infection
058.82 Human herpesvirus 7 infection
058.89 Other human herpesvirus infection

OTHER DISEASES DUE TO VIRUSES AND CHLAMYDIAE

070 Viral hepatitis

Includes: viral hepatitis (acute) (chronic)

The following fifth-digit subclassification is for use with categories 070.2 and 070.3:

0 acute or unspecified, without mention of hepatitis delta
1 acute or unspecified, with hepatitis delta
2 chronic, without mention of hepatitis delta
3 chronic, with hepatitis delta

070.0 Viral hepatitis A with hepatic coma
070.1 Viral hepatitis A without mention of hepatic coma
       Infectious hepatitis
070.2 Viral hepatitis B with hepatic coma
070.3 Viral hepatitis B without mention of hepatic coma
       Serum hepatitis
070.4 Other specified viral hepatitis with hepatic coma
    070.41 Acute hepatitis C with hepatic coma
    070.42 Hepatitis delta without mention of active hepatitis B disease with hepatic coma
        Hepatitis delta with hepatitis B carrier state
    070.43 Hepatitis E with hepatic coma
    070.44 Chronic hepatitis C with hepatic coma
    070.49 Other specified viral hepatitis with hepatic coma
070.5 Other specified viral hepatitis without mention of hepatic coma
    070.51 Acute hepatitis C without mention of hepatic coma
    070.52 Hepatitis delta without mention of active hepatitis B disease or hepatic coma
    070.53 Hepatitis E without mention of hepatic coma
    070.54 Chronic hepatitis C without mention of hepatic coma
    070.59 Other specified viral hepatitis without mention of hepatic coma
        Unspecified viral hepatitis with hepatic coma
070.9 Unspecified viral hepatitis without mention of hepatic coma
       Viral hepatitis NOS

072 Mumps

072.8 Mumps with unspecified complication
072.9 Mumps without mention of complication

TABULAR LIST: INFECTIOUS AND PARASITIC DISEASES (001–139)

075   **Infectious mononucleosis**
Glandular fever
Monocytic angina
Pfeiffer's disease

078   **Other diseases due to viruses and Chlamydiae**
Excludes: viral infection NOS (079.4–079.9)
078.0   *Molluscum contagiosum*
078.1   Viral warts
Viral warts due to human papillomavirus
078.10   Viral warts, unspecified
Verruca:
NOS
Vulgaris
Warts (infectious)
078.11   *Condyloma acuminatum*
Condyloma NOS
Gential warts NOS
078.12   Plantar wart
Verruca plantaris
078.19   Other specified genital viral warts
Common wart
Flat wart
Verruca plana

079   **Viral and chlamydial infection in conditions classified elsewhere and of unspecified site**
Codes in this category are used as an additional code to identify the viral agent in diseases classifiable elsewhere. Codes in this category also are used to classify virus infection of unspecified nature or site.
079.4   Human papillomavirus
079.5   Retrovirus
Excludes: human immunodeficiency virus, type 1 (HIV-1) (042)
human T-cell lymphotrophic virus, type III (HTLV-III) (042)
lymphadenopathy-associated virus (LAV) (042)
079.50   Retrovirus, unspecified
079.51   Human T-cell lymphotrophic virus, type I (HTLV-I)
079.52   Human T-cell lymphotrophic virus, type II (HTLV-II)
079.53   Human immunodeficiency virus, type 2 (HIV-2)
079.59   Other specified retrovirus
079.8   Other specified viral and chlamydial infections
079.82   SARS-associated coronavirus

079.83 Parvovirus B19
        Human parvovirus
        Parvovirus NOS
079.88 Other specified chlamydial infection
079.89 Other specified viral infection
079.9 Unspecified viral and chlamydial infections
079.98 Unspecified chlamydial infection
        Chlamydial infection NOS
079.99 Unspecified viral infection
        Viral infection NOS

SYPHILIS AND OTHER VENEREAL DISEASES

Excludes: urogenital trichomoniasis (131.0)

090 Congenital syphilis
090.0 Early congenital syphilis, symptomatic
       Any congenital syphilitic condition specified as early or manifest less
       than 2 years after birth

091 Early syphilis, symptomatic
091.0 Genital syphilis (primary)
       Genital chancre
091.1 Primary anal syphilis
091.2 Other primary syphilis
       Primary syphilis of:
            breast
            fingers
            lip
            tonsils
091.3 Secondary syphilis of skin or mucous membranes
       Condyloma latum
       Secondary syphilis of:
            anus
            mouth
            pharynx
            skin
            tonsils
            vulva
091.4 Adenopathy due to secondary syphilis
       Syphilitic adenopathy (secondary)
       Syphilitic lymphadenitis (secondary)
091.7 Secondary syphilis, relapse
       Secondary syphilis, relapse (treated) (untreated)
091.8 Other forms of secondary syphilis
       091.89 Other
091.9 Unspecified secondary syphilis

098 Gonococcal infections

098.0 Acute, lower genitourinary tract
Gonococcal:
Bartholinitis (acute)
urethritis (acute)
vulvovaginitis (acute)
Gonorrhea (acute):
NOS
genitourinary (tract) NOS

098.1 Acute, upper genitourinary tract
098.10 Gonococcal infection (acute) of upper genitourinary tract, site unspecified
098.11 Gonococcal cystitis (acute)
Gonorrhea (acute) of bladder
098.15 Gonococcal cervicitis (acute)
Gonorrhea (acute) of cervix
098.16 Gonococcal endometritis (acute)
Gonorrhea (acute) of uterus
098.17 Gonococcal salpingitis, specified as acute
098.19 Other

098.2 Chronic, lower genitourinary tract
Gonococcal specified as chronic or with duration of 2 months or more:
Bartholinitis
urethritis
vulvovaginitis
Gonorrhea specified as chronic or with duration of 2 months or more:
NOS
genitourinary (tract)
Any condition classifiable to 098.0 specified as chronic or with duration of 2 months or more

098.3 Chronic, upper genitourinary tract
Any condition classifiable to 098.1 stated as chronic or with a duration of 2 months or more
098.30 Chronic gonococcal infection of upper genitourinary tract, site unspecified
098.31 Gonococcal cystitis, chronic
Any condition classifiable to 098.11, specified as chronic
Gonorrhea of bladder, chronic
098.35 Gonococcal cervicitis, chronic
Any condition classifiable to 098.15, specified as chronic
Gonorrhea of cervix, chronic
098.36 Gonococcal endometritis, chronic
Any condition classifiable to 098.16, specified as chronic

098.37 Gonococcal salpingitis (chronic)
098.39 Other
098.7 Gonococcal infection of anus and rectum
Gonococcal proctitis
098.8 Gonococcal infection of other specified sites
098.86 Gonococcal peritonitis
098.89 Other
Gonococcemia

099 Other venereal diseases
099.0 Chancroid
Bubo (inguinal):
chancroidal
due to Hemophilus ducreyi
Chancre:
Ducrey's simple soft
Ulcus molle (cutis) (skin)
099.1 Lymphogranuloma venereum
Climatic or tropical bubo
(Durand-) Nicolas-Favre disease
Esthiomene
Lymphogranuloma inguinale
099.2 Granuloma inguinale
Donovanosis
Granuloma pudendi (ulcerating)
Granuloma venereum
Pudendal ulcer
099.3 Reiter's disease (syndrome)
099.4 Other nongonococcal urethritis (NGU)
099.40 Unspecified
Nonspecific urethritis
099.41 Chlamydia trachomatis
099.49 Other specified organism
099.5 Other venereal diseases due to *Chlamydia trachomatis*
Excludes: Lymphogranuloma venereum (099.1)
099.50 Unspecified site
099.52 Anus and rectum
099.53 Lower genitourinary sites
Excludes: urethra (099.41)
Use additional code to specify site of infection, such as:
cervix (616.0)
vagina and vulva (616.11)

099.54 Other genitourinary sites
Use additional code to specify site of infection, such as:
pelvic inflammatory disease NOS (614.9)
099.55 Unspecified genitourinary site
099.56 Peritoneum
099.59 Other specified site
099.8 Other specified venereal diseases

MYCOSES

110 Dermatophytosis
Includes: infection by species of Epidermophyton, Microsporum,
and Trichophyton Tinea
110.1 Of nail
Dermatophytic onychia
Tinea unguium
Onychomycosis
110.3 Of groin and perianal area
Dhobie itch
Eczema marginatum
Tinea cruris
110.8 Of other specified sites
Vulva

112 Candidiasis
Includes: infection by Candida species
Moniliasis
112.1 Of vulva and vagina
Candidal vulvovaginitis
Monilial vulvovaginitis
112.2 Of other urogenital sites
112.8 Of other specified sites
112.89 Of other specified sites
112.9 Of unspecified sites

OTHER INFECTIOUS AND PARASITIC DISEASES

131 Trichomoniasis
Includes: infection due to Trichomonas (vaginalis)
131.0 Urogenital trichomoniasis
131.00 Urogenital trichomoniasis, unspecified
Fluor (vaginalis) trichomonal or due to Trichomonas
(vaginalis)
Leukorrhea (vaginalis) trichomonal or due to Trichomonas
(vaginalis)

      131.01 Trichomonal vulvovaginitis
                Vaginitis, trichomonal or due to Trichomonas (vaginalis)
      131.02 Trichomonal urethritis
      131.09 Other
   131.8 Other specified sites
   131.9 Trichomoniasis, unspecified

132 Pediculosis and phthirus infestation
   132.2 Phthirus pubis (pubic louse)
            Pediculus pubis

NEOPLASMS (140–239)

All neoplasms are classified in this section, whether or not functionally active. An additional code from the section "Endocrine, Nutritional and Metabolic Diseases, and Immunity Disorders" may be used to identify such functional activity associated with any neoplasm.

MALIGNANT NEOPLASM OF DIGESTIVE ORGANS AND PERITONEUM

Excludes: carcinoma in situ (230.3–230.7)

150 Malignant neoplasm of esophagus
   150.8 Specified part
   150.9 Unspecified part

151 Malignant neoplasm of stomach
   151.8 Specified part
   151.9 Unspecified part

152 Malignant neoplasm of small intestine, including duodenum
   152.8 Specified part
   152.9 Unspecified part

153 Malignant neoplasm of colon
   153.5 Appendix
   153.9 Colon, unspecified

154 Malignant neoplasm of rectum, rectosigmoid junction, and anus
   154.0 Rectosigmoid junction
            Large colon and rectum
   154.1 Rectum
            Rectal ampulla
   154.2 Anal canal
            Anal sphincter
            Excludes: skin of anus (172.5, 173.5)

154.3 Anus, unspecified
Excludes: anus:
margin (172.5, 173.5)
skin (172.5, 173.50)
perianal skin (172.5, 173.5)
154.8 Other
Anorectum (junction)
Contiguous sites with rectosigmoid junction or rectum

155 Malignant neoplasm of liver and interhepatic bile ducts
155.0 Liver, primary
155.1 Intrahepatic bile ducts
155.2 Liver, not specified as primary or secondary

156 Malignant neoplasm of gallbladder and extrahepatic bile ducts
156.8 Specified sites
156.9 Biliary tract, part unspecified

157 Malignant neoplasm of pancreas
157.8 Specified sites
157.9 Unspecified sites

158 Malignant neoplasm of retroperitoneum and peritoneum
158.0 Retroperitoneum
Periadrenal tissue
Perinephric tissue
Perirenal tissue
Retrocecal tissue
158.8 Specified parts of peritoneum
Douglas' cul-de-sac
Mesentery
Mesoappendix
Mesocolon
Omentum
Peritoneum:
parietal
pelvic
Rectouterine pouch
Malignant neoplasm of contiguous or overlapping sites of
retroperitoneum and peritoneum whose point of origin cannot
be determined
158.9 Peritoneum, unspecified
peritoneal cavity

159 Malignant neoplasm of other and ill-defined sites within the digestive organs and peritoneum

    159.8 Other sites of digestive system and intra-adominal organs

          Contiguous sites with peritoneum

MALIGNANT NEOPLASM OF BONE, CONNECTIVE TISSUE, SKIN, AND BREAST

Excludes: carcinoma in situ:

        breast (233.0)

        skin (232.5–232.9)

171 Malignant neoplasm of connective and other soft tissue

    Excludes: connective tissue:

          Breast (174.0–74.89)

          Internal organs—code to malignant neoplasm of the site

          Uterine ligament (183.4)

    171.4 Thorax

        Connective tissue of axilla

    171.5 Abdomen

        Abdominal wall

        Connective tissue of abdomen

        Hypochondrium

        Excludes: peritoneum (158.8)

              retroperitoneum (158.0)

    171.6 Pelvis

        Axilla

        NEC

        Perineum

        Rectovaginal septum and wall

        Perineum

        Excludes: pelvic peritoneum (158.8)

              retroperitoneum (158.0)

              suterine ligament, any (183.3–183.5)

172 Malignant melanoma of skin

    Includes: melanocarcinoma

          melanoma in situ of skin

          melanoma (skin) NOS

    Excludes: skin of genital organs (184.0–184.9)

          sites other than skin-code to malignant neoplasm of the site

    172.5 Trunk

        Axilla

        Breast

        Perianal skin

        Perineum

        Umbilicus

        Excludes: anal canal (154.2)

              anus NOS (154.3)

172.8 Other specified sites of skin
       Malignant melanoma of contiguous or overlapping sites of skin
       whose point of origin cannot be determined
172.9 Melanoma of skin, site unspecified

173 Other malignant neoplasm of skin
Includes: malignant neoplasm of:
                  sebaceous glands
                  sudoriferous, sudoriparous glands
                  sweat glands
Excludes: malignant melanoma of skin (172.5–172.9)
                skin of genital organs (184.0–184.9)
173.5 Skin of trunk
       Axillary fold
       Perianal skin
       Skin of:
           abdominal wall
           anus
           breast
           mastectomy site
           perineum
       Umbilicus
       Excludes: anal canal (154.2)
                       anus NOS (154.3)
173.8 Other specified sites of skin
       Malignant neoplasm of contiguous or overlapping sites of skin
       whose point of origin cannot be determined
173.9 Skin, site unspecified
       Scar NEC

174 Malignant neoplasm of female breast
Includes: breast (female)
                connective tissue
                soft parts
                Paget's disease of:
                    breast
                    nipple
Use additional code to identify estrogen receptor status (V86.0, V86.1)
Excludes: skin of breast (172.5, 173.5)
174.0 Nipple and areola
174.1 Central portion
174.2 Upper-inner quadrant

174.3 Lower-inner quadrant

174.4 Upper-outer quadrant

174.5 Lower-outer quadrant

174.6 Axillary tail

174.8 Other specified sites of female breast
Ectopic sites
Inner breast
Lower breast
Midline of breast
Outer breast
Upper breast
Malignant neoplasm of contiguous or overlapping sites of breast
whose point of origin cannot be determined

174.9 Breast, unspecified

MALIGNANT NEOPLASM OF GENITOURINARY ORGANS

Excludes: carcinoma in situ (233.1–233.9)

179 Malignant neoplasm of uterus, part unspecified

180 Malignant neoplasm of cervix uteri
Includes: invasive malignancy (carcinoma)
Excludes: carcinoma in situ (233.1)

180.0 Endocervix (Internal os)
Cervical canal NOS
Endocervical canal or gland

180.1 Exocervix (External os)

180.8 Other specified sites of cervix
Cervical stump
Squamocolumnar junction of cervix
Malignant neoplasm of contiguous or overlapping sites of cervix
uteri whose point of origin cannot be determined

180.9 Cervix uteri, unspecified

181 Malignant neoplasm of placenta
Choriocarcinoma NOS
Chorioepithelioma NOS
Excludes: chorioadenoma (destruens) (236.1)
hydatidiform mole (630)
malignant (236.1)
invasive mole (236.1)

182 **Malignant neoplasm of body of uterus**
   Excludes: carcinoma in situ (233.2)
   182.0 Corpus uteri, except isthmus
      Cornu
      Endometrium
      Fundus
      Myometrium
   182.1 Isthmus
      Lower uterine segment
   182.8 Other specified sites of body of uterus
      Malignant neoplasm of contiguous or overlapping sites of body of
      uterus whose point of origin cannot be determined
      Excludes: uterus NOS (179)

183 **Malignant neoplasm of ovary and other uterine adnexa**
   Excludes: Douglas' cul-de-sac (158.8)
   183.0 Ovary
      Use additional code to identify any functional activity
   183.2 Fallopian tube
   183.3 Broad ligament
      Mesovarium
      Parovarian region
   183.4 Parametrium
      Uterine ligament NOS
      Uterosacral ligament
   183.5 Round ligament
   183.8 Other specified sites of uterine adnexa
      Tubo-ovarian or utero-ovarian
      Malignant neoplasm of contiguous or overlapping sites of ovary
      and other uterine adnexa whose point of origin cannot be
      determined
   183.9 Uterine adnexa, unspecified

184 **Malignant neoplasm of other and unspecified female genital organs**
   Excludes: carcinoma in situ (233.30–233.39)
   184.0 Vagina
      Gartner's duct
      Hymen
      Vaginal vault
   184.1 Labia majora
      Greater vestibular (Bartholin's) gland

184.2 Labia minora
184.3 Clitoris
184.4 Vulva, unspecified
External female genitalia NOS
Labia (skin)
Pudendum
184.8 Other specified sites of female genital organs
Malignant neoplasm of contiguous or overlapping sites of female
genital organs whose point of origin cannot be determined
184.9 Female genital organ, site unspecified
Female genitourinary tract NOS
Vesicovaginal

189 **Malignant neoplasm of kidney and other and unspecified urinary organs**
189.2 Ureter
189.3 Urethra

MALIGNANT NEOPLASM OF OTHER UNSPECIFIED SITES

Excludes: carcinoma in situ (234.8–234.9)

195 **Malignant neoplasm of other and ill-defined sites**
Includes: malignant neoplasms of contiguous sites, not elsewhere
classified, whose point of origin cannot be determined
Excludes: malignant neoplasm:
lymphatic and hematopoietic tissue (200.0–200.8)
secondary sites (197.8–198.0)
unspecified site (199.0–199.1)
195.2 Abdomen
Intra-abdominal NOS
195.3 Pelvis
Inguinal region NOS
Paravaginal
Pelvic floor
Perineum
Presacral region
Sacrococcygeal region
Sites overlapping systems within pelvis, as:
rectovaginal (septum)
rectovesical (septum)
195.8 Other specified sites
Abdominopelvic

197   Secondary malignant neoplasm of respiratory and digestive systems
  197.5 Large intestine and rectum
         Anorectum (junction)
         Anus, anal canal
         Appendix
         Large colon and rectum
  197.6 Retroperitoneum and peritoneum
         Douglas' cul-de-sac
         Mesoappendix
         Omentum
  197.8 Other digestive organs and spleen

198   Secondary malignant neoplasm of other specified sites
  198.1 Other urinary organs
  198.2 Skin
         Scar NEC
         Anus
         Axilla
         Breast
             Mastectomy site (skin)
  198.6 Ovary
  198.8 Other specified sites
         198.81 Breast
                 Areola
                 Connective tissue of breast
                 Nipple
                 Excludes: skin of breast (198.2)
         198.82 Genital organs
                 Adnexa
                 Bartholin's gland
                 Broad ligament
                 Cervix
                 Clitoris
                 Corpus uteri
                 Endocervix
                 Endometrium
                 Fallopian tube
                 Hymen
                 Isthmus
                 Labia (major, minor)
                 Round ligament
                 Squamocolumnar junction of cervix
                 Vagina
                 Vesicovaginal
                 Vulva

198.89 Other
Abdomen
Axilla, axillary
Connective tissue of:
    Axillary
    Abdomen
    NEC
    Pelvic floor
    Perineum
    Rectovaginal septum and wall
Lymph, lymphatic channels NEC
Paravaginal
Pelvic floor
Perineum
Rectovaginal septum

199 Malignant neoplasm without specification of site
199.0 Disseminated
Carcinomatosis unspecified site (primary) (secondary)
Generalized: cancer (malignancy) unspecified site (primary)
    (secondary)
Multiple cancer unspecified site (primary) (secondary)
199.1 Other
Cancer (carcinoma) (malignancy) unspecified site (primary)
(secondary)

MALIGNANT NEOPLASM OF LYMPHATIC AND HEMATOPOIETIC TISSUE
The following fifth-digit subclassification is for use with category 200:
0   unspecified site, extranodal and solid organ sites
3   intraabdominal lymph nodes
4   lymph nodes of axilla and upper limb
5   lymph nodes of inguinal region and lower limb
6   intrapelvic lymph nodes
8   lymph nodes of multiple sites

200 Lymphosarcoma and reticulosarcoma and other specified malignant tumors of lymphatic tissue
200.0 Reticulosarcoma
Lymphoma (malignant):
    histiocytic (diffuse):
        nodular
        pleomorphic cell type
    reticulum cell type
Reticulum cell sarcoma:
    NOS
    pleomorphic cell type

200.1 Lymphosarcoma
Lymphoblastoma (diffuse)
Lymphoma (malignant):
  lymphoblastic (diffuse)
  lymphocytic (cell type) (diffuse)
  lymphosarcoma type
Lymphosarcoma:
  NOS
  diffuse NOS
  lymphoblastic (diffuse)
  lymphocytic (diffuse)
  prolymphocytic
Excludes: lymphosarcoma:
  mixed cell type (200.8)
200.6 Anaplastic large cell lymphoma
200.7 Large cell lymphoma
200.8 Other named variants
Lymphoma (malignant):
  lymphoplasmacytoid type
  mixed lymphocytic-histiocytic (diffuse)
Lymphosarcoma, mixed cell type (diffuse)
Reticulolymphosarcoma (diffuse)

Benign Neoplasms

211 Benign neoplasm of other parts of digestive system
211.3 Colon
Appendix
Cecum
Ileocecal valve
Large intestine NOS
Excludes: rectosigmoid junction (211.4)
211.4 Rectum and anal canal
Anal canal or sphincter
Anorectum (junction)
Anus NOS
Large colon and rectum
Rectosigmoid junction
Excludes: anus:
  margin (216.5)
  skin (216.5)
  perianal skin (216.5)

211.8 Retroperitoneum and peritoneum
Douglas' cul-de-sac
Mesentery
Mesoappendix
Mesocolon
Omentum
Retroperitoneal tissue

214 Lipoma
Includes: angiolipoma
fibrolipoma
hibernoma
lipoma (fetal) (infiltrating) (intramuscular)
myelolipoma
myxolipoma
214.0 Skin and subcutaneous tissue of face
214.1 Other skin and subcutaneous tissue
214.3 Intra-abdominal organs
214.8 Other specified sites

215 Other benign neoplasm of connective and other soft tissue
Excludes: connective tissue of:
breast (217)
internal organ, except lipoma and hemangioma—code to
benign neoplasm of the site
lipoma (214.0–214.8)
215.5 Abdomen
Abdominal wall
Benign stromal tumors of abdomen
Hypochondrium
215.6 Pelvis
NEC
Pelvic floor
Perineum
Rectovaginal septum or wall
Excludes: uterine:
leiomyoma (218.9)
ligament, any (221.0)
215.8 Other specified sites
Pelvo-abdominal
215.9 Site unspecified
Connective tissue NEC
Lymph, lymphatic channels NEC

216 Benign neoplasm of skin
   Includes: blue nevus
                  dermatofibroma
                  hydrocystoma
                  pigmented nevus
                  syringoadenoma
                  syringoma
   Excludes: skin of genital organs (221.0–221.9)
   216.5 Skin of trunk
              Abdominal wall
              Axilla
              Anus
              Breast
              Perineum
              Umbilicus
              Excludes: anal canal (211.4)
                              anus NOS (211.4)
   216.8 Other specified sites of skin
              Skin, site unspecified
              Scar NEC

217 Benign neoplasm of breast
   Breast:
              areola
              nipple
              connective tissue
              glandular tissue
              soft parts
   Excludes: adenofibrosis (610.2)
                   benign cyst of breast (610.0)
                   fibrocystic disease (610.1)
                   skin of breast (216.5)

218 Uterine leiomyoma
   Includes: fibroid (bleeding) (uterine)
                   uterine fibromyoma (myoma)
   218.0 Submucous leiomyoma of uterus
   218.1 Intramural leiomyoma of uterus
              Interstitial leiomyoma of uterus
   218.2 Subserous leiomyoma of uterus
              Subperitoneal leiomyoma of uterus
   218.9 Leiomyoma of uterus, unspecified

219 Other benign neoplasm of uterus
219.0 Cervix uteri
Squamocolumnar junction of cervix
219.1 Corpus uteri
Endometrium
Fundus
Isthmus
Myometrium
219.8 Other specified parts of uterus
219.9 Uterus, part unspecified

220 Benign neoplasm of ovary
Use additional code to identify any functional activity (256.0–256.1)
Excludes: cyst:
corpus albicans (620.2)
corpus luteum (620.1)
endometrial (617.1)
follicular (atretic) (620.0)
graafian follicle (620.0)
ovarian NOS (620.2)
retention (620.2)

221 Benign neoplasm of other female genital organs
Includes: adenomatous polyp
benign teratoma
Excludes: cyst:
epoophoron (752.11)
fimbrial (752.11)
Gartner's duct (752.11)
parovarian (752.11)
221.0 Fallopian tube and uterine ligaments
Parametrium
Uterine ligament (broad) (round) (uterosacral)
221.1 Vagina
Hymen
221.2 Vulva
Clitoris
External female genitalia NOS
Greater vestibular (Bartholin's) gland
Labia (majora) (minora)
Pudendum
Excludes: Bartholin's (duct) (gland) cyst (616.2)
221.8 Other specified sites of female genital organs
Adnexa

221.9 Female genital organ, site unspecified
Female genitourinary tract NOS
Vesicovaginal

229 Benign neoplasm of other and unspecified sites
Lymph nodes
Axilla
Inguinal
Intra-abdominal
Intra-pelvic
Multiple sites
229.8 Other specified sites
Abdominopelvic
Axilla, axillary
Intra-abdominal
Paravaginal
Pelvic floor
Perineum
Rectovaginal septum
229.9 Site unspecified
Generalized
Disseminated

CARCINOMA IN SITU

Includes: Bowen's disease
erythroplasia
Queyrat's erythroplasia
Excludes: leukoplakia—*see* Alphabetic Index
230 Carcinoma in situ of digestive organs
230.3 Colon
Appendix
Cecum
Ileocecal valve
Large intestine NOS
Excludes: rectosigmoid junction (230.4)
230.4 Rectum
Rectosigmoid junction
Large colon and rectum
230.5 Anal canal
Anal sphincter
230.6 Anus, unspecified
Excludes: anus:
margin (232.5)
skin (232.5)
perianal skin (232.5)

230.7 Other and unspecified parts of intestine
      Anorectum (junction)
      Small intestine NOS

232 Carcinoma in situ of skin
    Includes: pigment cells
    Excludes: melanoma in situ of skin (172.0–172.9)
232.5 Skin of trunk
      Abdominal wall
      Anus
      Axilla
      Breast
      Perineum
      Umbilicus
      Excludes: anal canal (230.5)
                anus NOS (230.6)
                skin of genital organs (233.30–233.39, 233.5–233.6)
232.8 Other specified sites of skin
232.9 Skin, site unspecified
      Scar NEC

233 Carcinoma in situ of breast and genitourinary system
233.0 Breast
      Areola
      Connective tissue of breast
      Nipple
      Excludes: Paget's disease (174.0–174.9)
                skin of breast (232.5)
233.1 Cervix uteri
      adenocarcinoma in situ of cervix
      Cervical intraepithelial glandular neoplasia, grade III
      For additional information concerning coding for cervical neoplasms, see Appendix B.
      Cervical intraepithelial neoplasia III (CIN III)
      Severe dysplasia of cervix
      Excludes: cervical intraepithelial neoplasia II (CIN II) (622.12)
                cytologic evidence of malignancy without histologic confirmation (795.06)
                high grade squamous intraepithelial lesion (HGSIL) (795.04)
                moderate dysplasia of cervix (622.12)
233.2 Other and unspecified parts of uterus
      Corpus uteri
      Isthmus
      Endometrium

233.3 Other and unspecified female genital organs
    233.30 Unspecified female genital organ
    233.31 Vagina
        Hymen
        Severe dysplasia of vagina
        Vaginal intraepithelial neoplasia III (VAIN III)
    233.32 Vulva
        Bartholin's gland, clitoris
        Severe dysplasia of vulva
        Vulvar intraepithelial neoplasia III (VIN III)
    233.39 Other female genital organ
        Adnexa
        Broad ligament
        Fallopian tube
        Vesicovaginal

234 Carcinoma in situ of other and unspecified sites
    234.8 Other specified sites
        Abdominopelvic
        Axilla, axillary
        Intra-abdominal
        Pelvic floor
        Perineum
        Rectovaginal septum
    234.9 Site unspecified
        Carcinoma in situ NOS

Neoplasms of Uncertain Behavior

Categories 235–238 classify by site certain histomorphologically well-defined neoplasms, the subsequent behavior of which cannot be predicted from the present appearance.

235 Neoplasm of uncertain behavior of digestive and respiratory systems
    235.2 Stomach, intestines, and rectum
        Appendix
        Anorectum (junction)
        Large colon and rectum
        Small intestine
    235.4 Retroperitoneum and peritoneum
        Douglas' cul-de-sac
        Mesoappendix
        Omentum

235.5 Other and unspecified digestive organs
Anal:
    canal
    sphincter
Anorectal junction
Anus NOS
Connective tissue of retroperitoneum
Excludes: anus:
        margin (238.2)
        skin (238.2)
        perianal skin (238.2)

236 Neoplasm of uncertain behavior of genitourinary organs
236.0 Uterus
Cervix
Endometrium
Isthmus
Squamocolumnar junction of cervix
236.1 Placenta
Chorioadenoma (destruens)
Invasive mole
Malignant hydatid(iform) mole
236.2 Ovary
Use additional code to identify any functional activity
236.3 Other and unspecified female genital organs
Adnexa
Bartholin's gland
Broad ligament
Clitoris
Corpus uteri
Fallopian tube
Hymen
Labia (majora, minora)
Round ligament
Vagina
Vesicovaginal
Vulva
236.7 Bladder
236.9 Other and unspecified urinary organs
    236.90 Urinary organ, unspecified
    236.91 Kidney and ureter
    236.99 Other

238 **Neoplasm of uncertain behavior of other and unspecified sites and tissues**

238.1 Connective and other soft tissue
Abdomen
Axillary
Lymph, lymphatic channels NEC
Paravaginal
Pelvic floor
Perineum
Rectovaginal septum or wall

238.2 Skin
Abdominal wall
Anus
Axillary fold
Breast (skin)
Scar NEC

238.3 Breast
Areola
Nipple
Excludes: skin of breast (238.2)

238.8 Other specified sites
Abdominopelvic
Axilla
Intra-abdominal
Multiple sites
Paravaginal
Pelvic floor
Perineum
Rectovaginal septum

238.9 Site unspecified
Generalized
Disseminated

NEOPLASMS OF UNSPECIFIED NATURE

239 **Neoplasms of unspecified nature**

Category 239 classifies by site neoplasms of unspecified morphology and behavior. The term "mass," unless otherwise stated, is not to be regarded as a neoplastic growth.

Includes: "growth" NOS
neoplasm NOS
new growth NOS
tumor NOS

239.3 Breast
      Areola
      Breast connective tissue
      Nipple
239.4 Bladder
239.5 Other genitourinary organs
      Adnexa
      Broad ligament
      Cervix
      Clitoris
      Endometrium
      Fallopian tube
      Isthmus
      Hymen
      Labia (majora, minora)
      Ovary
      Squamocolumnar junction of cervix
      Vagina
      Vesicovaginal
      Vulva
239.8 Other specified sites
      Abdominopelvic
      Axilla, axillary
      Intra-abdominal
      Multiple sites secondary and unspecified
      Paravaginal
      Pelvic floor
      Perineum
      Rectovaginal septum
      239.89 Other specified sites
239.9 Site unspecified

ENDOCRINE, NUTRITIONAL, AND METABOLIC DISEASES AND IMMUNITY DISORDERS (240–279)

All neoplasms, whether functionally active or not, are classified in the "Neoplasms" section. Codes in this section (ie, 251–253, 256, 259) may be used to identify such functional activity associated with any neoplasm, or by ectopic endocrine tissue.

240 Simple and unspecified goiter
    240.0 Goiter, specified as simple
        Any condition classifiable to 240.9, specified as simple
    240.9 Goiter, unspecified
        Enlarged thyroid

244 Acquired hypothyroidism
244.0 Postsurgical hypothyroidism
244.1 Other postablative hypothyroidism
Hypothyroidism following therapy, such as irradiation
244.2 Iodine hypothyroidism
Hypothyroidism resulting from administration or ingestion of iodine
244.3 Other iatrogenic hypothyroidism

DISEASES OF OTHER ENDOCRINE GLANDS

249 Secondary diabetes mellitus
Includes: diabetes mellitus (due in) (in) (secondary) (with):
drug-induced or chemical induced infection

Use additional code to identify any associated insulin use (V58.67)

Excludes: gestational diabetes (648.8)
nonclinical diabetes (790.29)
Type I diabetes—see category 250
Type II diabetes—see category 250

The following fifth-digit subclassification is for use with category 249:
0 not stated as controlled, or unspecified
1 controlled
249.0 Secondary diabetes mellitus without mention of complication
Secondary diabetes mellitus without mention of complication or manifestation classifiable to 249.1–249.9
Secondary diabetes NOS
249.1 Secondary diabetes mellitus with ketoacidosis
Secondary diabetes mellitus with diabetes acidosis without mention of coma
Secondary diabetes mellitus with diabetic ketosis without mention of coma
249.2 Secondary diabetes mellitus with hyperosmolarity
Secondary diabetes mellitus with hypersmolar (nonketotic) coma
249.3 Secondary diabetes mellitus with other coma
Secondary diabetes mellitus with diabetic coma (with ketoacidosis)
Secondary diabetes mellitus with diabetic hypoglycemic coma
Secondary diabetes mellitus with insulin coma NOS
Excludes: secondary diabetes mellitus with hypersomolar coma (249.2)
249.4 Secondary diabetes mellitus with renal manifestations
Use additional code to identify manifestation
249.5 Secondary diabetes mellitus with opthalmic manifestations
Use additional code to identify manifestation
249.6 Secondary diabetes mellitus with neurological manifestations

Use additional code to identify manifestation

249.7 Secondary diabetes mellitus with peripheral circulatory disorders

Use additional code to identify manifestation

249.8 Secondary diabetes mellitus with other specified manifestations

Secondary diabetic hypoglycemia in diabetes mellitus

Secondary hypoglycemic shock in diabetes mellitus

Use additional code to identify manifestation

249.9 Secondary diabetes mellitus with unspecified complication

250 Diabetes mellitus

Excludes: gestational diabetes (648.8)

nonclinical diabetes (790.29)

The following fifth-digit subclassification is for use with category 250:

0 type II or unspecified type, not stated as uncontrolled

Fifth-digit 0 is for use for type II patients, even if the patient requires insulin

Use additional code, if applicable, for associated long-term (current) insulin use V58.67

1 type I (juvenile type), not stated as uncontrolled

2 type II or unspecified type, uncontrolled

Fifth-digit 2 is for use for type II patients, even if the patient requires insulin

Use additional code, if applicable, for associated long-term (current) insulin use V58.67

3 type I (juvenile type), uncontrolled

250.0 Diabetes mellitus without mention of complication

Diabetes mellitus without mention of complication or manifestation classifiable to 250.1–250.9

Diabetes (mellitus) NOS

250.1 Diabetes with ketoacidosis

Diabetic:

acidosis without mention of coma

ketosis without mention of coma

250.2 Diabetes with hyperosmolarity

Hyperosmolar (nonketotic) coma

250.3 Diabetes with other coma

Diabetic coma (with ketoacidosis)

Diabetic hypoglycemic coma

Insulin coma NOS

Excludes: diabetes with hyperosmolar coma (250.2)

250.4 Diabetes with renal manifestations

Use additional code to identify manifestation

250.5 Diabetes with ophthalmic manifestations
Use additional code to identify manifestation
250.6 Diabetes with neurological manifestations
Use additional code to identify manifestation
250.7 Diabetes with peripheral circulatory disorders
Use additional code to identify manifestation
250.8 Diabetes with other specified manifestations
Diabetic hypoglycemia NOS
Hypoglycemic shock NOS
250.9 Diabetes with unspecified complication

251 Other disorders of pancreatic internal secretion
251.0 Hypoglycemic coma
Iatrogenic hyperinsulinism
Nondiabetic insulin coma
Use additional E code to identify cause, if drug-induced
Excludes: hypoglycemic coma in diabetes mellitus (249.3, 250.3)
251.1 Other specified hypoglycemia
Hyperinsulinism:
NOS
ectopic
functional
Hyperplasia of pancreatic islet beta cells NOS
Excludes: hypoglycemia in diabetes mellitus (249.8, 250.8)
hypoglycemic coma (251.0)
251.2 Hypoglycemia, unspecified
Hypoglycemia:
NOS
reactive
spontaneous
Excludes: hypoglycemia:
with coma (251.0)
in diabetes mellitus (249.8, 250.8)

253 Disorders of pituitary gland and its hypothalamic control
253.1 Other and unspecified anterior pituitary hyperfunction
Nonpuerperal galactorrhea and amenorrhea
253.2 Panhypopituitarism
Postpartum pituitary cathexia
Postpartumpituitary necrosis
253.4 Other anterior pituitary disorders
Decrease function of ovary in hypopituitarism
Deficient FHS, LH, prolactin
Delayed menarche due to pituitary hypofunction
Insufficient gonadotropic hormone secretion

253.8 Other disorders of the pituitary and other syndromes of diencephalohypophysial origin

Report also infertility of pituitary-hypothalamic origin (628.1)

256 Ovarian dysfunction

256.0 Hyperestrogenism

256.1 Other ovarian hyperfunction

Hypersecretion of ovarian androgens

256.2 Postablative ovarian failure

Ovarian failure:

> iatrogenic
> postirradiation
> postsurgical

Use additional code for states associated with artificial menopause (627.4)

Excludes: acquired absence of ovary (V45.77)

> asymptomatic age-related (natural) postmenopausal status (V49.81)

256.3 Other ovarian failure

Use additional code for states associated with natural menopause (627.2)

Excludes: asymptomatic age-related (natural) postmenopausal status (V49.81)

256.31 Premature menopause

256.39 Other ovarian failure

> Delayed menarche
> Ovarian hypofunction
> Primary ovarian failure NOS

256.4 Polycystic ovaries

Isosexual virilization

Stein-Leventhal syndrome

256.8 Other ovarian dysfunction

256.9 Unspecified ovarian dysfunction

259 Other endocrine disorders

259.0 Delay in sexual development and puberty, not elsewhere classified

Delayed puberty

259.1 Precocious sexual development and puberty, not elsewhere classified

Sexual precocity:

> NOS
> constitutional
> cryptogenic
> idiopathic

OTHER METABOLIC AND IMMUNITY DISORDERS
Use additional code to identify any associated mental retardation

272 **Disorders of lipoid metabolism**
   272.4 Other an unspecified hyperlipidemia
       Alpha-lipoproteinemia
       Combined hyperlipidemia
       Hyperlipidemia NOS
       Hyperlipoproteinemia NOS

275 **Disorders of mineral metabolism**
   275.4 Disorders of calcium metabolism
       275.40 Unspecified disorder of calcium metabolism
       275.41 Hypocalcemia
       257.42 Hypercalcemia
       275.49 Other disorders of calcium metabolism
           Nephrocalcinosis
           Pseudohypoparathyroidism
           Pseudopseudohypoparathryoidism

276 **Disorders of fluid, electrolyte, and acid-base balance**
   276.0 Hyperosmolality and/or hypernatremia
       Sodium (Na) excess
       Sodium (Na) overload
   276.1 Hyposmolality and/or hyponatremia
       Sodium (Na) deficiency
   276.2 Acidosis
       NOS
       lactic
       metabolic
       respiratory
       Excludes: diabetic acidosis (249.1, 250.1)
   276.3 Alkalosis
       NOS
       metabolic
       respiratory
   276.4 Mixed acid-base balance disorder
       Hypercapnia with mixed acid-base disorder
   276.5 Volume depletion
       Excludes: hypovolemic shock:
                   postoperative (998.0)
                   traumatic (958.4)
       276.50 Volume depletion, unspecified
       276.51 Dehydration
       276.52 Hypovolemia
           Depletion of volume of plasma

276.6 Fluid overload
Fluid retention
Excludes: ascites (789.51–789.59)
localized edema (782.3)
276.7 Hyperpotassemia
Hyperkalemia
Potassium (K):
excess
intoxication
overload
276.8 Hypopotassemia
Hypokalemia
Potassium (K) deficiency
276.9 Electrolyte and fluid disorders not elsewhere classified
Electrolyte imbalance
Hyperchloremia
Hypochloremia
Excludes: electrolyte imbalance:
associated with hyperemesis gravidarum (643.1)
complicating labor and delivery (669.0)
following abortion and ectopic or molar
pregnancy (634–638 with fourth digit 4, 639.4)

277 **Other and unspecified disorders of metabolism**
277.0 Cystic fibrosis
Fibrocystic disease of the pancreas
Mucoviscidosis
277.00 Without mention of meconium ileus
Cystic fibrosis NOS
277.01 With meconium ileus
Meconium:
ileus (of newborn)
obstruction of intestine in mucoviscidosis
277.02 With pulmonary manifestations
Cystic fibrosis with pulmonary exacerbation
Use additional code to identify any infectious organism
present, such as:
pseudomonas (041.7)
277.03 With gastrointestinal manifestations
Excludes: with meconium ileus (277.01)
277.09 With other manifestations
277.7 Dysmetabolic syndrome X
Use additional code for associated manifestation, such as:
obesity (278.00-278.01)

278 Overweight, obesity, and other hyperalimentation
278.0 Overweight and obesity
Use additional code to identify Body Mass Index (BMI), if known
(V85.0–V85.54)
278.00 Obesity, unspecified
Obesity NOS
278.01 Morbid obesity
Severe obesity
278.02 Overweight

279 Disorders involving the immune mechanism
279.4 Autoimmune disease, not elsewhere classified
279.41 Autoimmune lymphoproliferative syndrome ALPS
279.49 Autoimmune disease, not elsewhere classified
Autoimmune disease NOS

DISEASES OF THE BLOOD AND BLOOD-FORMING ORGANS (280–289)

280 Iron deficiency anemias
Includes: anemia:
asiderotic
hypochromic-microcytic
sideropenic
Excludes: familial microcytic anemia (282.49)
280.0 Secondary to blood loss (chronic)
Normocytic anemia due to blood loss
Excludes: acute posthemorrhagic anemia (285.1)
280.1 Secondary to inadequate dietary iron intake
280.8 Other specified iron deficiency anemias
Paterson-Kelly syndrome
Plummer-Vinson syndrome
Sideropenic dysphagia
280.9 Iron deficiency anemia, unspecified
Anemia:
achlorhydric
chlorotic
idiopathic hypochromic
iron (Fe) deficiency NOS

281 Other deficiency anemias
281.0 Pernicious anemia
Anemia:
Addison's
Biermer's
congenital pernicious

Congenital intrinsic factor (Castle's) deficiency
281.1 Other vitamin B$_{12}$ deficiency anemia
Anemia:
    vegan's
    vitamin B$_{12}$ deficiency (dietary)
    due to selective vitamin B$_{12}$ malabsorption with proteinuria
Syndrome:
    Imerslund's
    Imerslund-Gräsbeck
281.2 Folate-deficiency anemia
Congenital folate malabsorption
Folate or folic acid deficiency anemia:
    NOS
    dietary
    drug-induced
Goat's milk anemia
Nutritional megaloblastic anemia (of infancy)
Use additional E code to identify drug
281.3 Other specified megaloblastic anemias, not elsewhere classified
Combined B$_{12}$ and folate-deficiency anemia
281.4 Protein-deficiency anemia
Amino-acid-deficiency anemia
281.8 Anemia associated with other specified nutritional deficiency
Scorbutic anemia
281.9 Unspecified deficiency anemia
Anemia:
    dimorphic
    macrocytic
    megaloblastic NOS
    nutritional NOS
    simple chronic

282 **Hereditary hemolytic anemias**
282.4 Thalassemias
Excludes: sickle-cell:
                    disease (282.60–282.69)
                    trait (282.5)
282.41 Sickle-cell thalassemia without crisis
Sickle-cell thalassemia NOS
Thalassemia Hb-S disease without crisis
282.42 Sickle-cell thalassemia with crisis
Sickle-cell thalassemia with vaso-occlusive pain
Thalassemia Hb-S disease with crisis
Use additional code for type of crisis
282.49 Other thalassemia
Cooley's anemia

Hb-Bart's disease
Hereditary leptocytosis
Mediterranean anemia (with other hemoglobinopathy)
Microdrepanocytosis
Thalassemia (alpha) (beta) (intermedia) (major) (minima) (minor) (mixed) (trait) (with other hemoglobinopathy)
Thalassemia NOS

282.5 Sickle-cell trait
Hb-AS genotype
Hemoglobin S (Hb-S) trait
Heterozygous:
    hemoglobin S
    Hb-S
Excludes: that with other hemoglobinopathy (282.60–282.69)
that with thalassemia (282.49)

282.6 Sickle-cell disease
Sickle-cell anemia
Excludes: sickle-cell thalassemia (282.41–282.42)
sickle-cell trait (282.5)

282.60 Sickle-cell disease, unspecified
Sickle-cell anemia NOS

282.61 Hb-SS disease without crisis

282.62 Hb-SS disease with crisis
Hb-SS disease with vaso-occlusive pain
Sickle-cell crisis NOS
Use additional code for type of crisis

282.63 Sickle-cell/Hb-C disease without crisis
Hb-S/Hb-C disease without crisis

282.64 Sickle-cell/HB-C disease with crisis
Hb-S/Hb-C disease with crisis
Sickle-cell/Hb-C disease with vaso-occlusive pain
Use additional code for types of crisis

282.68 Other sickle-cell disease without crisis
Hb-S/Hb-D disease without crisis
Hb-S/Hb-E disease without crisis
Sickle-cell/Hb-D disease without crisis
Sickle-cell/Hb-E disease without crisis

282.69 Other sickle-cell disease with crisis
Hb-S/Hb-D disease with crisis
Hb-S/Hb-E disease with crisis
Sickle-cell/Hb-D disease with crisis
Sickle-cell/Hb-E disease with crisis
Other sickle-cell disease with vaso-occlusive pain
Use additional code for type of crisis

284 Aplastic anemia

284.0 Constitutional aplastic anemia

    284.01 Constitutional red blood cell aplasia

        Aplasia, (pure) red cell:

           congenital

           primary

           Blackfan-Diamond syndrome

           Familial hypoplastic anemia

    284.09 Other constitutional aplastic anemia

284.8 Other specified aplastic anemias

    284.81 Red cell aplasia (acquired)

    284.89 Other specified aplastic anemia (due to):

        chronic systemic disease

        drugs

        infection

        radiation

        toxic (paralytic)

284.9 Aplastic anemia, unspecified

    Anemia:

        aplastic (idiopathic) NOS

        aregenerative

        hypoplastic NOS

        nonregenerative

        Medullary hypoplasia

285 Other and unspecified anemias

285.1 Acute posthemorrhagic anemia

    Anemia due to acute blood loss

    Excludes: anemia due to chronic blood loss (280.0)

               blood loss anemia NOS (280.0)

285.2 Anemia in chronic illness

    Anemia in (due to) (with) chronic illness

    285.21 Anemia in chronic kidney disease

        Anemia in end stage renal disease

        Erythropoietin-resistant anemia (EPO resistant anemia)

    285.22 Anemia in neoplastic disease

    285.29 Anemia of other chronic disease

        Anemia in other chronic illness

285.3 Antineoplastic chemotherapy induced anemia

    Anemia due to antineoplastic chemotherapy

    Excludes: anemia due to drug NEC – code to type of anemia

        anemia in neoplastic disease (285.22)

        aplastic anemia due to antineoplastic chemotherapy (284.89)

286 Coagulation defects
286.0 Congenital factor VIII disorder
Antihemophilic globulin (AHG) deficiency
Factor VIII (functional) deficiency
Hemophilia:
  NOS
  A
  classical
  familial
  hereditary
Subhemophilia
Excludes: factor VIII deficiency with vascular defect (286.4)
286.1 Congenital factor IX disorder
Christmas disease
Deficiency:
  factor IX (functional)
  plasma thromboplastin component (PTC)
Hemophilia B
286.2 Congenital factor XI deficiency
Hemophilia C
Plasma thromboplastin antecedent (PTA) deficiency
Rosenthal's disease
286.3 Congenital deficiency of other clotting factors
Congenital afibrinogenemia
Deficiency:
  AC globulin factor:
    I (fibrinogen)
    II (prothrombin)
    V (labile)
    VII (stable)
    X (Stuart-Prower)
    XII (Hageman)
    XIII (fibrin stabilizing)
  Laki-Lorand factor
  proaccelerin
Disease:
  Owren's
  Stuart-Prower
Dysfibrinogenemia (congenital)
Dysprothrombinemia (constitutional)
Hypoproconvertinemia
Hypoprothrombinemia (hereditary)
Parahemophilia

286.4 von Willebrand's disease
Angiohemophilia (A) (B)
Constitutional thrombopathy
Factor VIII deficiency with vascular defect
Pseudohemophilia type B
Vascular hemophilia
von Willebrand's (-Jürgens') disease
Excludes: factor VIII deficiency:
NOS (286.0)
with functional defect (286.0)

286.5 Hemorrhagic disorder due to circulating anticoagulants
Antithrombinemia
Antithromboplastinemia
Antithromboplastino-genemia
Hyperheparinemia
Increase in:
anti-VIIIa
anti-IXa
anti-Xa
anti-XIa
antithrombin
Systemic lupus erythematosus (SLE) inhibitor

286.6 Defibrination syndrome
Afibrinogenemia, acquired
Consumption coagulopathy
Diffuse or disseminated intravascular coagulation (DIC syndrome)
Fibrinolytic hemorrhage, acquired
Hemorrhagic fibrinogenolysis
Pathologic fibrinolysis
Purpura:
fibrinolytic
fulminans
Excludes: that complicating:
abortion (634–638 with fourth digit 1, 639.1)
pregnancy or the puerperium (641.3, 666.3)

286.7 Acquired coagulation factor deficiency
Deficiency of coagulation factor due to:
liver disease
vitamin K deficiency
Hypoprothrombinemia, acquired

286.9 Other and unspecified coagulation defects
Defective coagulation NOS
Deficiency, coagulation factor NOS
Delay, coagulation
Disorder:
coagulation
hemostasis
Excludes: abnormal coagulation profile (790.92)
that complicating:
abortion (634–638 with fourth digit 1,
639.1)
pregnancy or the puerperium (641.3,
666.3)

287 Purpura and other hemorrhagic conditions
Excludes: purpura fulminans (286.6)
allergic purpura
287.2 Other nonthrombocytopenic purpuras)
287.3 Primary thrombocytopenia
287.30 Primary thrombocytopenia, unspecified
Megakaryocytic hypoplasia
287.31 Immune thrombocytopenic purpura
287.32 Evans' syndrome
287.33 Congenital and hereditary thrombocytopenic purpura
287.39 Other primary thrombocytopenia
287.4 Secondary thrombocytopenia
Posttransfusion purpura
Thrombocytopenia (due to):
dilutional
drugs
extracorporeal circulation of blood
massive blood transfusion
platelet alloimmunization
287.5 Thrombocytopenia, unspecified

MENTAL DISORDERS (290–319)

PSYCHOSES

293 Transient mental disorders due to conditions classified elsewhere
293.9 Unspecified transient organic mental disorder in conditions classified
elsewhere
Puerperal delirium

296 **Episodic mood disorders**
Includes: episodic affective disorders
Excludes: neurotic depression (300.4)

The following fifth-digit subclassification is for use with categories 296.0–296.3:
0   unspecified
1   mild
2   moderate
3   severe, without mention of psychotic behavior
4   severe, specified as with psychotic behavior
5   in partial or unspecified remission
6   in full remission

296.0   Bipolar I disorder, single manic episode
        Puerperal, single episode or unspecified
296.2   Major depressive disorder, single episode
        Climacteric depression, single episode or unspecified
        Menopausal depression, single episode or unspecified
296.3   Major depressive disorder, recurrent episode
        Any condition classifiable to 296.2, stated to be recurrent
        Excludes: depression NOS (311)
                        reactive depression (neurotic) (300.4)
296.9   Other and unspecified episodic mood disorder
        296.99   Other specified episodic mood disorder
                 Mood swings:
                     brief compensatory
                     rebound

297 **Delusional disorders**
297.2   Paraphrenia
        Climeractic, menopausal paraphrenia
        Involutional paranoid state
        Late paraphrenia

Neurotic Disorders, Personality Disorders, and Other Nonpsychotic Mental Disorders

300   Anxiety, dissociative and somatoform disorders
      300.0   Anxiety states
              Excludes: anxiety in:
                              acute stress reaction (308.0)
                              transient adjustment reaction (309.24)
                              psychophysiological disorders (306.5)
                              separation anxiety (309.21)

300.00 Anxiety state, unspecified
Anxiety:
    neurosis
    reaction
    state (neurotic)
Atypical anxiety disorder
300.01 Panic disorder without agoraphobia
Panic:
    attack
    state
300.02 Generalized anxiety disorder
300.09 Other
300.1 Dissociative, conversion and factitious disorders
300.11 Conversion disorder
False pregnancy
300.3 Obsessive-compulsive disorders
300.4 Dysthymic disorder
Anxiety depression
Depression with anxiety
Depressive reaction
Neurotic depressive state
Reactive depression
Excludes: adjustment reaction with depressive symptoms (309.0–309.1)
depression NOS (311)
300.9 Unspecified nonpsychotic mental disorder
Suicidal tendencies
Self-mutilation
Nervous collapse

302 Sexual deviations and disorders
302.7 Psychosexual dysfunction
Excludes: decreased sexual desire NOS (799.81)
normal transient symptoms from ruptured hymen
transient or occasional failures of erection due to fatigue, anxiety, alcohol, or drugs
302.70 Psychosexual dysfunction, unspecified
302.71 Hypoactive sexual desire disorder
Excludes: decreased sexual desire NOS (799.81)
302.72 With inhibited sexual excitement
Female sexual arousal disorder
Frigidity
Impotence
302.73 Female orgasic disorder
302.76 Dyspareunia, psychogenic
With other specified psychosexual dysfunctions
302.79 Sexual aversion disorder

303 **Alcohol dependence syndrome**
Use additional code to identify any associated condition, as:
    drug dependence (304.0–304.9)
    physical complications of alcohol, such as:
        epilepsy (345.0–345.9)
        gastritis (535.3)
Excludes: drunkenness NOS (305.0)

The following fifth-digit subclassification is for use with category 303:
0   unspecified
1   continuous
2   episodic
3   in remission

303.0 Acute alcoholic intoxication
        Acute drunkenness in alcoholism
303.9 Other and unspecified alcohol dependence
        Chronic alcoholism
        Dipsomania

304 **Drug dependence**
Excludes: nondependent abuse of drugs (305.1–305.9)

The following fifth-digit subclassification is for use with category 304:
0   unspecified
1   continuous
2   episodic
3   in remission

304.0 Opioid type dependence
        Heroin
        Meperidine
        Methadone
        Morphine
        Opium
        Opium alkaloids and their derivatives
        Synthetics with morphine-like effects
304.1 Sedative or hypnotic or anxiolytic dependence
        Barbiturates
        Nonbarbiturate sedatives and tranquilizers with a similar effect:
            chlordiazepoxide
            diazepam
            glutethimide
            meprobamate
            methaqualone

304.2 Cocaine dependence
Coca leaves and derivatives
304.3 Cannabis dependence
Hashish
Hemp
Marihuana
304.4 Amphetamine and other psychostimulant dependence
Methylphenidate
Phenmetrazine
304.5 Hallucinogen dependence
Dimethyltryptamine (DMT)
Lysergic acid diethylamide (LSD) and derivatives
Mescaline
Psilocybin
304.6 Other specified drug dependence
Absinthe addiction
Glue sniffing
Inhalant dependence
Phencyclidine dependence
Excludes: tobacco dependence (305.1)
304.7 Combinations of opioid type drug with any other
304.8 Combinations of drug dependence excluding opioid type drug
304.9 Unspecified drug dependence
Drug addiction NOS
Drug dependence NOS

305 Nondependent abuse of drugs
Includes cases where a person, for whom no other diagnosis is possible, has come under medical care because of the maladaptive effect of a drug on which he or she is not dependent and that he or she has taken on his or her own initiative to the detriment of his or her health or social functioning.
Excludes: alcohol dependence syndrome (303.0–303.9)
drug dependence (304.0–304.9)

The following fifth-digit subclassification is for use with codes 305.0, 305.2–305.9
0   unspecified
1   continuous
2   episodic
3   in remission
305.0 Alcohol abuse
Drunkenness NOS
Excessive drinking of alcohol NOS
"Hangover" (alcohol)
Inebriety NOS
Excludes: acute alcohol intoxication in alcoholism (303.0)

305.1 Tobacco use disorder
Tobacco dependence
Excludes: history of tobacco use (V15.82)
Smoking complicating pregnancy (649.0)

305.2 Cannabis abuse

305.3 Hallucinogen abuse
Acute intoxication from hallucinogens ("bad trips")
LSD reaction

305.4 Sedative or hypnotic or anxiolytic abuse

305.5 Opioid abuse

305.6 Cocaine abuse

305.7 Amphetamine or related acting sympathomimetic abuse

305.8 Antidepressant type abuse

305.9 Other, mixed, or unspecified drug abuse
Caffeine intoxication
Inhalant abuse
"Laxative habit"
Misuse of drugs NOS
Nonprescribed use of drugs or patent medicinals
Phencyclidine abuse

306 Physiological malfunction arising from mental factors
Includes: psychogenic:
physical symptoms not involving tissue damage
physiological manifestations not involving tissue damage
Excludes: hysteria (300.11)
physical symptoms secondary to a psychiatric disorder
classified elsewhere

306.5 Genitourinary
Excludes: frigidity (302.72)
psychogenic dyspareunia (302.76)

306.50 Psychogenic genitourinary malfunction, unspecified

306.51 Psychogenic vaginismus
Functional vaginismus

306.52 Psychogenic dysmenorrhea

306.53 Psychogenic dysuria

306.59 Other

307 Special symptoms or syndromes, not elsewhere classified
This category is intended for use if the psychopathology is manifested by a single specific symptom or group of symptoms which is not part of an organic illness or other mental disorder classifiable elsewhere.
Excludes: those due to mental disorders classified elsewhere
those of organic origin

307.1 Anorexia nervosa
Excludes: eating disturbance NOS (307.50)
feeding problem, nonorganic origin (307.59)
loss of appetite (783.0)
of nonorganic origin (307.59)
307.5 Other and unspecified disorders of eating
Excludes: anorexia nervosa (307.1)
of unspecified cause (783.0)
vomiting NOS (787.03)
307.50 Eating disorder, unspecified
Eating disorder NOS
307.51 Bulimia nervosa
Overeating of nonorganic origin
307.52 Pica
Perverted appetite of nonorganic origin
307.53 Rumination disorder
Regurgitation, of nonorganic origin, of food with
reswallowing
Excludes: obsessional rumination (300.3)
307.54 Psychogenic vomiting
307.59 Other

308 **Acute reaction to stress**
Includes: catastrophic stress
combat fatigue
gross stress reaction (acute)
transient disorders in response to exceptional physical or
mental stress which usually subside within hours or days
Excludes: adjustment reaction or disorder (309.0–309.2)
chronic stress reaction (309.1–309.2)
308.0 Predominant disturbance of emotions
Anxiety as acute reaction to exceptional (gross) stress
Emotional crisis as acute reaction to exceptional (gross) stress
Panic state as acute reaction to exceptional (gross) stress
308.1 Predominant disturbance of consciousness
Fugues as acute reaction to exceptional (gross) stress
308.2 Predominant psychomotor disturbance
Agitation states as acute reaction to exceptional (gross) stress
Stupor as acute reaction to exceptional (gross) stress
308.3 Other acute reactions to stress
Acute situational disturbance
308.4 Mixed disorders as reaction to stress
308.9 Unspecified acute reaction to stress

309 Adjustment reaction
Includes: adjustment disorders
            reaction (adjustment) to chronic stress
Excludes: acute reaction to major stress (308.0–308.9)
            neurotic disorders (300.0–300.9)
309.0 Adjustment disorder with depressed mood
       grief reaction
       Excludes: affective psychoses (296.0–296.9)
                  neurotic depression (300.4)
                  prolonged depressive reaction (309.1)
309.1 Prolonged depressive reaction
       Excludes: affective psychoses (296.0–296.9)
                  brief depressive reaction (309.0)
                  neurotic depression (300.4)
309.2 With predominant disturbance of other emotions
       309.21 Separation anxiety disorder
       309.22 Emancipation disorder of adolescence and early adult life
       309.24 Adjustment disorder with anxiety
       309.28 Adjustment disorder with mixed anxiety and depressed
               mood
               Adjustment reaction with anxiety and depression
       309.29 Other
               Culture shock

311 Depressive disorder, not elsewhere classified
Depressive disorder NOS
Depressive state NOS
Depression NOS
Excludes: acute reaction to major stress with depressive symptoms
            (308.0)
            affective psychoses (296.0–296.9)
            brief depressive reaction (309.0)
            depressive states associated with stressful events
            (309.0–309.1)
            neurotic depression (300.4)
            prolonged depressive adjustment reaction (309.1)

DISEASES OF THE NERVOUS SYSTEM AND SENSE ORGANS (320–389)

INFLAMMATORY DISEASES OF THE CENTRAL NERVOUS SYSTEM

320 Bacterial meningitis

Includes: Bacterial:
arachnoiditis
leptomeningitis
meningitis
meningoencephalitis
meningomyelitis
pachymeningitis

320.0 Hemophilus meningitis
320.1 Pneumococcal meningitis
320.2 Streptococcal meningitis
320.3 Staphylococcal meningitis
320.7 Meningitis in other bacterial diseases classified elsewhere
Code first underlying disease

HEREDITARY AND DEGENERATIVE DISEASES OF THE CENTRAL NERVOUS SYSTEM

Excludes: multiple sclerosis (340)

331 Other cerebral degenerations

331.0 Alzheimer's disease
331.8 Other cerebral degeneration
331.83 mild cognitive impairment, so stated

332 Parkinson's disease

332.0 Paralysis agitans
Parkinsonism or Parkinson's disease:
NOS
idiopathic
primary

338 Pain, not elsewhere classified

Use additional code to identify:
pain associated with psychological factors (307.89)

Excludes: generalized pain (780.96)
headache syndromes (339.00–339.89)
migraines (346.0–346.9)
localized pain, unspecified type—code to pain by site
pain disorder exclusively attributed to psychological factors (307.80)
vulvar vestibulitis (625.71)
vulvodynia (625.70-625.79)

338.1 Acute pain
    338.11 Acute pain due to trauma
    338.18 Other acute postoperative pain
         Postoperative pain NOS
    338.19 Other acute pain
         Excludes: neoplasm related acute pain (338.3)
338.2 Chronic pain
    Excludes: neoplasm related chronic pain (338.3)
    338.21 Chronic pain due to trauma
    338.28 Other chronic postoperative pain
    338.29 Other chronic pain
338.3 Neoplasm related pain (acute) (chronic)
    Cancer associated pain
    Pain due to malignancy (primary) (secondary)
    Tumor associated pain
338.4 Chronic pain syndrome
    Chronic pain associated with significant psychosocial dysfunction

OTHER HEADACHE SYNDROMES

339 Other headache syndromes
Excludes: headache:
    NOS (784.0)
    migraine (346.0–346.9)
339.0 Cluster headaches and other trigeminal autonomic cephalgias
    TACS
    339.00 Cluster headache syndrome, unspecified
         Ciliary neuralgia
         Cluster headache NOS
         Histamine cephalgia
         Lower half migraine
         Migrainous neuralgia
    339.01 Episodic cluster headache
    339.02 Chronic cluster headache
    339.03 Episodic paroxysmal hemicrania
         Paroxysmal hemicrania NOS
    339.04 Chronic paroxysmal hemicrania
    339.05 Short lasting unilateral neuralgiform headache with
         conjunctival injection and tearing
           SUNCT
    339.09 Other trigeminal autonomic cephalgias

339.1 Tension type headache
Excludes: tension headache NOS (307.81)
         tension headache related to psychological factors (307.81)
    339.10 Tension type headache, unspecified
    339.11 Episodic tension type headache
    339.12 Chronic tension type headache
339.2 Post-traumatic headache
    339.20 Post-traumatic headache, unspecified
    339.21 Acute post-traumatic headache
    339.22 Chronic post-traumatic headache
339.3 Drug induced headache, not elsewhere classified
    Medication overuse headache
    Rebound headache
339.4 Complicated headache syndromes
    339.41 Hemicrania continua
    339.42 New daily persistant headache
        NDPH
    339.43 Primary thunderlcap headache
    339.44 Other complicated headache syndrome
339.8 Other specified headache syndromes
    339.81 Hypnic headache
    339.82 Headache associated with sexual activity
    Orgasmic headache
    Preorgasmic headache
    339.83 Primary cough headache
    338.84 Primary exertional headache
    339.85 Primary stabbing headache
    339.89 Other specified headache syndromes

OTHER DISORDERS OF THE CENTRAL NERVOUS SYSTEM

340 Multiple sclerosis
Disseminated or multiple sclerosis:
    NOS
    brain stem
    cord
    generalized

345 Epilepsy and recurrent seizures
The following fifth-digit subclassification is for use with categories 345.0, 345.1, and 345.8:
    0 without mention of intractable epilepsy
    1 with intractable epilepsy

345.0 Generalized nonconvulsive epilepsy
    Absences:
        atonic
        typical
    Minor epilepsy
    Petit mal
    Pykno-epilepsy
    Seizures:
        akinetic
        atonic
345.1 Generalized convulsive epilepsy
    Epileptic seizures:
        clonic
        myoclonic
        tonic
        tonic-clonic
    Grand mal
    Major epilepsy
    Progressive myoclonic epilepsy
    Unverricht-Lundborg disease
    Excludes: convulsions:
                NOS (780.39)
                infantile (780.39)
345.2 Petit mal status
    Epileptic absence status
345.3 Grand mal status
    Status epilepticus NOS
345.9 Epilepsy, unspecified
    Recurrent seizures NOS
    Seizure disorders NOS
    Excludes: convulsive seizure or fit NOS (780.3)

346 Migraine
Excludes: headache:
        NOS (784.0)
        syndromes (339.00–339.89)
The following fifth-digit subclassification is for use with category 346:
0   without mention of intractable migraine without mention of status migrainosus
1   with intractable migraine, so stated, without mention of status migrainosus
2   without mention of intractable migraine with status migrainosus
3   with intractable migraine, so stated, with status migrainos

346.0 Migraine with aura
Basilar migraine
Classic migraine
Migraine triggered seizures
Migraine with acute-onset aura
Migraine with aura without headache (migraine equivalents)
Migraine with prolonged aura
Migraine with typical aura
Retinal migraine
Excludes: persistant migraine aura (346.5, 346.6)
346.1 Migraine without aura
Common migraine
346.2 Variants of migraine, not elsewhere classified
Abdominal migraine
Cyclical vomiting associated with migraine
Ophthalmoplegic migraine
Periodic headache syndromes in child or adolescent
Excludes: cyclical vomiting NOS (536.2)
psychogenic cyclical vomiting (306.4)
346.3 Hemiplegic migraine
Familial migraine
Sporadic migraine
346.4 Menstrual migraine
Menstrual headache
Menstrually related migraine
Premenstrual headache
Premenstrual migraine
Pure menstrual migraine
346.5 Persistant migraine aura without cerebral infarction
Persistent migraine aura NOS
346.6 Persistent migraine aura with cerebral infarction
346.7 Chronic migraine without aura
Transformed migraine without aura
346.8 Other forms of migraine
346.9 Migraine, unspecified

354 Mononeuritis of upper limb and mononeuritis multiplex
354.0 Carpal tunnel syndrome

DISEASES OF THE CIRCULATORY SYSTEM (390–459)

Excludes: that complicating pregnancy, childbirth, or the puerperium (642.0–642.9)
that involving coronary vessels (410.00–414.9)

401 Essential hypertension
    Includes: high blood pressure
               hyperpiesia
               hyperpiesis
               hypertension (arterial) (essential) (primary) (systemic)
               hypertensive vascular:
                    degeneration
                    disease
    Excludes: elevated blood pressure without diagnosis of hypertension (796.2)
    401.0 Malignant
    401.1 Benign
    401.9 Unspecified

402 Hypertensive heart disease
    Use additional code to specify type of heart failure.
    Includes: hypertensive:
                    cardiomegaly
                    cardiopathy
                    cardiovascular disease
                    heart (disease) (failure)
    402.0 Malignant
        402.00 Without heart failure
        402.01 With heart failure
    402.1 Benign
        402.10 Without heart failure
        402.11 With heart failure
    402.9 Unspecified
        402.90 Without heart failure
        402.91 With heart failure

403 Hypertensive chronic kidney disease
    Includes: arteriolar nephritis
               arteriosclerosis of:
                    kidney
                    renal arterioles
               arteriosclerotic nephritis (chronic) (interstitial)
               hypertensive:
                    nephropathy
                    renal failure
                    uremia (chronic)

Excludes: acute kidney failure (584.5–584.9)
renal disease stated as not due to hypertension

The following fifth-digit subclassification is for use with category 403:
0 with chronic kidney disease stage I–IV or unspecified
1 with chronic kidney disease stage V or end stage renal disease

403.0 Malignant
403.1 Benign
403.9 Unspecified

410 Acute myocardial infarction
Includes: cardiac infarction
coronary (artery):
embolism
occlusion
rupture
thrombosis
infarction of heart, myocardium, or ventricle
rupture of heart, myocardium, or ventricle
ST elevation (STEMI) and non-ST elevation (NSTEMI) myocardial infarction

The following fifth-digit subclassification is for use with category 410:
0 episode of care unspecified
1 initial episode of care (newly diagnosed myocardial infarction)
2 subsequent episode of care (admitted for further observation, evaluation or treatment for myocardial infarction less than 8 weeks old)

410.8 Specified site
410.9 Unspecified site

413 Angina pectoris
413.0 Angina decubitus
413.1 Prinzmetal angina
413.9 Other and unspecified angina pectoris

420 Acute pericarditis
Includes: acute:
mediastinopericarditis
myopericarditis
pericardial effusion
pleuropericarditis
pneumopericarditis
420.0 Acute pericarditis in diseases classified elsewhere
Code first underlying disease

420.9 Other and unspecified acute pericarditis
    420.90 Acute pericarditis, unspecified
    420.91 Acute idiopathic pericarditis
    420.99 Other

427 **Cardiac dysrhythmias**
Excludes: that complicating:
        abortion (634–638 with fourth digit 7, 639.8)
        ectopic or molar pregnancy (639.8)
        labor or delivery (668.1, 669.4)
427.0 Paroxysmal supraventricular tachycardia
    Paroxysmal tachycardia:
       atrial (PAT)
       atrioventricular (AV)
       junctional
       nodal
427.1 Paroxysmal ventricular tachycardia
    Ventricular tachycardia (paroxysmal)
427.2 Paroxysmal tachycardia, unspecified
    Bouveret-Hoffmann syndrome
    Paroxysmal tachycardia:
       NOS
       essential
427.3 Atrial fibrillation and flutter
    427.31 Atrial fibrillation
    427.32 Atrial flutter
427.4 Ventricular fibrillation and flutter
    427.41 Ventricular fibrillation
    427.42 Ventricular flutter
427.5 Cardiac arrest
    Cardiorespiratory arrest
427.6 Premature beats
    427.60 Premature beats, unspecified
       Ectopic beats
       Extrasystoles
       Extrasystolic arrhythmia
       Premature contractions or systoles NOS
    427.61 Supraventricular premature beats
       Atrial premature beats, contractions, or systoles
    427.69 Other
       Ventricular premature beats, contractions, or systoles

427.8   Other specified cardiac dysrhythmias
   427.81   Sinoatrial node dysfunction
      Sinus bradycardia:
         persistent
         severe
      Syndrome:
         sick sinus
         tachycardia-bradycardia
      Excludes: sinus bradycardia NOS (427.89)
   427.89   Other
      Rhythm disorder:
         coronary sinus
         ectopic
         nodal
      Wandering (atrial) pacemaker
      Excludes: tachycardia NOS (785.0)
427.9   Cardiac dysrhythmia, unspecified
      Arrhythmia (cardiac) NOS

429   Ill-defined descriptions and complications of heart disease
429.2   Cardiovascular disease, unspecified
      Arteriosclerotic cardiovascular disease (ASCVD)
      Cardiovascular arteriosclerosis
      Cardiovascular:
         degeneration (with mention of arteriosclerosis)
         disease (with mention of arteriosclerosis)
         sclerosis (with mention of arteriosclerosis)
      Use additional code to identify presence of arteriosclerosis
      Excludes: that due to hypertension (402.0–402.9)

DISEASES OF **A**RTERIES, **A**RTERIOLES, AND **C**APILLARIES

440   Atherosclerosis
   Includes: arteriolosclerosis
      arteriosclerosis (obliterans) (senile)
      arteriosclerotic vascular disease
      atheroma
      degeneration:
         arterial
         arteriovascular
         vascular
      endarteritis deformans or obliterans
      senile:
         arteritis
         endarteritis

440.9   Generalized and unspecified atherosclerosis
Arteriosclerotic vascular disease NOS
Excludes: arteriosclerotic cardiovascular disease (ASCVD) (429.2)

443 Other peripheral vascular disease
443.0   Raynaud's syndrome
Raynaud's:
   disease
   phenomenon (secondary)
Use additional code to identify gangrene (785.4)
443.9   Peripheral vascular disease, unspecified
Intermittent claudication NOS
Peripheral:
   angiopathy NOS
   vascular disease NOS
Spasm of artery

446 Polyarteritis nodosa and allied conditions
446.0   Polyarteritis nodosa
446.1   Acute febrile mucocutaneous lymph node syndrome (MCLS)

DISEASES OF VEINS AND LYMPHATICS, AND OTHER DISEASES OF CIRCULATORY SYSTEM

451 Phlebitis and thrombophlebitis
Includes: endophlebitis
   inflammation, vein
   periphlebitis
   suppurative phlebitis
Excludes: that complicating:
   abortion (634–638 with fourth digit 7, 639.8)
   ectopic or molar pregnancy (639.8)
   pregnancy, childbirth, or the puerperium
   (671.0–671.9)
   that due to or following:
   implant or catheter device (996.61–996.62)
   infusion, perfusion, or transfusion (999.2)
451.0   Of superficial vessels of lower extremities
Saphenous vein (greater) (lesser)
451.1   Of deep vessels of lower extremities
   451.11   Femoral vein (deep) (superficial)
   451.19   Other
      Femoropopliteal vein
      Popliteal vein
      Tibial vein
451.2   Of lower extremities, unspecified

453   Other venous embolism and thrombosis
   453.4 Acute venus embolism and thrombosis of deep vessels of lower extremity
         453.40   Acute venous embolism and thrombosis of unspecified deep
                  vessels of lower extremity
                  Deep vein thrombosis (DVT) NOS
         453.41   Acute venous embolism and thrombosis of deep vessels of
                  proximal lower extremity
                  Femoral
                  Iliac
                  Popliteal
                  Thigh
                  Upper leg NOS
         453.42   Acute venous embolism and thrombosis of deep vessels of
                  distal lower extremity
                  Calf
                  Lower leg NOS
                  Peroneal
                  Tibial
   453.5 Chronic venous embolism and thrombosis of deep vessels of lower
          extremity
   Use additional code, if applicable, for associated long-term (current) use of
   anticoagulants (V58.61)
   Excludes: personal history of venous thrombosis and embolism (V12.51)
         453.50 Chronic venous embolism and thrombosis of
                unspecified deep vessels of lower extremity
         453.51 Chronic venous embolism and thrombosis of
                deep vessels of proximal lower extremity
         453.52 Chronic venous embolism and thrombosis of
                deep vessels of distal lower extremity
   453.8 Of other specified veins
   453.9 Of unspecified sited Embolism of vein Thrombosis (vein)

454   Varicose veins of lower extremities
   Excludes: that complicating pregnancy, childbirth, or the puerperium (671.0)
   454.0 With ulcer
          Varicose ulcer (lower extremity, any part)
          Varicose veins with ulcer of lower extremity (any part) or of
          unspecified site
          Any condition classifiable to 454.9 with ulcer or specified as ulcerated
   454.1 With inflammation
          Stasis dermatitis
          Varicose veins with inflammation of lower extremity (any part) or of
          unspecified site
          Any condition classifiable to 454.9 with inflammation or specified as
          inflamed

454.2 With ulcer and inflammation
Varicose veins with ulcer and inflammation of lower extremity (any part) or of unspecified site
Any condition classifiable to 454.9 with ulcer and inflammation

454.8 With other complications
Edema
Pain
Swelling

454.9 Asymptomatic varicose veins
Phlebectasia of lower extremity (any part) or of unspecified site
Varicose veins NOS
Varicose veins of lower extremity (any part) or of unspecified site
Varix of lower extremity (any part) or of unspecified site

455 Hemorrhoids

Includes: hemorrhoids (anus) (rectum)
piles
varicose veins, anus or rectum

Excludes: that complicating pregnancy, childbirth, or the puerperium (671.8)

455.0 Internal hemorrhoids without mention of complication

455.1 Internal thrombosed hemorrhoids

455.2 Internal hemorrhoids with other complication
Internal hemorrhoids:
bleeding
prolapsed
strangulated
ulcerated

455.3 External hemorrhoids without mention of complication

455.4 External thrombosed hemorrhoids

455.5 External hemorrhoids with other complication
External hemorrhoids:
bleeding
prolapsed
strangulated
ulcerated

455.6 Unspecified hemorrhoids without mention of complication
Hemorrhoids NOS

455.7 Unspecified thrombosed hemorrhoids
Thrombosed hemorrhoids, unspecified whether internal or external

455.8 Unspecified hemorrhoids with other complication
Hemorrhoids, unspecified whether internal or external:
bleeding
prolapsed
strangulated
ulcerated

455.9 Residual hemorrhoidal skin tags
      Skin tags, anus or rectum

456 Varicose veins of other sites
456.5 Pelvic varices
      Varices of broad ligament
456.6 Vulval varices
      Varices of perineum
      Excludes: that complicating pregnancy, childbirth, or the puerperium
                (671.1)

457 Noninfectious disorders of lymphatic channels
457.0 Postmastectomy lymphedema syndrome
      Elephantiasis due to mastectomy
      Obliteration of lymphatic vessel due to mastectomy

458 Hypotension
Includes: hypopiesis
Excludes: cardiovascular collapse (785.50)
           maternal hypotension syndrome (669.2)
           shock (785.50–785.59)
458.1 Chronic hypotension
      Permanent idiopathic hypotension
458.2 Iatrogenic hypotension
      458.21 Hypotension of hemodialysis
            Intra-dialytic hypotension
      458.29 Other iatrogenic hypotension
            Postoperative hypotension
458.8 Other specified hypotension
458.9 Hypotension, unspecified
      Hypotension (arterial) NOS

459 Other disorders of circulatory system
459.0 Hemorrhage, unspecified
      Rupture of blood vessel NOS
      Spontaneous hemorrhage NEC
      Excludes: hemorrhage:
                gastrointestinal NOS (578.9)
                nontraumatic hematoma of soft tissue (729.92)
                secondary or recurrent following trauma (958.2)
459.1 Postphlebitic syndrome
      Chronic venous hypertension due to deep vein thrombosis
      459.10 Postphlebitic syndrome without complications
            Asymptomatic postphlebitic syndrome
            Postphlebitic syndrome NOS

459.11 Postphlebitic syndrome with ulcer
459.12 Postphlebitic syndrome with inflammation
459.13 Postphlebitic syndrome with ulcer and inflammation
459.19 Postphlebitic syndrome with other complication
459.2 Compression of vein
Stricture of vein
Vena cava syndrome (inferior) (superior)
459.9 Unspecified circulatory system disorder

DISEASES OF THE RESPIRATORY SYSTEM (460–519)

Use additional code to identify infectious organism.

ACUTE RESPIRATORY INFECTIONS

Excludes: pneumonia and influenza (480.0–488)

460 Acute nasopharyngitis (common cold)
Coryza (acute)
Nasal catarrh, acute
Nasopharyngitis:
  NOS
  acute
  infective NOS
Rhinitis:
  acute
  infective
Excludes: nasopharyngitis, chronic (472.2)
    pharyngitis:
      acute or unspecified (462)
      chronic (472.1)
    rhinitis:
      allergic (477.0–477.8)
      chronic or unspecified (472.0)
    sore throat:
      acute or unspecified (462)
      chronic (472.1)

461 Acute sinusitis
Includes: abscess, acute, of sinus (accessory) (nasal)
    empyema, acute, of sinus (accessory) (nasal)
    infection, acute, of sinus (accessory) (nasal)
    inflammation, acute, of sinus (accessory) (nasal)
    suppuration, acute, of sinus (accessory) (nasal)
Excludes: chronic or unspecified sinusitis (473.0–473.9)
461.0 Maxillary
Acute antritis

461.1 Frontal
461.2 Ethmoidal
461.3 Sphenoidal
461.8 Other acute sinusitis
Acute pansinusitis
461.9 Acute sinusitis, unspecified
Acute sinusitis NOS

462 Acute pharyngitis
Acute sore throat NOS
Pharyngitis (acute):
    NOS
    gangrenous
    infective
    phlegmonous
    pneumococcal
    staphylococcal
    suppurative
    ulcerative
Sore throat (viral) NOS
Viral pharyngitis
Excludes: abscess:
        chronic pharyngitis (472.1)
        infectious mononucleosis (075)
      that specified as (due to):
        gonococcus (098.6)
        influenza (487.1)
        septic (034.0)
        streptococcal (034.0)

465 Acute upper respiratory infections of multiple or unspecified sites
Excludes: upper respiratory infection due to:
        influenza (487.1)
        Streptococcus (034.0)
465.0 Acute laryngopharyngitis
465.8 Other multiple sites
Multiple URI
465.9 Unspecified site
Acute URI NOS
Upper respiratory infection (acute)

466 Acute bronchitis and bronchiolitis
Includes: that with:
        bronchospasm
        obstruction

466.0 Acute bronchitis
      Bronchitis, acute or subacute:
         fibrinous
         membranous
         pneumococcal
         purulent
         septic
         viral
         with tracheitis
      Croupous bronchitis
      Tracheobronchitis, acute
      Excludes: acute bronchitis with chronic obstructive pulmonary disease (491.22)

466.1 Acute bronchiolitis
      Bronchiolitis (acute)
      Capillary pneumonia
      466.11 Acute bronchiolitis due to respiratory syncytial virus (RSV)
      466.19 Acute bronchiolitis due to other infectious organisms
           Use additional code to identify organism

472 **Chronic pharyngitis and nasopharyngitis**

472.0 Chronic rhinitis
      Ozena
      Rhinitis:
         NOS
         atrophic
         granulomatous
         hypertrophic
         obstructive
         purulent
         ulcerative
      Excludes: allergic rhinitis (477.0–477.8)

472.1 Chronic pharyngitis
      Chronic sore throat
      Pharyngitis:
         atrophic
         granular (chronic)
         hypertrophic

472.2 Chronic nasopharyngitis
      Excludes: acute or unspecified nasopharyngitis (460)

473 **Chronic sinusitis**
      Includes: abscess (chronic) of sinus (accessory) (nasal)
            empyema (chronic) of sinus (accessory) (nasal)

infection (chronic) of sinus (accessory) (nasal)
suppuration (chronic) of sinus (accessory) (nasal)
Excludes: acute sinusitis (461.0–461.9)
473.0 Maxillary
Antritis (chronic)
473.1 Frontal
473.2 Ethmoidal
473.3 Sphenoidal
473.8 Other chronic sinusitis
Pansinusitis (chronic)
473.9 Unspecified sinusitis (chronic)
Sinusitis (chronic) NOS

476 Chronic laryngitis and laryngotracheitis
476.0 Chronic laryngitis
Laryngitis:
catarrhal
hypertrophic
sicca
476.1 Chronic laryngotracheitis
Laryngitis, chronic, with tracheitis (chronic)
Tracheitis, chronic, with laryngitis
Excludes: chronic tracheitis (491.8)

477 Allergic rhinitis
Includes: allergic rhinitis (nonseasonal) (seasonal)
hay fever
spasmodic rhinorrhea
Excludes: allergic rhinitis with asthma (bronchial) (493.0)
477.0 Due to pollen
Pollinosis
477.1 Due to food
477.2 Due to animal (cat) (dog) hair and dander
477.8 Due to other allergen
477.9 Cause unspecified
Pneumonia and Influenza

480 Viral pneumonia
480.0 Pneumonia due to adenovirus
480.1 Pneumonia due to respiratory syncytial virus
480.2 Pneumonia due to parainfluenza virus
480.3 Pneumonia due to SARS-associated coronavirus
480.8 Pneumonia due to other virus not elsewhere classified
Excludes: influenza with pneumonia, any form (487.0)
pneumonia complicating viral diseases classified
elsewhere (484.8)

480.9 Viral pneumonia, unspecified

481 Pneumococcal pneumonia (*Streptococcus pneumoniae* pneumonia)
Lobar pneumonia, organism unspecified

482 Other bacterial pneumonia
482.0 Pneumonia due to *Klebsiella pneumoniae*
482.1 Pneumonia due to Pseudomonas
482.2 Pneumonia due to *Hemophilus influenzae (H. influenzae)*
482.3 Pneumonia due to Streptococcus
 Excludes: *Streptococcus pneumoniae* pneumonia (481)
 482.30 Streptococcus, unspecified
 482.31 Group A
 482.32 Group B
 482.39 Other Streptococcus
482.4 Pneumonia due to Staphylococcus
 482.40 Pneumonia due to Staphylococcus, unspecified
 482.41 Methicillin susceptible pneumonia due to
   Staphylococcus aureus
    MSSA pneumonia
    Pneumonia due to Staphylococcus aureus
    NOS
 482.42 Methicillin resistant pneumonia due to
   Staphylococcus aureus
 482.49 Other Staphylococcus pneumonia
482.8 Pneumonia due to other specified bacteria
 Excludes: pneumonia complicating infectious disease classified
   elsewhere (484.8)
 482.81 Anaerobes
   Gram-negative anaerobes
   Bacteroides (melaninogenicus)
 482.82 *Escherichia coli (E. coli)*
 482.83 Other gram-negative bacteria
   Gram-negative pneumonia NOS
   Proteus
   Serratia marcescens
   Excludes: gram-negative anaerobes (482.81)
 482.89 Other specified bacteria
482.9 Bacterial pneumonia unspecified

483 Pneumonia due to other specified organism
483.0 *Mycoplasma pneumoniae*
   Eaton's agent
   Pleuropneumonia-like organisms (PPLO)
483.1 Chlamydia
483.8 Other specified organism

484 Pneumonia in infectious diseases classified elsewhere
Excludes: influenza with pneumonia, any form (487.0)
484.8 Pneumonia in other infectious diseases classified elsewhere
Code first underlying disease
Excludes: pneumonia in:
tuberculosis (011.6)
varicella (052.1)

485 Bronchopneumonia, organism unspecified
Bronchopneumonia:
hemorrhagic
terminal
Pleurobronchopneumonia
Pneumonia:
lobular
segmental
Excludes: bronchiolitis (acute) (466.11–466.19)
chronic (491.8)

486 Pneumonia, organism unspecified
Excludes: influenza with pneumonia, any form (487.0)

487 Influenza
Excludes: *Hemophilus influenzae (H. influenzae)*:
infection NOS (041.5)
meningitis (320.0)
487.0 With pneumonia
Influenza with pneumonia, any form
Influenzal:
bronchopneumonia
pneumonia
Use additional code to identify the type of pneumonia (480.0–480.9,
481, 482.0–482.9, 483.0–483.8, 485)
487.1 With other respiratory manifestations
Influenza NOS
Influenzal:
laryngitis
pharyngitis
respiratory infection (upper) (acute)
487.8 With other manifestations
Encephalopathy due to influenza
Influenza with involvement of gastrointestinal tract
488 Influenza due to certain identified influenza viruses
Excludes: influenza caused by unspecified influenza viruses (487.0- 487.8)
488.0 Influenza due to identified avian influenza virus
Avian influenza

Bird flu
Influenza A/H5N1
488.1 Influenza due to identified novel H1N1 influenza virus
2009 H1N1 [swine] influenza virus
Novel 2009 influenza H1N1
Novel H1N1 influenza
Novel influenza A/H1N1
Swine flu

CHRONIC OBSTRUCTIVE PULMONARY DISEASE AND ALLIED CONDITIONS

490 Bronchitis, not specified as acute or chronic
Bronchitis NOS:
catarrhal
with tracheitis NOS
Tracheobronchitis NOS
Excludes: bronchitis:
allergic NOS (493.9)
asthmatic NOS (493.9)

491 Chronic bronchitis
Excludes: chronic obstructive asthma (493.2)
491.0 Simple chronic bronchitis
Catarrhal bronchitis, chronic
Smokers' cough
491.1 Mucopurulent chronic bronchitis
Bronchitis (chronic) (recurrent):
fetid
mucopurulent
purulent
491.2 Obstructive chronic bronchitis
Bronchitis:
emphysematous
obstructive (chronic) (diffuse)
Bronchitis with:
chronic airway obstruction
emphysema
Excludes: asthmatic bronchitis (acute) (NOS) 493.9
chronic obstructive asthma 493.2
491.20 Without exacerbation
Emphysema with chronic bronchitis
491.21 With (acute) exacerbation
Acute exacerbation of chronic obstructive pulmonary
disease) (COPD)
Decompensated chronic obstructive pulmonary disease
(COPD)

Decompensated chronic obstructive pulmonary disease
(COPD) with exacerbation
Excludes: chronic obstructive asthma with acute
exacerbation 493.2
491.22   With acute bronchitis
491.8   Other chronic bronchitis
Chronic:
tracheitis
tracheobronchitis
491.9   Unspecified chronic bronchitis

492   Emphysema
492.0   Emphysematous bleb
Giant bullous emphysema
Ruptured emphysematous bleb
Tension pneumatocele
Vanishing lung
492.8   Other emphysema
Emphysema (lung or pulmonary):
NOS
centriacinar
centrilobular
obstructive
panacinar
panlobular
unilateral
vesicular
Excludes: emphysema:
with chronic bronchitis (491.20–491.22)
compensatory (518.2)
surgical (subcutaneous) (998.81)

493   Asthma
Excludes: wheezing NOS (786.07)

The following fifth-digit subclassification is for use with category
493.0–493.2, 493.9:
0   unspecified
1   with status asthmaticus
2   with (acute) exacerbation

493.0   Extrinsic asthma
Asthma:
allergic with stated cause
atopic
childhood

hay

platinum

Hay fever with asthma

Excludes: asthma, allergic NOS (493.9)

493.1 Intrinsic asthma

Late-onset asthma

493.2 Chronic obstructive asthma

Asthma with chronic obstructive pulmonary disease (COPD)

Chronic asthmatic bronchitis

Excludes: acute bronchitis (466.0)

chronic obstructive bronchitis (491.20–491.22)

493.8 Other forms of asthma

493.81 Exercise induced bronchospasm

493.82 Cough variant asthma

493.9 Asthma, unspecified

Asthma (bronchial) (allergic NOS)

Bronchitis:

allergic

asthmatic

494 Bronchiectasis

Bronchiectasis (fusiform) (postinfectious) (recurrent)

Bronchiolectasis

Excludes: tuberculous bronchiectasis (current disease) (011.5)

494.0 Bronchiectasis without acute exacerbation

494.1 Bronchiectasis with acute exacerbation

496 Chronic airway obstruction, not elsewhere classified

Chronic:

nonspecific lung disease

obstructive lung disease

obstructive pulmonary disease (COPD) NOS

This code is not to be used with any code from categories 491–493

Excludes: chronic obstructive lung disease (COPD) specified (as) (with):

asthma (493.2)

bronchiectasis (494.0)

bronchitis (with emphysema) (491.20–491.22)

emphysema (492.0–492.8)

DISEASES OF THE DIGESTIVE SYSTEM (520–579)

DISEASES OF ESOPHAGUS, STOMACH, AND DUODENUM

532 Duodenal ulcer

Includes: erosion (acute) of duodenum

Ulcer (peptic):

duodenum
postpyloric
Excludes: peptic ulcer NOS (533.0–533.9)

The following fifth-digit subclassification is for use with category 532:
0   without mention of obstruction
1   with obstruction

532.0 Acute with hemorrhage
532.1 Acute with perforation
532.2 Acute without mention of hemorrhage or perforation
532.4 Chronic or unspecified with hemorrhage
532.5 Chronic or unspecified with perforation
532.6 Chronic or unspecified with hemorrhage and perforation
532.7 Chronic without mention of hemorrhage or perforation
532.9 Unspecified as acute or chronic, without mention of hemorrhage or
        perforation

533 Peptic ulcer, site unspecified
Includes: gastroduodenal ulcer NOS
            Peptic ulcer NOS
            Stress ulcer NOS
Excludes: Peptic ulcer: duodenal (532.0–532.9)

The following fifth-digit subclassification is for use with category 532:
0   without mention of obstruction
1   with obstruction

533.0 Acute with hemorrhage
533.1 Acute with perforation
533.2 Acute with hemorrhage and perforation
533.3 Acute without mention of hemorrhage and perforation
533.4 Chronic or unspecified with hemorrhage
533.5 Chronic or unspecified with perforation
533.6 Chronic or unspecified with hemorrhage and perforation
533.7 Chronic without mention of hemorrhage or perforation
533.9 Unspecified as acute or chronic, without mention of hemorrhage
        or perforation

535 Gastritis and duodenitis
The following fifth-digit subclassification is for use with category 535:
0   without mention of hemorrhage
1   with hemorrhage

535.0 Acute gastritis
535.1 Atrophic gastritis

Gastritis:
    atrophic-hyperplastic
    chronic (atrophic)
535.2 Gastric mucosal hypertrophy
    Hypertrophic gastritis
535.3 Alcoholic gastritis
535.4 Other specified gastritis
    Gastritis:
    allergic
    bile induced
    irritant
    superficial
    toxic
    Excludes: cosinophilic gastritis (535.7)
535.5 Unspecified gastritis and gastroduodenitis
    Duodenitis
535.6 Duodenitis
535.7 Eosinophilic gastritis

APPENDICITIS

540 Acute appendicitis
540.0 With generalized peritonitis
    Appendicitis (acute) with: perforation, peritonitis (generalized), rupture:
    fulminating
    gangrenous
    obstructive
    Cecitis (acute) with: perforation, peritonitis (generalized), rupture
    Rupture of appendix
    Excludes: acute appendicitis with peritoneal abscess (540.1)
540.1 With peritoneal abscess
    Abscess of appendix
    With generalized peritonitis
540.9 Without mention of peritonitis

541 Appendicitis, unqualified

542 Other appendicitis
    Appendicitis:
    chronic
    recurrent
    relapsing
    subacute
    Excludes: hyperplasia (lymphoid) of appendix (543.0)

543 Other diseases of appendix
543.0 Hyperplasia of appendix (lymphoid)
543.9 Other and unspecified diseases of appendix
Appendicular or appendiceal:
colic
concretion
fistula
Diverticulum of appendix
Fecalith of appendix
Intussusception of appendix
Mucocele of appendix
Stercolith of appendix

HERNIA OF ABDOMINAL CAVITY
Includes: hernia:
acquired
congenital, except diaphragmatic or
hiatal

550 Inguinal hernia
Includes: bubonocele
inguinal hernia (direct) (double) (indirect) (oblique)
(sliding)
The following fifth-digit subclassification is for use with category 550:
0   unilateral or unspecified (not specified as recurrent)
Unilateral NOS
1   unilateral or unspecified, recurrent
2   bilateral (not specified as recurrent)
Bilateral NOS
3   bilateral, recurrent

550.0 Inguinal hernia, with gangrene
Inguinal hernia with gangrene (and obstruction)
550.1 Inguinal hernia, with obstruction, without mention of gangrene
Inguinal hernia with mention of incarceration, irreducibility, or
strangulation
550.9 Inguinal hernia, without mention of obstruction or gangrene
Inguinal hernia NOS

OTHER DISEASES OF INTESTINES AND PERITONEUM
564 Functional digestive disorders, not elsewhere classified
564.0 Constipation
564.00 Constipation, unspecified
564.01 Slow transit constipation
564.02 Outlet dysfunction constipation
564.09 Other constipation

564.1 Irritable bowel syndrome
Irritable colon
Spastic colon

564.5 Functional diarrhea
Excludes: diarrhea NOS (787.91)

564.9 Unspecified functional disorder of intestine
Functional bowel disease

565 Anal fissure and fistula

565.0 Anal fissure
Excludes: anal sphincter tear (healed) (non-traumatic) (old) (569.43)

565.1 Anal fistula
Fistula:
anorectal
rectal
rectum to skin
Excludes: fistula of rectum to internal organs—*see* Alphabetic Index
ischiorectal fistula (566)
rectovaginal fistula (619.1)

566 Abscess of anal and rectal regions

Abscess:
ischiorectal
perianal
perirectal
Cellulitis:
anal
perirectal
rectal
Ischiorectal fistula

567 Peritonitis and retroperitoneal infection

Excludes: peritonitis:
pelvic (614.5, 614.7)
puerperal (670)
with or following:
abortion (634–638 with fourth digit 0, 639.0)
appendicitis (540.0–540.1)
ectopic or molar pregnancy (639.0)

567.1 Pneumococcal peritonitis

567.2 Other suppurative peritonitis
567.21 Peritonitis (acute) generalized

567.22 Peritoneal abscess
Abscess (of):
abdominopelvic
omentum
peritoneum
567.23 Spontaneous bacterial peritonitis
Excludes: bacterial peritonitis NOS (567.29)
567.29 Other suppurative peritonitis
567.3 Retroperitoneal infections
567.31 Psoas muscle abscess
567.38 Other retroperitoneal abscess
567.39 Other retroperitoneal infections
567.8 Other specified peritonitis
567.81 Choleperitonitis
567.82 Sclerosing mesenteritis
567.89 Other specified peritonitis
567.9 Unspecified peritonitis
Peritonitis:
NOS
of unspecified cause

568 Other disorders of peritoneum
568.0 Peritoneal adhesions (postoperative) (postinfection)
Adhesions (of):
abdominal (wall)
diaphragm
intestine
mesenteric
Adhesions (of):
omentum
stomach
Adhesive bands
Excludes: adhesions, pelvic (614.6)
568.8 Other specified disorders of peritoneum
568.81 Hemoperitoneum (nontraumatic)
568.82 Peritoneal effusion (chronic)
Excludes: ascites NOS (789.51–789.59)
568.89 Other
Peritoneal:
cyst
granuloma
568.9 Unspecified disorder of peritoneum

569 Other disorders of intestine

569.0 Anal and rectal polyp
Anal and rectal polyp NOS
Excludes: adenomatous anal and rectal polyp (211.4)

569.1 Rectal prolapse
Procidentia:
anus (sphincter)
rectum (sphincter)
Proctoptosis
Prolapse:
anal canal
rectal mucosa
Excludes: prolapsed hemorrhoids (455.2, 455.5)

569.2 Stenosis of rectum and anus
Stricture of anus (sphincter)

569.3 Hemorrhage of rectum and anus
Excludes: gastrointestinal bleeding NOS (578.9)
melena (578.1)

569.4 Other specified disorders of rectum and anus
569.41 Ulcer of anus and rectum
Solitary ulcer of anus (sphincter) or rectum (sphincter)
Stercoral ulcer of anus (sphincter) or rectum (sphincter)

569.42 Anal or rectal pain

569.43 Anal sphincter tear (healed) (old)
Tear of anus, non-traumatic
Use additional code for any associated fecal incontinence (787.6)
Excludes: anal fissure (565.0)
anal sphincter tear (healed) (old) complicating delivery (654.8)

569.44 Dysplasia of anus
Anal intraepithelial neoplasia I and II (AIN I and II) (histologically confirmed)
Dysplasia of anus NOS
Mild and moderate dysplasia of anus (histologically confirmed)
Excludes: abnormal results from anal cytologic examination without histologic confirmation (796.70–796.79)
anal intraepithelial neoplasia III (230.5, 230.6)
carcinoma in situ of anus (230.5, 230.6)
HGSIL of anus (796.74)
severe dysplasia of anus (230.5, 230.6)

569.49 Other
Granuloma of rectum (sphincter)
Rupture of rectum (sphincter)
Hypertrophy of anal papillae
Proctitis NOS
Excludes: fistula of rectum to:
internal organs—*see* Alphabetic Index
skin (565.1)
hemorrhoids (455.0–455.9)
incontinence of sphincter ani (787.6)

569.5 Abscess of intestine
Excludes: appendiceal abscess (540.1)

569.6 Colostomy and enterostomy complications
569.60 Colostomy and enterostomy complication, unspecified
569.61 Infection of colostomy or enterostomy
569.62 Mechanical complication of colostomy and enterostomy
569.69 Other complication

573   Other disorders of liver

573.0 Chronic passive congestion of liver
573.3 Hepatitis, unspecified
Toxic (noninfectious) hepatitis
Use additional E code to identify cause
573.4 Hepatic infarction
573.8 Other specified disorders of liver
Hepatoptosis
573.9 Unspecified disorder of liver

578   Gastrointestinal hemorrhage

Excludes: that with mention of gastritis and duodenitis (535.0–535.6)
578.0 Hematemesis
Vomiting of blood
578.1 Blood in stool
Melena
Excludes: melena of the newborn (772.4, 777.3)
occult blood (792.1)
578.9 Hemorrhage of gastrointestinal tract, unspecified
Gastric hemorrhage
Intestinal hemorrhage

DISEASES OF THE GENITOURINARY SYSTEM (580–629)

NEPHRITIS, NEPHROTIC SYNDROME, AND NEPHROSIS

Excludes: hypertensive renal disease (403.00–403.91)

584 Acute renal failure
    Excludes: following labor and delivery (669.3)
             posttraumatic (958.5)
             that complicating:
                abortion (634–638 with fourth digit 3, 639.3)
                ectopic or molar pregnancy (639.3)
    584.5 With lesion of tubular necrosis
    584.6 With lesion of renal cortical necrosis
    584.7 With lesion of renal medullary (papillary) necrosis
    584.8 With other specified pathological lesion in kidney
    584.9 Acute renal failure, unspecified
             Acute kidney injury (nontraumatic)

OTHER DISEASES OF URINARY SYSTEM

590 Infections of kidney
    Use additional code to identify organism, such as *Escherichia coli (E. coli)*
    (041.4)
    590.1 Acute pyelonephritis
        590.10 Without lesions of renal medullary necrosis
        590.11 With lesion of renal medullary necrosis

591 Hydronephrosis
    Excludes: congenital hydronephrosis (753.29)

592 Calculus of kidney and ureter
    592.0 Calculus of kidney
    592.1 Calculus of ureter
    592.9 Urinary calculus, unspecified

595 Cystitis
    Use additional code to identify organism, such as *Escherichia coli (E. coli)*
    (041.4)
    595.0 Acute cystitis
        Excludes: trigonitis (595.3)
    595.1 Chronic interstitial cystitis
        Hunner's ulcer
        Panmural fibrosis of bladder
        Submucous cystitis

595.2 Other chronic cystitis
Chronic cystitis NOS
Subacute cystitis
Excludes: trigonitis (595.3)
595.3 Trigonitis
Follicular cystitis
Trigonitis (acute) (chronic)
Urethrotrigonitis
595.8 Other specified types of cystitis
595.81 Cystitis cystica
595.82 Irradiation cystitis
Use additional E to identify cause
595.89 Other
Abscess of bladder
Cystitis:
bullous
emphysematous
glandularis
595.9 Cystitis, unspecified

596 Other disorders of bladder
Use additional code to identify urinary incontinence (625.6, 788.30–788.39)
596.0 Bladder neck obstruction
Contracture, obstruction, or stenosis (acquired) of bladder neck or
vesicourethral orifice
596.3 Diverticulum of bladder
Diverticulitis of bladder
596.4 Atony of bladder
High compliance bladder
Hypotonicity of bladder
Inertia of bladder
Excludes: neurogenic bladder (596.54)
596.5 Other functional disorders of bladder
596.51 Hypertonicity of bladder
Hyperactivity
Overactive bladder
596.52 Low bladder compliance
596.53 Paralysis of bladder
596.54 Neurogenic bladder NOS
596.55 Detrusor sphincter dyssynergia
596.59 Other functional disorder of bladder
Detrusor instability

597 Urethritis, not sexually transmitted, and urethral syndrome

597.0 Urethral abscess

Abscess of:

bulbourethral gland

Cowper's gland

Littré's gland

Abscess:

periurethral

urethral (gland)

Periurethral cellulitis

Excludes: urethral caruncle (599.3)

597.8 Other urethritis

597.80 Urethritis, unspecified

597.81 Urethral syndrome NOS

597.89 Other

Adenitis, Skene's glands

Cowperitis

Meatitis, urethral

Ulcer, urethra (meatus)

Verumontanitis

Excludes: trichomonal (131.02)

598 Urethral stricture

Use additional code to identify urinary incontinence (625.6, 788.30–788.39)

Excludes: congenital stricture of urethra and urinary meatus (753.6)

598.0 Urethral stricture due to infection

598.00 Due to unspecified infection

598.01 Due to infective diseases classified elsewhere

Code first underlying disease, as: gonococcal infection (098.2)

598.1 Traumatic urethral stricture

Stricture of urethra:

late effect of injury

postobstetric

Excludes: postoperative following surgery on genitourinary tract (598.2)

598.2 Postoperative urethral stricture

Postcatheterization stricture of urethra

598.8 Other specified causes of urethral stricture

598.9 Urethral stricture, unspecified

599 Other disorders of urethra and urinary tract

599.0 Urinary tract infection, site not specified
Excludes: Candidiasis of urinary tract (112.2)
Use additional code to identify organism, such as *Escherichia coli (E. coli)* (041.4)

599.1 Urethral fistula
Fistula:
urethroperineal
urethrorectal
Urinary fistula NOS
Excludes: fistula:
urethrovaginal (619.0)
urethrovesicovaginal (619.0)

599.2 Urethral diverticulum

599.3 Urethral caruncle
Polyp of urethra

599.4 Urethral false passage

599.5 Prolapsed urethral mucosa
Prolapse of urethra
Urethrocele
Excludes: urethrocele (618.03, 618.09, 618.2–618.4)

599.6 Urinary obstruction
Use additional code to identify urinary incontinence (625.6, 788.30–788.39)
599.60 Urinary obstruction, unspecified
Obstructive uropathy NOS
Urinary (tract) obstruction NOS
599.69 Urinary obstruction, not elsewhere classified

599.7 Hematuria
Hematuria (benign) (essential)
Excludes: hemoglobinuria (791.2)
599.70 Hematuria, unspecified
599.71 Gross hematuria
599.72 Microscopic hematuria

599.8 Other specified disorders of urethra and urinary tract
Use additional code to identify urinary incontinence (625.6, 788.30–788.39)
Excludes: symptoms and other conditions classifiable to 788.0–788.2, 788.4–788.9, 791.0–791.9
599.81 Urethral hypermobility
599.82 Intrinsic (urethral) sphincter deficiency (ISD)
599.83 Urethral instability

599.84   Other specified disorders of urethra
Rupture of urethra (nontraumatic)
Urethral:
cyst
granuloma
599.89   Other specified disorders of urinary tract
Unspecified disorder of urethra and urinary tract

606   Infertility, male

606.0   Azoospermia
Absolute infertility
Infertility due to:
germinal (cell) aplasia
spermatogenic arrest (complete)
606.1   Oligospermia
Infertility due to:
germinal cell desquamation
hypospermatogenesis
incomplete spermatogenic arrest
606.8   Infertility due to extratesticular causes
Infertility due to:
drug therapy
infection
obstruction of efferent ducts
radiation
systemic disease
606.9   Male infertility, unspecified

DISORDERS OF BREAST

610   Benign mammary dysplasias

610.0   Solitary cyst of breast
Cyst (solitary) of breast
610.1   Diffuse cystic mastopathy
Chronic cystic mastitis
Cystic breast
Fibrocystic disease of breast
610.2   Fibroadenosis of breast
NOS
chronic
cystic
diffuse
periodic
segmental

610.3 Fibrosclerosis of breast
610.4 Mammary duct ectasia
    Comedomastitis
    Duct ectasia
    Mastitis:
        periductal
        plasma cell
610.8 Other specified benign mammary dysplasias
    Mazoplasia
    Sebaceous cyst of breast
610.9 Benign mammary dysplasia, unspecified

611 Other disorders of breast
Excludes: that associated with lactation or the puerperium (675.0–676.9)
611.0 Inflammatory disease of breast
    Abscess (acute) (chronic) (nonpuerperal) of:
        areola
        breast
    Mammillary fistula
    Mastitis (acute) (subacute) (nonpuerperal):
        NOS
        infective
        retromammary
        submammary
    Excludes: carbuncle of breast (680.2)
                chronic cystic mastitis (610.1)
611.1 Hypertrophy of breast
    Gynecomastia
    Hypertrophy of breast:
        NOS
        massive pubertal
    Excludes: disproportion or reconstructed breast (612.1)
611.2 Fissure of nipple
611.3 Fat necrosis of breast
    Fat necrosis (segmental) of breast
    Code first breast necrosis due to breast graft (996.79)
611.4 Atrophy of breast
611.5 Galactocele
611.6 Galactorrhea not associated with childbirth
611.7 Signs and symptoms in breast
    611.71 Mastodynia
            Pain in breast
    611.72 Lump or mass in breast

611.79 Other
Induration of breast
Inversion of nipple
Nipple discharge
Retraction of nipple
611.8 Other specified disorders of breast
611.81 Ptosis of breast
Excludes: ptosis of native breast in relation to reconstructed breast (612.1)
611.82 Hypoplasia of breast
Micromastia
Excludes: congenital absence of breast (757.6)
hypoplasia of native breast in relation to reconstructed breast (612.1)
611.83 Capsular contracture of breast implant
611.89 Other specified disorders of the breast
Hematoma (nontraumatic) of breast
Infarction of breast
Occlusion of breast duct
Subinvolution of breast (postlactational) (postpartum)
611.9 Unspecified breast disorder

612 Deformity and disproportion of reconstructed breast
612.0 Deformity of reconstructed breast
Contour irregularity in reconstructed breast
Excess tissue in reconstructed breast
Misshapen reconstructed breast
612.1 Disproportion of reconstructed breast
Breast asymmetry between native breast and reconstructed breast
Disproportion between native breast and reconstructed breast

INFLAMMATORY DISEASE OF FEMALE PELVIC ORGANS

Use additional code to identify organism, such as Staphylococcus (041.1), or Streptococcus (041.0)
Excludes: that associated with pregnancy, abortion, childbirth, or the puerperium (630–676.9)

614 Inflammatory disease of ovary, fallopian tube, pelvic cellular tissue, and peritoneum
Excludes: endometritis (615.0–615.9)
major infection following delivery (670.0-670.8)
that complicating:
abortion (634–638 with fourth digit 0, 639.0)
ectopic or molar pregnancy (639.0)
pregnancy or labor (646.6)

614.0 Acute salpingitis and oophoritis
Any condition classifiable to 614.2, specified as acute or subacute
614.1 Chronic salpingitis and oophoritis
Hydrosalpinx
Salpingitis:
   follicularis
   isthmica nodosa
Any condition classifiable to 614.2, specified as chronic
614.2 Salpingitis and oophoritis not specified as acute, subacute, or
   chronic
Abscess (of):
   fallopian tube
   ovary
   tubo-ovarian
Oophoritis
Perioophoritis
Perisalpingitis
Pyosalpinx
Salpingitis
Salpingo-oophoritis
Tubo-ovarian inflammatory disease
Excludes: gonococcal infection (chronic) (098.37)
                acute (098.17)
                tuberculous (016.6)
614.3 Acute parametritis and pelvic cellulitis
Acute inflammatory pelvic disease
Any condition classifiable to 614.4, specified as acute
614.4 Chronic or unspecified parametritis and pelvic cellulitis
Abscess (of):
   broad ligament chronic or NOS
   parametrium chronic or NOS
   pelvis, female chronic or NOS
   pouch of Douglas chronic or NOS
Chronic inflammatory pelvic disease
Pelvic cellulitis
Excludes: tuberculous (016.7)
614.5 Acute or unspecified pelvic peritonitis
614.6 Pelvic peritoneal adhesions (postoperative) (postinfection)
Adhesions:
   peritubal
   tubo-ovarian
Use additional code to identify any associated infertility (628.2)
614.7 Other chronic pelvic peritonitis
Excludes: tuberculous (016.7)

614.8 Other specified inflammatory disease of pelvic organs and tissues
614.9 Unspecified inflammatory disease of female pelvic organs and tissues
       Pelvic infection or inflammation NOS
       Pelvic inflammatory disease (PID)

615 Inflammatory diseases of uterus, except cervix
   Excludes: following delivery (670.0-670.8)
                  hyperplastic endometritis (621.30–621.35)
                  that complicating:
                      abortion (634–638 with .0, 639.0)
                      ectopic or molar pregnancy (639.0)
                      pregnancy or labor (646.6)
615.0 Acute
       Any condition classifiable to 615.9, specified as acute or subacute
615.1 Chronic
       Any condition classifiable to 615.9, specified as chronic
615.9 Unspecified inflammatory disease of uterus
       Endometritis
       Endomyometritis
       Metritis
       Myometritis
       Perimetritis
       Pyometra
       Uterine abscess

616 Inflammatory disease of cervix, vagina, and vulva
   Excludes: that complicating:
                  abortion (634–638 with fourth digit 0, 639.0)
                  ectopic or molar pregnancy (639.0)
                  pregnancy, childbirth, or the puerperium (646.6)
616.0 Cervicitis and endocervicitis
       Cervicitis with or without mention of erosion or ectropion
       Endocervicitis with or without mention of erosion or ectropion
       Nabothian (gland) cyst or follicle
       Excludes: erosion or ectropion without mention of cervicitis
                  (622.0)
616.1 Vaginitis and vulvovaginitis
       Excludes: vulvar vestibulitis (625.71)
       616.10 Vaginitis and vulvovaginitis, unspecified
               Vaginitis:
                   NOS
                   postirradiation
               Vulvitis NOS
               Vulvovaginitis NOS

Use additional code to identify organism, such as
Escherichia coli (E. coli) (041.4), Staphylococcus
(041.1), or Streptococcus (041.0)
Excludes: noninfective leukorrhea (623.5)
postmenopausal or senile vaginitis (627.3)

616.11 Vaginitis and vulvovaginitis in diseases classified elsewhere
Code first underlying disease
Excludes: herpetic vulvovaginitis (054.11)
monilial vulvovaginitis (112.1)
trichomonal vaginitis or vulvovaginitis (131.01)

616.2 Cyst of Bartholin's gland
Bartholin's duct cyst

616.3 Abscess of Bartholin's gland
Vulvovaginal gland abscess

616.4 Other abscess of vulva
Abscess of vulva
Carbuncle of vulva
Furuncle of vulva

616.5 Ulceration of vulva

616.50 Ulceration of vulva, unspecified
Ulcer NOS of vulva

616.51 Ulceration of vulva in diseases classified elsewhere
Code first underlying disease, as tuberculosis (016.7)
Excludes: vulvar ulcer (in):
gonococcal (098.0)
herpes simplex (054.12)
syphilitic (091.0)

616.8 Other specified inflammatory diseases of cervix, vagina, and vulva
Excludes: noninflammatory disorders of:
cervix (622.0–622.9)
vagina (623.0–623.9)
vulva (624.0–624.9)

618.81 Mucositis (ulcerative) of cervix, vagina, and vulva
Use additional E code to identify adverse effects of therapy,
such as:
antineoplastic and immunosuppressive drugs (E930.7,
E933.1)
radiation therapy (E879.2)

616.89 Other inflammatory disease of cervix, vagina and vulva
Caruncle, vagina or labium
Ulcer, vagina

616.9 Unspecified inflammatory disease of cervix, vagina, and vulva

OTHER DISORDERS OF FEMALE GENITAL TRACT

617 Endometriosis

617.0 Endometriosis of uterus
Adenomyosis
Endometriosis:
 cervix
 internal
 myometrium
Excludes: stromal endometriosis (236.0)

617.1 Endometriosis of ovary
Chocolate cyst of ovary
Endometrial cystoma of ovary

617.2 Endometriosis of fallopian tube

617.3 Endometriosis of pelvic peritoneum
Endometriosis:
 broad ligament
 cul-de-sac (Douglas')
 parametrium
 round ligament

617.4 Endometriosis of rectovaginal septum and vagina

617.5 Endometriosis of intestine
Endometriosis:
 appendix
 colon
 rectum

617.6 Endometriosis in scar of skin

617.8 Endometriosis of other specified sites
Endometriosis:
 bladder
 lung
 umbilicus
 vulva

617.9 Endometriosis, site unspecified

618 Genital prolapse

Use additional code to identify urinary incontinence (625.6, 788.31, 788.33–788.39)
Excludes: that complicating pregnancy, labor, or delivery (654.4)

618.0 Prolapse of vaginal walls without mention of uterine prolapse
 Excludes: that with uterine prolapse (618.2–618.4)
   enterocele (618.6)
   vaginal vault prolapse following hysterectomy (618.5)

 618.00 Unspecified prolapse of vaginal walls
  Vaginal prolapse NOS

618.01 Cystocele, midline
Cystocele NOS
618.02 Cystocele, lateral
Paravaginal
618.03 Urethrocele
618.04 Rectocele
618.05 Perineocele
618.09 Other prolapse of vaginal walls without mention of uterine prolapse
Cystourethrocele

618.1 Uterine prolapse without mention of vaginal wall prolapse
Descensus uteri
Uterine prolapse:
NOS
complete
first degree
second degree
third degree
Excludes: that with mention of cystocele, urethrocele, or rectocele (618.2–618.4)

618.2 Uterovaginal prolapse, incomplete
618.3 Uterovaginal prolapse, complete
618.4 Uterovaginal prolapse, unspecified
618.5 Prolapse of vaginal vault after hysterectomy
618.6 Vaginal enterocele, congenital or acquired
Pelvic enterocele, congenital or acquired
618.7 Old laceration of muscles of pelvic floor
618.8 Other specified genital prolapse
618.81 Incompetence or weakening of pubocervical tissue
618.82 Incompetence of weakening of rectovaginal tissue
618.83 Pelvic muscle wasting
Diffuse atrophy of pelvic muscles and anal sphincter
618.84 Cervical stump prolapse
618.89 Other specified genital prolapse
618.9 Unspecified genital prolapse
Incompetence or weakening of pelvic fundus
Relaxation of vaginal outlet or pelvis

619 Fistula involving female genital tract
619.0 Urinary-genital tract fistula
Fistula:
cervicovesical
ureterovaginal
urethrovaginal
urethrovesicovaginal

Fistula:
    uteroureteric
    uterovesical
    vesicocervicovaginal
    vesicovaginal

619.1 Digestive-genital tract fistula
Fistula:
    intestinouterine
    intestinovaginal
    rectovaginal
    rectovulval
    sigmoidovaginal
    uterorectal

619.2 Genital tract-skin fistula
Fistula:
    uterus to abdominal wall
    vaginoperineal

619.8 Other specified fistulas involving genital tract
Fistula:
    cervix
    cul-de-sac (Douglas')
    uterus
    vagina

619.9 Unspecified fistula involving female genital tract

620 Noninflammatory disorders of ovary, fallopian tube, and broad ligament
Excludes: hydrosalpinx (614.1)

620.0 Follicular cyst of ovary
Cyst of graafian follicle

620.1 Corpus luteum cyst or hematoma
Corpus luteum hemorrhage or rupture
Lutein cyst

620.2 Other and unspecified ovarian cyst
Cyst of ovary:
    NOS
    corpus albicans
    retention NOS
    serous
    theca-lutein
Simple cystoma of ovary
Excludes: cystadenoma (benign) (serous) (220)
         developmental cysts (752.0)
         neoplastic cysts (220)
         polycystic ovaries (256.4)
         Stein-Leventhal syndrome (256.4)

620.3 Acquired atrophy of ovary and fallopian tube
Senile involution of ovary

620.4 Prolapse or hernia of ovary and fallopian tube
Displacement of ovary and fallopian tube
Salpingocele

620.5 Torsion of ovary, ovarian pedicle, or fallopian tube
Torsion:
  accessory tube
  hydatid of Morgagni

620.6 Broad ligament laceration syndrome
Masters-Allen syndrome

620.7 Hematoma of broad ligament
Hematocele, broad ligament

620.8 Other noninflammatory disorders of ovary, fallopian tube, and
broad ligament
Cyst of broad ligament or fallopian tube
Polyp of broad ligament or fallopian tube
Infarction of ovary or fallopian tube
Rupture of ovary or fallopian tube
Hematosalpinx of ovary or fallopian tube
Excludes: hematosalpinx in ectopic pregnancy (639.2)
peritubal adhesions (614.6)
torsion of ovary, ovarian pedicle, or fallopian
tube (620.5)

620.9 Unspecified noninflammatory disorder of ovary, fallopian tube,
and broad ligament

621 Disorders of uterus, not elsewhere classified

621.0 Polyp of corpus uteri
Polyp:
  endometrium
  uterus NOS
Excludes: cervical polyp NOS (622.7)

621.1 Chronic subinvolution of uterus
Excludes: puerperal (674.8)

621.2 Hypertrophy of uterus
Bulky or enlarged uterus
Excludes: puerperal (674.8)

621.3 Endometrial hyperplasia
621.30 Endometrial hyperplasia, unspecified
Endometrial hyperplasia NOS
Hyperplasia (adenomatous) (cystic) (glandular) of endometrium
Hyperplastic endometritis
621.31 Simple endometrial hyperplasia without atypia
Excludes: benign endometrial hyperplasia (621.34)

621.32 Complex endometrial hyperplasia without atypia
Excludes: benign endometrial hyperplasia (621.34)
621.33 Endometrial hyperplasia with atypia
Excludes: endometrial intraepithelial neoplasia [EIN] (621.35)
621.34 Benign endometrial hyperplasia
621.35 Endometrial intraepithelial neoplasia [EIN]
Excludes: malignant neoplasm of endometrium with
endometrial intraepithelial neoplasia [EIN] (182.0)

621.4 Hematometra
Hemometra
Excludes: that in congenital anomaly (752.2–752.3)

621.5 Intrauterine synechiae
Adhesions of uterus
Band(s) of uterus

621.6 Malposition of uterus
Anteversion of uterus
Retroflexion of uterus
Retroversion of uterus
Excludes: malposition complicating pregnancy, labor, or
delivery (654.3–654.4)
prolapse of uterus (618.1–618.4)

621.7 Chronic inversion of uterus
Excludes: current obstetrical trauma (665.2)
prolapse of uterus (618.1–618.4)

621.8 Other specified disorders of uterus, not elsewhere classified
Atrophy, acquired of uterus
Cyst of uterus
Fibrosis NOS of uterus
Old laceration (postpartum) of uterus
Ulcer of uterus
Excludes: endometriosis (617.0)
fistulas (619.0–619.8)
inflammatory diseases (615.0–615.9)

621.9 Unspecified disorder of uterus

622 **Noninflammatory disorders of cervix**
Excludes: abnormality of cervix complicating pregnancy, labor, or delivery
(654.5–654.6)
fistula (619.0–619.8)

622.0 Erosion and ectropion of cervix
Eversion of cervix
Ulcer of cervix
Excludes: that in chronic cervicitis (616.0)

622.1 Dysplasia of cervix (uteri)
For additional information concerning reporting cervical dysplasia, see

TABULAR LIST: DISEASES OF THE GENITOURINARY SYSTEM (580–629)

Appendix B.

Excludes: abnormal results from cervical cytologic examination
without histologic confirmation (795.00–795.09)
carcinoma in situ of cervix (233.1)
cervical intraepithelial neoplasia III (CIN III) (233.1)
HGSIL of cervix (795.04)

622.10 Dysplasia of cervix, unspecified
Anaplasia of cervix
Cervical atypism
Cervical dysplasia NOS

622.11 Mild dysplasia of cervix
Cervical intraepithelial neoplasia I (CIN I)

622.12 Moderate dysplasia of cervix
Cervical intraepithelial neoplasia (CIN II)
Excludes: carcinoma in situ of cervix (233.1)
cervical intraepithelial neoplasia III
(CIN III) (233.1)
severe dysplasia (233.1)

622.2 Leukoplakia of cervix (uteri)
Excludes: carcinoma in situ of cervix (233.1)

622.3 Old laceration of cervix
Adhesions of cervix
Band(s) of cervix
Cicatrix (postpartum) of cervix
Excludes: current obstetrical trauma (665.3)

622.4 Stricture and stenosis of cervix
Atresia (acquired) of cervix
Contracture of cervix
Occlusion of cervix
Pinpoint os uteri
Excludes: congenital (752.49)
that complicating labor (654.6)

622.5 Incompetence of cervix
Excludes: complicating pregnancy (654.5)

622.6 Hypertrophic elongation of cervix

622.7 Mucous polyp of cervix
Polyp NOS of cervix
Excludes: adenomatous polyp of cervix (219.0)

622.8 Other specified noninflammatory disorders of cervix
Atrophy (senile) of cervix
Cyst of cervix
Fibrosis of cervix
Hemorrhage of cervix

    Excludes: endometriosis (617.0)
             fistula (619.0–619.8)
             inflammatory diseases (616.0)
622.9 Unspecified noninflammatory disorder of cervix

623 **Noninflammatory disorders of vagina**
    Excludes: abnormality of vagina complicating pregnancy, labor, or
             delivery (654.7)
             congenital absence of vagina (752.49)
             congenital diaphragm or bands (752.49)
             fistulas involving vagina (619.0–619.8)
623.0 Dysplasia of vagina
      Mild and moderate dysplasia of vagina
      Vaginal intraepithelial neoplasia I and II (VAIN I and II)
      Excludes: abnormal results from vaginal cytological examination
               histologic confirmation (795.10–795.19)
               carcinoma in situ of vagina (233.31)
               HGSIL of vagina (795.14)
               severe dysplasia of vagina (233.31)
               vaginal intraepithelial neoplasia III (VAIN III) (233.31)
623.1 Leukoplakia of vagina
623.2 Stricture or atresia of vagina
      Adhesions (postoperative) (postradiation) of vagina
      Occlusion of vagina
      Stenosis, vagina
      Excludes: congenital atresia or stricture (752.49)
623.3 Tight hymenal ring
      Rigid hymen acquired or congenital
      Tight hymenal ring acquired or congenital
      Tight introitus acquired or congenital
      Excludes: imperforate hymen (752.42)
623.4 Old vaginal laceration
      Excludes: old laceration involving muscles of pelvic floor
               (618.7)
623.5 Leukorrhea, not specified as infective
      Leukorrhea NOS of vagina
      Vaginal discharge NOS
      Excludes: trichomonal (131.00)
623.6 Vaginal hematoma
      Excludes: current obstetrical trauma (665.7)
623.7 Polyp of vagina
623.8 Other specified noninflammatory disorders of vagina
      Cyst of vagina
      Hemorrhage of vagina
623.9 Unspecified noninflammatory disorder of vagina

624   Noninflammatory disorders of vulva and perineum
Excludes: abnormality of vulva and perineum complicating pregnancy,
labor, or delivery (654.8)
condyloma acuminatum (078.11)
fistulas involving:
perineum—*see* Alphabetic Index
vulva (619.0–619.8)
vulval varices (456.6)
vulvar involvement in skin conditions (691–709)

624.0   Dystrophy of vulva
Excludes: carcinoma in situ of vulva (233.32)
severe dysplasia of vulva (233.32)
vulvar intraepithelial neoplasia III (VIN III) 233.32

624.01   Vulvar intraepithelial neoplasia (VIN I)
Mild dysplasia of vulva

624.02   Vulvar intraepithelial neoplasia (VIN II)
Moderate dysplasia of vulva

624.09   Other dystrophy of vulva
Kraurosis of vulva
Leukoplakia of vulva

624.1   Atrophy of vulva

624.2   Hypertrophy of clitoris
Excludes: that in endocrine disorders (256.1)

624.3   Hypertrophy of labia
Hypertrophy of vulva NOS

624.4   Old laceration or scarring of vulva

624.5   Hematoma of vulva
Excludes: that complicating delivery (664.5)

624.6   Polyp of labia and vulva

624.8   Other specified noninflammatory disorders of vulva and perineum
Cyst of vulva
Edema of vulva
Stricture of vulva

624.9   Unspecified noninflammatory disorder of vulva and perineum

625   Pain and other symptoms associated with female genital organs
625.0   Dyspareunia
Excludes: psychogenic dyspareunia (302.76)

625.1   Vaginismus
Colpospasm
Vulvismus
Excludes: psychogenic vaginismus (306.51)

625.2   Mittelschmerz
Intermenstrual pain
Ovulation pain

625.3 Dysmenorrhea
Painful menstruation
Excludes: psychogenic dysmenorrhea (306.52)

625.4 Premenstrual tension syndromes
Menstrual molimen
Premenstrual dysphoric disorder
Premenstrual syndrome
Premenstrual tension NOS

625.5 Pelvic congestion syndrome
Congestion-fibrosis syndrome
Taylor's syndrome

625.6 Stress incontinence
Excludes: mixed incontinence (788.33)

625.7 Vulvodynia
  625.70 Vulvodynia unspecified
Vulvodynia NOS
  625.71 Vulvar vestibulitis
  625.79 Other vulvodynia

625.8 Other specified symptoms associated with genital organs

625.9 Unspecified symptom associated with genital organs

626 Disorders of menstruation and other abnormal bleeding from genital tract
Excludes: menopausal and premenopausal bleeding (627.0)
pain and other symptoms associated with menstrual cycle (625.2–625.4)
postmenopausal bleeding (627.1)

626.0 Absence of menstruation
Amenorrhea (primary) (secondary)

626.1 Scanty or infrequent menstruation
Hypomenorrhea
Oligomenorrhea

626.2 Excessive or frequent menstruation
Heavy periods
Menometrorrhagia
Menorrhagia
Polymenorrhea
Excludes: premenopausal (627.0)
that in puberty (626.3)

626.3 Puberty bleeding
Excessive bleeding associated with onset of menstrual periods
Pubertal menorrhagia

626.4 Irregular menstrual cycle
Irregular:
bleeding NOS
menstruation
periods
626.5 Ovulation bleeding
Regular intermenstrual bleeding
626.6 Metrorrhagia
Bleeding unrelated to menstrual cycle
Irregular intermenstrual bleeding
626.7 Postcoital bleeding
626.8 Other
Dysfunctional or functional uterine hemorrhage NOS
Menstruation:
retained
suppression of
626.9 Unspecified

627 **Menopausal and postmenopausal disorders**
Excludes: asymptomatic age-related (natural) postmenopausal status
(V49.81)
627.0 Premenopausal menorrhagia
Excessive bleeding associated with onset of menopause
Menorrhagia:
climacteric
menopausal
preclimacteric
627.1 Postmenopausal bleeding
627.2 Symptomatic menopausal or female climacteric states
Symptoms, such as flushing, sleeplessness, headache, lack of
concentration, associated with the menopause
627.3 Postmenopausal atrophic vaginitis
Senile (atrophic) vaginitis
627.4 Symptomatic states associated with artificial menopause
Postartificial menopause syndromes
Any condition classifiable to 627.1, 627.2, or 627.3, which follows
induced menopause
627.8 Other specified menopausal and postmenopausal disorders
Excludes: premature menopause NOS (256.31)
627.9 Unspecified menopausal and postmenopausal disorder

628 **Infertility, female**
Includes: primary and secondary sterility
628.0 Associated with anovulation
Anovulatory cycle
Use additional code for any associated Stein-Leventhal syndrome (256.4)

628.1 Of pituitary-hypothalamic origin
Code first underlying disease, as:
adiposogenital dystrophy (253.8)
anterior pituitary disorder (253.1–253.4)
628.2 Of tubal origin
Infertility associated with congenital anomaly of tube
Tubal:
block
occlusion
stenosis
Use additional code for any associated peritubal adhesions (614.6)
628.3 Of uterine origin
Infertility associated with congenital anomaly of uterus
Nonimplantation
Use additional code for any associated tuberculous endometritis
(016.7)
628.4 Of cervical or vaginal origin
Infertility associated with:
anomaly or cervical mucus
congenital structural anomaly
dysmucorrhea
628.8 Of other specified origin
628.9 Of unspecified origin

629 **Other disorders of genital organs**
629.0 Hematocele, not elsewhere classified
Excludes: hematocele or hematoma:
broad ligament (620.7)
fallopian tube (620.8)
that associated with ectopic pregnancy
(633.00–633.91)
uterus (621.4)
vagina (623.6)
vulva (624.5)
629.1 Hydrocele, canal of Nuck
Cyst of canal of Nuck (acquired)
Excludes: congenital (752.41)
629.2 Female genital mutilation status
Female circumcision status
Female genital cutting
629.20 Female genital mutilation status, unspecified
Female genital mutilation status NOS
629.21 Female genital mutilation Type I status
Clitorectomy status

629.22 Female genital mutilation Type II status
Clitorectomy with excision of labia minora status
629.23 Female genital mutilation Type III status
Infibulation status
629.29 Other female genital mutilation status
Female genital mutilation Type IV status
629.8 Other specified disorders of female genital organs
629.81 Habitual aborter without current pregnancy
Excludes: habitual aborter without current pregnancy (646.3)
629.89 Other specified disorders of female genital organs
629.9 Unspecified disorder of female genital organs

COMPLICATIONS OF PREGNANCY, CHILDBIRTH, AND THE PUERPERIUM (630–679)

For additional information concerning codes for abortions and stillbirths, see Appendix A.

ECTOPIC AND MOLAR PREGNANCY

Use additional code from category 639 to identify any complications

630 Hydatidiform mole
Trophoblastic disease NOS
Vesicular mole
Excludes: chorioadenoma (destruens) (236.1)
chorionepithelioma (181)
malignant hydatidiform mole (236.1)

631 Other abnormal product of conception
Blighted ovum
Mole:
NOS
carneous
fleshy
stone

632 Missed abortion
Early fetal death before completion of 22 weeks' gestation with retention of dead fetus
Retained products of conception, not following spontaneous or induced abortion or delivery
Excludes: failed induced abortion (638.0–638.9)
fetal death (intrauterine) (late) (656.4)
missed delivery (656.4)
that with abnormal product of conception (630, 631)

633 Ectopic pregnancy
Includes: ruptured ectopic pregnancy
633.0 Abdominal pregnancy
Intraperitoneal pregnancy
633.00 Abdominal pregnancy without intrauterine pregnancy
633.01 Abdominal pregnancy with intrauterine pregnancy
633.1 Tubal pregnancy
Fallopian pregnancy
Rupture of (fallopian) tube due to pregnancy
Tubal abortion
633.10 Tubal pregnancy without intrauterine pregnancy
633.11 Tubal pregnancy with intrauterine pregnancy
633.2 Ovarian pregnancy
633.20 Ovarian pregnancy without intrauterine pregnancy
633.21 Ovarian pregnancy with intrauterine pregnancy
633.8 Other ectopic pregnancy
Pregnancy:
cervical
combined
cornual
intraligamentous
mesometric
mural
633.80 Other ectopic pregnancy without intrauterine pregnancy
633.81 Other ectopic pregnancy with intrauterine pregnancy
633.9 Unspecified ectopic pregnancy
633.90 Unspecified ectopic pregnancy without intrauterine pregnancy
633.91 Unspecified ectopic pregnancy with intrauterine pregnancy

OTHER PREGNANCY WITH ABORTIVE OUTCOME
The following fifth-digit subdivisions are for use with categories 634–637
Requires fifth digit to identify stage:
0 unspecified
1 incomplete
2 complete
634 Spontaneous abortion
Includes: miscarriage
spontaneous abortion
634.0 Complicated by genital tract and pelvic infection
634.1 Complicated by delayed or excessive hemorrhage
634.2 Complicated by damage to pelvic organs or tissues
634.3 Complicated by renal failure
634.4 Complicated by metabolic disorder

634.5 Complicated by shock
634.6 Complicated by embolism
634.7 With other specified complications
634.8 With unspecified complication
634.9 Without mention of complication

635 Legally induced abortion
Includes: abortion or termination of pregnancy:
  elective
  therapeutic
Excludes: menstrual extraction or regulation (V25.3)
635.0 Complicated by genital tract and pelvic infection
635.1 Complicated by delayed or excessive hemorrhage
635.2 Complicated by damage to pelvic organs or tissues
635.3 Complicated by renal failure
635.4 Complicated by metabolic disorder
635.5 Complicated by shock
635.6 Complicated by embolism
635.7 With other specified complications
635.8 With unspecified complication
635.9 Without mention of complication

637 Unspecified abortion
Includes: retained products of conception following abortion
637.0 Complicated by genital tract and pelvic infection
637.1 Complicated by delayed or excessive hemorrhage
637.2 Complicated by damage to pelvic organs or tissues
637.3 Complicated by renal failure
637.4 Complicated by metabolic disorder
637.5 Complicated by shock
637.6 Complicated by embolism
637.7 With other specified complications
637.8 With unspecified complications
637.9 Without mention or complication

638 Failed attempted abortion
Includes: failure of attempted induction of (legal) abortion
Excludes: incomplete abortion (634.0–635.9)
638.0 Complicated by genital tract and pelvic infection
638.1 Complicated by delayed or excessive hemorrhage
638.2 Complicated by damage to pelvic organs or tissues
638.3 Complicated by renal failure

638.4 Complicated by metabolic disorder
638.5 Complicated by shock
638.6 Complicated by embolism
638.7 With other specified complications
638.8 With unspecified complication
638.9 Without mention of complication

639 Complications following abortion and ectopic and molar pregnancies
This category is used to report separately complications for ectopic or molar pregnancies or pregnancies with abortive outcomes; for example:
a) when the patient is seen for treatment of a complication; the ectopic, molar, or abortive pregnancy itself having been dealt with during a previous episode of care
b) when a complication occurred immediately following treatment of the ectopic, molar, or abortive pregnancy (same episode of care) but the complication cannot be identified at fourth digit level.

639.0 Genital tract and pelvic infection
Endometritis following conditions classifiable to 630–638
Parametritis following conditions classifiable to 630–638
Pelvic peritonitis following conditions classifiable to 630–638
Salpingitis following conditions classifiable to 630–638
Salpingo-oophoritis following conditions classifiable to 630–638
Sepsis NOS following conditions classifiable to 630–638
Septicemia NOS following conditions classifiable to 630–638
Excludes: urinary tract infection (639.8)
639.1 Delayed or excessive hemorrhage
Afibrinogenemia following conditions classifiable to 630–638
Defibrination syndrome following conditions classifiable to 630–638
Intravascular hemolysis following conditions classifiable to 630–638
639.2 Damage to pelvic organs and tissues
Laceration, perforation, or tear of:
bladder following conditions classifiable to 630–638
bowel following conditions classifiable to 630–638
broad ligament following conditions classifiable to 630–638
cervix following conditions classifiable to 630–638
periurethral tissue following conditions classifiable to 630–638
uterus following conditions classifiable to 630–638
vagina following conditions classifiable to 630–638

639.3 Kidney failure
Oliguria following conditions classifiable to 630–638
Renal (kidney):
    failure (acute) following conditions classifiable to
    630–638
    shutdown following conditions classifiable to 630–638
    tubular necrosis following conditions classifiable to
    630–638
Uremia following conditions classifiable to 630–638

639.4 Metabolic disorders
Electrolyte imbalance following conditions classifiable to 630–638

639.5 Shock
Circulatory collapse following conditions classifiable to 630–638
Shock (postoperative) (septic) following conditions classifiable to
630–638

639.6 Embolism
Embolism:
    NOS following conditions classifiable to 630–638
    air following conditions classifiable to 630–638
    amniotic fluid following conditions classifiable to 630–638
    blood-clot following conditions classifiable to 630–638
    fat following conditions classifiable to 630–638
    pulmonary following conditions classifiable to 630–638
    pyemic following conditions classifiable to 630 638
    septic following conditions classifiable to 630–638
    soap following conditions classifiable to 630–638

639.8 Other specified complications following abortion or ectopic and
molar pregnancy
Acute yellow atrophy or necrosis of liver following conditions
classifiable to 630–638
Cardiac arrest or failure following conditions classifiable to
630–638
Cerebral anoxia following conditions classifiable to 630–638
Urinary tract infection following conditions classifiable to
630–638

639.9 Unspecified complication following abortion or ectopic and molar
pregnancy
Complication(s) not further specified following conditions classifiable
to 630–638

COMPLICATIONS MAINLY RELATED TO PREGNANCY

Includes: the listed conditions even if they arose or were present during labor, delivery, or the puerperium

For information concerning diagnostic coding for ultrasound procedures, see Appendix C.

The following fifth-digit subclassification is for use with categories 640–649 to denote the current episode of care:

0   unspecified as to episode of care or not applicable
1   delivered, with or without mention of antepartum condition
     Antepartum condition with delivery
     Delivery NOS (with mention of antepartum complication during current episode of care)
     Intrapartum obstetric condition (with mention of antepartum complication during current episode of care)
     Pregnancy, delivered (with mention of antepartum complication during current episode of care)
2   Delivered, with mention of postpartum complication
     Delivery with mention of puerperal complication during current episode of care
3   Antepartum condition or complication (patient is still pregnant at end of episode of care)
4   Postpartum condition or complication (patient delivered during previous episode of care)
     Postpartum or puerperal obstetric condition or complication following delivery that occurred:
          during previous episode of care
          outside hospital, with subsequent admission for observation or care

640 Hemorrhage in early pregnancy
Requires fifth digit; valid digits are in [brackets] under each code. See beginning of section 640–649 for definitions.
Includes: hemorrhage before completion of 22 weeks' gestation
640.0   Threatened abortion
[0,1,3]
640.8   Other specified hemorrhage in early pregnancy
[0,1,3]
640.9   Unspecified hemorrhage in early pregnancy
[0,1,3]

641 Antepartum hemorrhage, abruptio placentae, and placenta previa
Requires fifth digit; valid digits are in [brackets] under each code. See beginning of section 640–649 for definitions.

641.0   Placenta previa without hemorrhage
[0,1,3] Low implantation of placenta without hemorrhage
       Placenta previa noted:
           during pregnancy without hemorrhage
           before labor (and delivered by cesarean delivery) without
           hemorrhage
641.1   Hemorrhage from placenta previa
[0,1,3] Low-lying placenta NOS or with hemorrhage (intrapartum)
       Placenta previa:
           incomplete NOS or with hemorrhage (intrapartum)
           marginal NOS or with hemorrhage (intrapartum)
           partial NOS or with hemorrhage (intrapartum)
           total NOS or with hemorrhage (intrapartum)
       Excludes: hemorrhage from vasa previa (663.5)
641.2   Premature separation of placenta
[0,1,3] Ablatio placentae
       Abruptio placentae
       Accidental antepartum hemorrhage
       Couvelaire uterus
       Detachment of placenta (premature)
       Premature separation of normally implanted placenta
641.3   Antepartum hemorrhage associated with coagulation defects
[0,1,3] Antepartum or intrapartum hemorrhage associated with:
       afibrinogenemia
       hyperfibrinolysis
       hypofibrinogenemia
       Excludes: coagulation defects not associated with antepartum hem-
           orrhage (649.3)
641.8   Other antepartum hemorrhage
[0,1,3] Antepartum or intrapartum hemorrhage associated with:
       trauma
       uterine leiomyoma
641.9   Unspecified antepartum hemorrhage
[0,1,3] Hemorrhage:
       antepartum NOS
       intrapartum NOS
       of pregnancy NOS

642 Hypertension complicating pregnancy, childbirth, and the puerperium
       Requires fifth digit; valid digits are in [brackets] under each code. See begin-
       ning of section 640–649 for definitions.
642.0   Benign essential hypertension complicating pregnancy, childbirth,
[0–4]   and the puerperium
       Hypertension:
           benign essential specified as complicating, or as a reason
           for obstetric care during pregnancy, childbirth, or the puerperium

chronic NOS specified as complicating, or as a reason for obstetric care during pregnancy, childbirth, or the puerperium

essential specified as complicating, or as a reason for obstetric care during pregnancy, childbirth, or the puerperium

pre-existing NOS specified as complicating, or as a reason for obstetric care during pregnancy, childbirth, or the puerperium

642.1 Hypertension secondary to renal disease, complicating pregnancy,
[0–4] childbirth, and the puerperium

Hypertension secondary to renal disease, specified as complicating, or as a reason for obstetric care during pregnancy, childbirth, or the puerperium

642.2 Other pre-existing hypertension complicating pregnancy, childbirth,
[0–4] and the puerperium

Hypertensive:

heart and chronic kidney disease specified as complicating, or as a reason for obstetric care during pregnancy, childbirth, or the puerperium

heart disease specified as complicating, or as a reason for obstetric care during pregnancy, childbirth, or the puerperium

chronic kidney disease specified as complicating, or as a reason for obstetric care during pregnancy, childbirth, or the puerperium

Malignant hypertension specified as complicating, or as a reason for obstetric care during pregnancy, childbirth, or the puerperium

642.3 Transient hypertension of pregnancy
[0–4] Gestational hypertension

Transient hypertension, so described, in pregnancy, childbirth, or the puerperium

642.4 Mild or unspecified pre-eclampsia
[0–4] Hypertension in pregnancy, childbirth, or the puerperium, not specified as pre-existing, with either albuminuria or edema, or both; mild or unspecified

Pre-eclampsia:
    NOS
    mild
Toxemia (pre-eclamptic):
    NOS
    mild

Excludes: albuminuria in pregnancy, without mention of hypertension (646.2)

edema in pregnancy, without mention of hypertension (646.1)

642.5 Severe pre-eclampsia
[0–4] Hypertension in pregnancy, childbirth, or the puerperium, not
specified as pre-existing, with either albuminuria or edema, or
both; specified as severe
Pre-eclampsia, severe
Toxemia (pre-eclamptic), severe

642.6 Eclampsia
[0–4] Toxemia:
eclamptic
with convulsions

642.7 Pre-eclampsia or eclampsia superimposed on pre-existing hyper
[0–4] tension
Conditions classifiable to 642.4–642.6, with conditions classifiable
to 642.0–642.2

642.9 Unspecified hypertension complicating pregnancy, childbirth, or
the puerperium
[0–4] Hypertension NOS, without mention of albuminuria or edema,
complicating pregnancy, childbirth, or the puerperium

643 Excessive vomiting in pregnancy
Requires fifth digit; valid digits are in [brackets] under each code. See beginning of section 640–649 for definitions.
Includes: hyperemesis arising during pregnancy
vomiting:
persistent arising during pregnancy
vicious arising during pregnancy
hyperemesis gravidarum

643.0 Mild hyperemesis gravidarum
[0,1,3] Hyperemesis gravidarum, mild or unspecified, starting before the
end of the 22nd week of gestation

643.1 Hyperemesis gravidarum with metabolic disturbance
[0,1,3] Hyperemesis gravidarum, starting before the end of the 22nd week
of gestation, with metabolic disturbance, such as:
carbohydrate depletion
dehydration
electrolyte imbalance

643.2 Late vomiting of pregnancy
[0,1,3] Excessive vomiting starting after 22 completed weeks of gestation

643.8 Other vomiting complicating pregnancy
[0,1,3] Vomiting due to organic disease or other cause, specified as complicat
ing pregnancy, or as a reason for obstetric care during pregnancy
Use additional code to specify cause

643.9 Unspecified vomiting of pregnancy
[0,1,3] Vomiting as a reason for care during pregnancy, length of gestation
unspecified

644 Early or threatened labor
Requires fifth digit; valid digits are in [brackets] under each code. See beginning of section 640–649 for definitions.
644.0   Threatened premature labor
[0,3]   Premature labor after 22 weeks, but before 37 completed weeks of gestation without delivery
  Excludes: that occurring before 22 completed weeks of gestation (640.0)
644.1   Other threatened labor
[0,3]   False labor:
  NOS without delivery
  after 37 completed weeks of gestation without delivery
  Threatened labor NOS without delivery
644.2   Early onset of delivery
[0–1]   Onset (spontaneous) of delivery before 37 completed weeks of gestation
  Premature labor with onset of delivery before 37 completed weeks of gestation

645 Late pregnancy
Requires fifth digit; valid digits are in [brackets] under each code. See beginning of section 640–649 for definitions.
645.1   Post term pregnancy
[0,1,3] Pregnancy over 40 completed weeks to 42 completed weeks gestation
645.2   Prolonged pregnancy
[0,1,3] Pregnancy which has advanced beyond 42 completed weeks of gestation

646 Other complications of pregnancy, not elsewhere classified
Use additional code(s) to further specify complication. Requires fifth digit; valid digits are in [brackets] under each code. See beginning of section 640–649 for definitions.
646.0   Papyraceous fetus
[0,1,3]
646.1   Edema or excessive weight gain in pregnancy, without mention of
[0–4]   hypertension
  Gestational edema
  Maternal obesity syndrome
  Excludes: that with mention of hypertension (642.0–642.9)
646.2   Unspecified renal disease in pregnancy, without mention of hyper-
[0–4]   tension
  Albuminuria in pregnancy or the puerperium, without mention of hypertension

Nephropathy NOS in pregnancy or the puerperium, without mention of hypertension
Renal disease NOS in pregnancy or the puerperium, without mention of hypertension
Uremia in pregnancy or the puerperium, without mention of hypertension
Gestational proteinuria in pregnancy or the puerperium, without mention of hypertension
Excludes: that with mention of hypertension (642.0–642.9)

646.3 Habitual aborter
[0,1,3] **Excludes:** with current abortion (634.0–634.9)
without current pregnancy (629.81)

646.4 Peripheral neuritis in pregnancy
[0–4]

646.5 Asymptomatic bacteriuria in pregnancy
[0–4]

646.6 Infections of genitourinary tract in pregnancy
[0–4] Conditions classifiable to 590, 595, 597, 599.0, 616 complicating pregnancy, childbirth, or the puerperium
Conditions classifiable to 614.0–614.5, 614.7–614.9, 615 complicating pregnancy or labor
Excludes: major puerperal infection (670.0-670.8)

646.7 Liver disorders in pregnancy
[0,1,3] Acute yellow atrophy of liver (obstetric) (true) of pregnancy
Icterus gravis of pregnancy
Necrosis of liver of pregnancy
Excludes: hepatorenal syndrome following delivery (674.8)
viral hepatitis (647.6)

646.8 Other specified complications of pregnancy
[0–4] Fatigue during pregnancy
Herpes gestationis
Insufficient weight gain of pregnancy

646.9 Unspecified complication of pregnancy
[0,1,3]

647 Infectious and parasitic conditions in the mother classifiable elsewhere, but complicating pregnancy, childbirth, or the puerperium
Use additional code(s) to further specify complication. Requires fifth digit; valid digits are in [brackets] under each code. See beginning of section 640–649 for definitions.
Includes: the listed conditions when complicating the pregnant state, aggravated by the pregnancy, or when a main reason for obstetric care

Excludes: those conditions in the mother known or suspected to
have affected the fetus (655.0–655.9)

647.0   Syphilis
[0–4]   Conditions classifiable to 091–097
647.1   Gonorrhea
[0–4]   Conditions classifiable to 098
647.2   Other venereal diseases
[0–4]   Conditions classifiable to 099
647.3   Tuberculosis
[0–4]   Conditions classifiable to 010–016
647.4   Malaria
[0–4]   Conditions classifiable to 084
647.5   Rubella
[0–4]   Conditions classifiable to 056
647.6   Other viral diseases
[0–4]   Conditions classifiable to 042, 050–055, 057–079, 795.05, 795.15,
796.75
647.8   Other specified infectious and parasitic diseases
[0–4]
647.9   Unspecified infection or infestation
[0–4]

**648   Other current conditions in the mother classifiable elsewhere, but
complicating pregnancy, childbirth, or the puerperium**
Use additional code(s) to identify the condition. Requires fifth digit; valid digits are in [brackets] under each code. See beginning of section 640–649 for
definitions.

Includes: the listed conditions when complicating the pregnant
state, aggravated by the pregnancy, or when a main
reason for obstetric care
Excludes: those conditions in the mother known or suspected to
have affected the fetus (655.0–655.9)

648.0   Diabetes mellitus
[0–4]   Conditions classifiable to 249, 250
Excludes: gestational diabetes (648.8)
648.1   Thyroid dysfunction
[0–4]   Conditions classifiable to 240–246
648.2   Anemia
[0–4]   Conditions classifiable to 280–285
648.3   Drug dependence
[0–4]   Conditions classifiable to 304
648.4   Mental disorders
[0–4]   Conditions classifiable to 293–303, 305.0, 305.2–305.9, 306–316,
317, 319

648.5 Congenital cardiovascular disorders
[0–4]
648.6 Other cardiovascular diseases
[0–4] Conditions classifiable to 410–429
Excludes: cerebrovascular disorders in the puerperium (674.0)
peripartum cardiomyopathy (674.5)
venous complications (671.0–671.9)
648.7 Bone and joint disorders of back, pelvis, and lower limbs
[0–4] Conditions classifiable to 724, and those classifiable to 714–716 or
727–738 specified as affecting the lower limbs
648.8 Abnormal glucose tolerance
[0–4] Conditions classifiable to 790.2–790.29
Gestational diabetes
Use additional code, if applicable, for associated long-term (current)
insulin use (V58.67)
648.9 Other current conditions classifiable elsewhere
[0–4] Conditions classifiable to 440–459, 795.01–795.04, 795.06,
795.10–795.14, 795.16, 796.70–796.74, 796.76

649 **Other conditions or status of the mother complicating pregnancy, childbirth, or the puerperium**
Requires fifth digit; valid digits are in [brackets] under each code. See beginning of section 640–649 for definitions.
649.0 Tobacco use disorder complicating pregnancy, childbirth,
[0–4] or the puerperium
Smoking complicating pregnancy, childbirth, or the puerperium
649.1 Obesity complicating pregnancy, childbirth, or the puerperium
[0–4] Use additional code to identify the obesity (278.00, 278.01)
649.2 Bariatric surgery status complicating pregnancy, childbirth, or the
puerperium
[0–4] Gastric banding status complicating pregnancy, childbirth, or the
puerperium
Gastric bypass status for obesity complicating pregnancy, childbirth, or
the puerperium
Obesity surgery status complicating pregnancy, childbirth, or the
puerperium
649.3 Coagulation defects complicating pregnancy, childbirth, or
[0–4] the puerperium
Conditions classifiable to 286, 287, 289
Use additional code to identify the specific coagulation defect (286.0–
286.9, 287.0-287.9, 289.0-289.9)
Excludes: coagulation defects causing antepartum hemorrhage
(641.3)
postpartum coagulation defects (666.3)

649.4   Epilepsy complicating pregnancy, childbirth, or the
[0–4]   puerperium
Conditions classifiable to 345
Use additional code to identify the specific type of epilepsy (345.00–345.91)
Excludes: eclampsia (642.6)
649.5   Spotting complicating pregnancy
[0,1,3] **Excludes:** antepartum hemorrhage (641.0–641.9)
hemorrhage in early pregnancy (640.0–640.9)
649.6   Uterine size date discrepancy
[0–4]   **Excludes:** suspected problem with fetal growth not found (V89.04)
649.7   Cervical shortening
[0,1,3] **Excludes:** suspected cervical shortening not found (V89.05)

NORMAL DELIVERY AND OTHER INDICATIONS FOR CARE IN PREGNANCY, LABOR, AND DELIVERY

The following fifth-digit subclassification is for use with categories 651–659 to denote the current episode of care:
0   unspecified as to episode of care or not applicable
1   delivered, with or without mention of antepartum condition
2   delivered, with mention of postpartum complication
3   antepartum condition or complication (patient still pregnant at end of episode of care)
4   postpartum condition or complication (patient delivered during previous episode of care)

650   Normal delivery
Delivery requiring minimal or no assistance, with or without episiotomy, without fetal manipulation (eg, rotation version) or instrumentation (forceps) of a spontaneous, cephalic, vaginal, full-term, single, live-born infant. This code is for use as a single diagnostic code and is not to be used with any other code in the range 630–676.
Use additional code to indicate outcome of delivery (V27.0)
Excludes: breech delivery (assisted) (spontaneous) NOS (652.2)
delivery by vacuum extractor, forceps, cesarean section, or breech extraction, without specified complication (669.5–669.7)

651   Multiple gestation
Requires fifth digit; valid digits are in [brackets] under each code. See beginning of section 650–659 for definitions.
651.0   Twin pregnancy
[0,1,3] **Excludes:** fetal conjoined twins (678.1)

651.1 Triplet pregnancy
[0,1,3]
651.2 Quadruplet pregnancy
[0,1,3]
651.3 Twin pregnancy with fetal loss and retention of one fetus
[0,1,3]
651.4 Triplet pregnancy with fetal loss and retention of one or more
[0,1,3] fetus(es)
651.5 Quadruplet pregnancy with fetal loss and retention of one or more
[0,1,3] fetus(es)
651.6 Other multiple pregnancy with fetal loss and retention of one or
[0,1,3] more fetus(es)
651.7 Multiple gestation following (elective) fetal reduction
[0,1,3] Fetal reduction of multiple fetuses reduced to single fetus
651.8 Other specified multiple gestation
[0,1,3]
651.9 Unspecified multiple gestation
[0,1,3]

652 Malposition and malpresentation of fetus
Requires fifth digit; valid digits are in [brackets] under each code. See beginning of section 650–659 for definitions.
Code first any associated obstructed labor (660.0)
652.0 Unstable lie
[0,1,3]
652.1 Breech or other malpresentation successfully converted to cephalic
[0,1,3] presentation
       Cephalic version NOS
652.2 Breech presentation without mention of version
[0,1,3] Attempted version, unsuccessful
       Breech delivery (assisted) (spontaneous) NOS
       Buttocks presentation
       Complete breech
       Frank breech
       Excludes: footling presentation (652.8)
                    incomplete breech (652.8)
652.3 Transverse or oblique presentation
[0,1,3] Oblique lie
       Transverse lie
       Excludes: transverse arrest of fetal head (660.3)
652.4 Face or brow presentation
[0,1,3] Mentum presentation

652.5 High head at term
[0,1,3] Failure of head to enter pelvic brim
652.6 Multiple gestation with malpresentation of one fetus or more
[0,1,3]
652.7 Prolapsed arm
[0,1,3]
652.8 Other specified malposition or malpresentation
[0,1,3] Compound presentation
652.9 Unspecified malposition or malpresentation
[0,1,3]

653 Disproportion
Requires fifth digit; valid digits are in [brackets] under each code. See beginning of section 650–659 for definitions. Code first any associated obstructed labor (660.1)
653.0 Major abnormality of bony pelvis, not further specified
[0,1,3] Pelvic deformity NOS
653.1 Generally contracted pelvis
[0,1,3] Contracted pelvis NOS
653.2 Inlet contraction of pelvis
[0,1,3] Inlet contraction (pelvis)
653.3 Outlet contraction of pelvis
[0,1,3] Outlet contraction (pelvis)
653.4 Fetopelvic disproportion
[0,1,3] Cephalopelvic disproportion NOS
        Disproportion of mixed maternal and fetal origin, with normally
            formed fetus
653.5 Unusually large fetus causing disproportion
[0,1,3] Disproportion of fetal origin with normally formed fetus
        Fetal disproportion NOS
        Excludes: that when the reason for medical care was
            concern for the fetus (656.6)
653.6 Hydrocephalic fetus causing disproportion
[0,1,3] **Excludes:** that when the reason for medical care was
            concern for the fetus (655.0)
653.7 Other fetal abnormality causing disproportion
[0,1,3] Fetal:
        ascites
        hydrops
        myelomeningocele
        sacral teratoma
        tumor
        Excludes: conjoined twins causing disproportion (678.1)
653.8 Disproportion of other origin
[0,1,3] **Excludes:** shoulder (girdle) dystocia (660.4)

TABULAR LIST: COMPLICATIONS OF PREGNANCY, CHILDBIRTH, AND THE PUERPERIUM (630–679)

653.9   Unspecified disproportion
[0,1,3]

654   Abnormality of organs and soft tissues of pelvis
Requires fifth digit; valid digits are in [brackets] under each code. See beginning of section 650–659 for definitions.
Includes: the listed conditions during pregnancy, childbirth, or the
puerperium
Excludes: trauma to perineum or acquired abnormality of vulva complicating
current delivery (664.0–664.9)
Code first any associated obstructed labor (660.2)
654.0   Congenital abnormalities of uterus
[0–4]   Double uterus
Uterus bicornis
654.1   Tumors of body of uterus
[0–4]   Uterine fibroids
654.2   Previous cesarean delivery
[0,1,3]   Uterine scar from previous cesarean delivery
654.3   Retroverted and incarcerated gravid uterus
[0–4]
654.4   Other abnormalities in shape or position of gravid uterus and of
[0–4]   neighboring structures
Cystocele
Pelvic floor repair
Pendulous abdomen
Prolapse of gravid uterus
Rectocele
Rigid pelvic floor
654.5   Cervical incompetence
[0–4]   Presence of Shirodkar suture with or without mention of cervical
incompetence
654.6   Other congenital or acquired abnormality of cervix
[0–4]   Cicatricial cervix
Polyp of cervix
Previous surgery to cervix
Rigid cervix (uteri)
Stenosis or stricture of cervix
Tumor of cervix
654.7   Congenital or acquired abnormality of vagina
[0–4]   Previous surgery to vagina
Septate vagina
Stenosis of vagina (acquired) (congenital)
Stricture of vagina
Tumor of vagina

654.8 Congenital or acquired abnormality of vulva
       Anal sphincter tear (healed) (old) complicating delivery
[0–4] Fibrosis of perineum
       Persistent hymen
       Previous surgery to perineum or vulva
       Rigid perineum
       Tumor of vulva
       Excludes: varicose veins of vulva (671.1)
                      anal sphincter tear (healed) (old) not associated with delivery (569.43)
654.9 Other and unspecified
[0–4] Uterine scar NEC

655 **Known or suspected fetal abnormality affecting management of mother**
       Requires fifth digit; valid digits are in [brackets] under each code. See beginning of section 650–659 for definitions.
       Includes: the listed conditions in the fetus as a reason for observation or obstetrical care of the mother, or for termination of pregnancy
655.0 Central nervous system malformation in fetus
[0,1,3] Fetal or suspected fetal:
         anencephaly
         hydrocephalus
         spina bifida (with myelomeningocele)
655.1 Chromosomal abnormality in fetus
[0,1,3]
655.2 Hereditary disease in family possibly affecting fetus
[0,1,3]
655.3 Suspected damage to fetus from viral disease in the mother
[0,1,3] Suspected damage to fetus from maternal rubella
655.4 Suspected damage to fetus from other disease in the mother
[0,1,3] Suspected damage to fetus from maternal:
         alcohol addiction
         listeriosis
         toxoplasmosis
655.5 Suspected damage to fetus from drugs
[0,1,3]
655.6 Suspected damage to fetus from radiation
[0,1,3]
655.7 Decreased fetal movements
[0,1,3]

655.8   Other known or suspected fetal abnormality, not elsewhere
[0,1,3] classified
    Suspected damage to fetus from:
      environmental toxins
      intrauterine contraceptive device
655.9   Unspecified
[0,1,3]

656   **Other known or suspected fetal and placental problems affecting management of mother**
Requires fifth digit; valid digits are in [brackets] under each code. See beginning of section 650–659 for definitions.
Excludes: fetal hematologic condition (678.0)
            suspected placental problems not found (V89.02)
656.0   Fetal–maternal hemorrhage
[0,1,3] Leakage (microscopic) of fetal blood into maternal circulation
656.1   Rhesus isoimmunization
[0,1,3] Anti-D [Rh] antibodies
    Rh incompatibility
656.2   Isoimmunization from other and unspecified blood-group incompatibility
[0,1,3] ABO isoimmunization
656.3   Fetal distress
[0,1,3] Fetal metabolic acidemia
    Excludes: abnormal fetal acid-base balance (656.8)
             abnormality in fetal heart rate or rhythm (659.7)
             fetal bradycardia (659.7)
             fetal tachycardia (659.7)
             meconium in liquor (656.8)
656.4   Intrauterine death
[0,1,3] Fetal death:
    NOS
    after completion of 22 weeks' gestation
    late
    Missed delivery
    Excludes: missed abortion (632)
656.5   Poor fetal growth
[0,1,3] "Light-for-dates"
    "Placental insufficiency"
    "Small-for-dates"
656.6   Excessive fetal growth
[0,1,3] "Large-for-dates"

656.7   Other placental conditions
[0,1,3]   Abnormal placenta
    Placental infarct
    Excludes: placental polyp (674.4)
               placentitis (658.4)
656.8   Other specified fetal and placental problems
[0,1,3]   Abnormal acid-base balance
    Intrauterine acidosis
    Lithopedian
    Meconium in liquor
    Subchorionic hematoma
656.9   Unspecified fetal and placental problem
[0,1,3]

657   Polyhydramnios
[0,1,3]   Hydramnios
Excludes: suspected polyhydramnios not found (V89.01)
Requires fifth digit; valid digits are in [brackets] under each code. See beginning of section 650–659 for definitions. Use 0 as fourth digit for category 657.

658   Other problems associated with amniotic cavity and membranes
Requires fifth digit; valid digits are in [brackets] under each code. See beginning of section 650–659 for definitions.
Excludes: amniotic fluid embolism (673.1)
        suspected problems with amniotic cavity and membranes not
        found (V89.01)
658.0   Oligohydramnios
[0,1,3]   Oligohydramnios without mention of rupture of membranes
658.1   Premature rupture of membranes
[0,1,3]   Rupture of amniotic sac less than 24 hours prior to the onset of
    labor
658.2   Delayed delivery after spontaneous or unspecified rupture of
[0,1,3]   membranes
    Prolonged rupture of membranes NOS
    Rupture of amniotic sac 24 hours or more prior to the onset of
    labor
658.3   Delayed delivery after artificial rupture of membranes
[0,1,3]
658.4   Infection of amniotic cavity
[0,1,3]   Amnionitis
    Chorioamnionitis
    Membranitis
    Placentitis

658.8   Other
[0,1,3] Amnion nodosum
        Amniotic cyst
658.9   Unspecified
[0,1,3]

659   **Other indications for care or intervention related to labor and delivery, not elsewhere classified**
Requires fifth digit; valid digits are in [brackets] under each code. See beginning of section 650–659 for definitions.
659.0   Failed mechanical induction
[0,1,3] Failure of induction of labor by surgical or other instrumental
        methods
659.1   Failed medical or unspecified induction
[0,1,3] Failed induction NOS
        Failure of induction of labor by medical methods, such as oxytocic
        drugs
659.2   Maternal pyrexia during labor, unspecified
[0,1,3]
659.3   Generalized infection during labor
[0,1,3] Septicemia during labor
659.4   Grand multiparity
[0,1,3] **Excludes:** supervision only, in pregnancy (V23.3)
        without current pregnancy (V61.5)
659.5   Elderly primigravida
[0,1,3] First pregnancy in a woman who will be 35 years of age or older at
        expected date of delivery
        Excludes: supervision only, in pregnancy (V23.81)
659.6   Elderly multigravida
[0,1,3] Second or more pregnancy in a woman who will be 35 years of age
        or older at expected date of delivery
        Excludes: elderly primigravida (659.5)
                     supervision only, in pregnancy (V23.82)
659.7   Abnormality in fetal heart rate or rhythm
[0,1,3] Depressed fetal heart tones
        Fetal:
            bradycardia
            tachycardia
        Fetal heart rate decelerations
        Nonreassuring fetal heart rate or rhythm
659.8   Other specified indications for care or intervention related to labor
[0,1,3] and delivery
        Pregnancy in a female less than 16 years of age at expected date of
        delivery
        Very young maternal age

659.9   Unspecified indication for care or intervention related to labor and
[0,1,3]   delivery

COMPLICATIONS OCCURRING MAINLY IN THE COURSE OF LABOR AND DELIVERY

The following fifth-digit subclassification is for use with categories 660–669 to denote the current episode of care:

0   unspecified as to episode of care or not applicable
1   delivered, with or without mention of antepartum condition
2   delivered, with mention of postpartum complication
3   antepartum condition or complication (patient still pregnant at end of episode of care)
4   postpartum condition or complication (patient delivered during previous episode of care)

660   Obstructed labor

Requires fifth digit; valid digits are in [brackets] under each code. See beginning of section 660–669 for definitions.

660.0   Obstruction caused by malposition of fetus at onset of labor
[0,1,3]   Any condition classifiable to 652, causing obstruction during labor
          Use additional code from 652.0–652.9 to identify condition
660.1   Obstruction by bony pelvis
[0,1,3]   Any condition classifiable to 653, causing obstruction during labor
          Use additional code from 653.0–653.9 to identify condition
660.2   Obstruction by abnormal pelvic soft tissues
[0,1,3]   Prolapse of anterior lip of cervix
          Any condition classifiable to 654, causing obstruction during labor
          Use additional code from 654.0–654.9 to identify condition
660.3   Deep transverse arrest and persistent occipitoposterior position
[0,1,3]
660.4   Shoulder (girdle) dystocia
[0,1,3]   Impacted shoulders
660.5   Locked twins
[0,1,3]
660.6   Failed trial of labor, unspecified
[0,1,3]   Failed trial of labor, without mention of condition or suspected condition
660.7   Failed forceps or vacuum extractor, unspecified
[0,1,3]   Application of ventouse or forceps, without mention of condition
660.8   Other causes of obstructed labor
[0,1,3]   Use additional code to identify condition
660.9   Unspecified obstructed labor
[0,1,3]   Dystocia:
              NOS
              fetal NOS
              maternal NOS

661 Abnormality of forces of labor
Requires fifth digit; valid digits are in [brackets] under each code. See beginning of section 660–669 for definitions.

661.0 Primary uterine inertia
[0,1,3] Failure of cervical dilation
Hypotonic uterine dysfunction, primary
Prolonged latent phase of labor

661.1 Secondary uterine inertia
[0,1,3] Arrested active phase of labor
Hypotonic uterine dysfunction, secondary

661.2 Other and unspecified uterine inertia
Atony of uterus without hemorrhage
Excludes: atony of uterus with hemorrhage (666.1)
postpartum atony of uterus without hemorrhage (669.8)

[0,1,3] Desultory labor
Irregular labor
Poor contractions
Slow slope active phase of labor

661.3 Precipitate labor
[0,1,3]

661.4 Hypertonic, incoordinate, or prolonged uterine contractions
[0,1,3] Cervical spasm
Contraction ring (dystocia)
Dyscoordinate labor
Hourglass contraction of uterus
Hypertonic uterine dysfunction
Incoordinate uterine action
Retraction ring (Bandl's) (pathological)
Tetanic contractions
Uterine dystocia NOS
Uterine spasm

661.9 Unspecified abnormality of labor
[0,1,3]

662 Long labor
Requires fifth digit; valid digits are in [brackets] under each code. See beginning of section 660–669 for definitions.

662.0 Prolonged first stage
[0,1,3]

662.1 Prolonged labor, unspecified
[0,1,3]

662.2 Prolonged second stage
[0,1,3]

662.3 Delayed delivery of second twin, triplet, etc.
[0,1,3]

663 Umbilical cord complications

Requires fifth digit; valid digits are in [brackets] under each code. See beginning of section 660–669 for definitions.

663.0 Prolapse of cord
[0,1,3] Presentation of cord
663.1 Cord around neck, with compression
[0,1,3] Cord tightly around neck
663.2 Other and unspecified cord entanglement, with compression
[0,1,3] Entanglement of cords of twins in mono-amniotic sac
    Knot in cord (with compression)
663.3 Other and unspecified cord entanglement, without mention of
[0,1,3] compression
663.4 Short cord
[0,1,3]
663.5 Vasa previa
[0,1,3]
663.6 Vascular lesions of cord
[0,1,3] Bruising of cord
    Hematoma of cord
    Thrombosis of vessels of cord
663.8 Other umbilical cord complications
[0,1,3] Velamentous insertion of umbilical cord
663.9 Unspecified umbilical cord complication
[0,1,3]

664 Trauma to perineum and vulva during delivery

Requires fifth digit; valid digits are in [brackets] under each code. See beginning of section 660–669 for definitions.

Includes: damage from instruments
    that from extension of episiotomy
664.0 First-degree perineal laceration
[0,1,4] Perineal laceration, rupture, or tear involving:
    fourchette
    hymen
    labia
    skin
    vagina
    vulva
664.1 Second-degree perineal laceration
[0,1,4] Perineal laceration, rupture, or tear (following episiotomy)
    involving:
      pelvic floor
      perineal muscles
      vaginal muscles
    Excludes: that involving anal sphincter (664.2)

664.2   Third-degree perineal laceration
[0,1,4] Perineal laceration, rupture, or tear (following episiotomy) involving:
anal sphincter
rectovaginal septum
sphincter NOS
Excludes: that with anal or rectal mucosal laceration
(664.3)
anal sphincter tear during delivery not associated with
third-degree perineal laceration (664.6)
664.3   Fourth-degree perineal laceration
[0,1,4] Perineal laceration, rupture, or tear as classifiable to 664.2 and
involving also:
anal mucosa
rectal mucosa
664.4   Unspecified perineal laceration
[0,1,4] Central laceration
664.5   Vulval and perineal hematoma
[0,1,4]
664.6   Anal sphincter tear complicating delivery, not associated with
third-degree perineal laceration
Excludes: third-degree perineal laceration (664.2)
664.8   Other specified trauma to perineum and vulva
[0,1,4]
664.9   Unspecified trauma to perineum and vulva
[0,1,4]

665   Other obstetrical trauma
Requires fifth digit; valid digits are in [brackets] under each code. See beginning of section 660–669 for definitions.
Includes: damage from instruments
665.0   Rupture of uterus before onset of labor
[0,1,3]
665.1   Rupture of uterus during labor
[0,1]   Rupture of uterus NOS
665.2   Inversion of uterus
[0,2,4]
665.3   Laceration of cervix
[0,1,4]
665.4   High vaginal laceration
[0,1,4] Laceration of vaginal wall or sulcus without mention of perineal
laceration
665.5   Other injury to pelvic organs
[0,1,4] Injury to:
bladder
urethra

665.6 Damage to pelvic joints and ligaments
[0,1,4] Avulsion of inner symphyseal cartilage
Damage to coccyx
Separation of symphysis (pubis)

665.7 Pelvic hematoma
[0–2,4] Hematoma of vagina

665.8 Other specified obstetrical trauma
[0–4]

665.9 Unspecified obstetrical trauma
[0–4]

666 Postpartum hemorrhage

Requires fifth digit; valid digits are in [brackets] under each code. See beginning of section 660–669 for definitions.

666.0 Third-stage hemorrhage
[0,2,4] Hemorrhage associated with retained, trapped, or adherent placenta
Retained placenta NOS

666.1 Other immediate postpartum hemorrhage
[0,2,4] Atony of uterus with hemorrhage
Hemorrhage within the first 24 hours following delivery of placenta
Postpartum hemorrhage (atonic) NOS
Postpartum atony of uterus with hemorrhage

Excludes: Atony of uterus without hemorrhage (661.2)
Postpartum atony of uterus without hemorrhage (669.8)

666.2 Delayed and secondary postpartum hemorrhage
[0,2,4] Hemorrhage:
after the first 24 hours following delivery
associated with retained portions of placenta or membranes
Postpartum hemorrhage specified as delayed or secondary
Retained products of conception NOS, following delivery

666.3 Postpartum coagulation defects
[0,2,4] Postpartum:
afibrinogenemia
fibrinolysis

667 Retained placenta without hemorrhage

Requires fifth digit; valid digits are in [brackets] under each code. See beginning of section 660–669 for definitions.

667.0 Retained placenta without hemorrhage
[0,2,4] Placenta accreta without hemorrhage
Retained placenta:
NOS without hemorrhage
total without hemorrhage

667.1 Retained portions of placenta or membranes, without hemorrhage
[0,2,4] Retained products of conception following delivery, without hemorrhage

668 Complications of the administration of anesthetic or other sedation in labor and delivery
Use additional code(s) to further specify complication. Requires fifth digit; valid digits are in [brackets] under each code. See beginning of section 660–669 for definitions.

Includes: complications arising from the administration of a general or local anesthetic, analgesic, or other sedation in labor and delivery

668.0 Pulmonary complications
[0–4] Inhalation (aspiration) of stomach contents or secretions following anesthesia or other sedation in labor or delivery
Mendelson's syndrome following anesthesia or other sedation in labor or delivery
Pressure collapse of lung following anesthesia or other sedation in labor or delivery

668.1 Cardiac complications
[0–4] Cardiac arrest or failure following anesthesia or other sedation in labor and delivery

668.2 Central nervous system complications
[0–4] Cerebral anoxia following anesthesia or other sedation in labor and delivery

668.8 Other complications of anesthesia or other sedation in labor and
[0–4] delivery

668.9 Unspecified complication of anesthesia and other sedation
[0–4]

669 Other complications of labor and delivery, not elsewhere classified
Requires fifth digit; valid digits are in [brackets] under each code. See beginning of section 660–669 for definitions.

669.0 Maternal distress
[0–4] Metabolic disturbance in labor and delivery

669.1 Shock during or following labor and delivery
[0–4] Obstetric shock

669.2 Maternal hypotension syndrome
[0–4]

669.3 Acute kidney failure following labor and delivery
[0,2,4]

669.4 Other complications of obstetrical surgery and procedures
[0–4] Cardiac:
arrest following cesarean or other obstetrical surgery or procedure, including delivery NOS
failure following cesarean or other obstetrical surgery or procedure, including delivery NOS

Cerebral anoxia following cesarean or other obstetrical surgery or procedure, including delivery NOS
Excludes: complications of obstetrical surgical wounds (674.1–674.3)

669.5 Forceps or vacuum extractor delivery without mention of
[0,1] indication
Delivery by ventouse, without mention of indication

669.6 Breech extraction, without mention of indication
[0,1] **Excludes:** breech delivery NOS (652.2)

669.7 Cesarean delivery, without mention of indication
[0,1] Elective cesarean delivery

669.8 Other complications of labor and delivery
[0–4]

669.9 Unspecified complication of labor and delivery
[0–4]

COMPLICATIONS OF THE PUERPERIUM

Categories 671 and 673–676 include the listed conditions even if they occur during pregnancy or childbirth. The following fifth-digit subclassification is for use with categories 670–676 to denote the current episode of care:
0 unspecified as to episode of care or not applicable
1 delivered, with or without mention of antepartum condition
2 delivered, with mention of postpartum complication
3 antepartum condition or complication (patient still pregnant at end of episode of care)
4 postpartum condition or complication (patient delivered during previous episode of care)

670 Major puerperal infection
[0,2,4] Requires fifth digit; valid digits are in [brackets] under each code. See beginning of section 670–676 for definitions.
Excludes: infection following abortion (639.0)
minor genital tract infection following delivery (646.6)
puerperal pyrexia NOS (672)
puerperal fever NOS (672)
puerperal pyrexia of unknown origin (672)
urinary tract infection following delivery (646.6)

670.0 Major puerperal infection, unspecified
[0,2,4]

670.1 Puerperal endometritis
[0,2,4]

670.2 Puerperal sepsis
[0,2,4] Puerperal pyemia

670.3 Puerperal septic thrombophlebitis
[0,2,4]

TABULAR LIST: COMPLICATIONS OF PREGNANCY, CHILDBIRTH, AND THE PUERPERIUM (630–679)

670.8 Other major puerperal infection
[0,2,4] Puerperal:
pelvic cellulitis
peritonitis
salpingitis

671 Venous complications in pregnancy and the puerperium
Requires fifth digit; valid digits are in [brackets] under each code. See beginning of section 670–676 for definitions.
Excludes: personal history of venous complications prior to pregnancy, such as:
thrombophlebitis (V12.52)
thrombosis and embolism (V12.51)
671.0 Varicose veins of legs
[0–4] Varicose veins NOS
671.1 Varicose veins of vulva and perineum
[0–4]
671.2 Superficial thrombophlebitis
Phlebitis NOS
[0–4] Thrombophlebitis (superficial)
Thrombosis NOS
671.3 Deep phlebothrombosis, antepartum
[0,1,3] Deep-vein thrombosis, antepartum
Use additional code to identify the deep vein thrombosis
(453.40-453.42, 453.50-453.52, 453.72-453.79, 453.82-453.89)
Use additional code for long term (current) use of anticoagulants, if applicable (V58.61)
671.4 Deep phlebothrombosis, postpartum
[0,2,4] Deep-vein thrombosis, postpartum
Pelvic thrombophlebitis, postpartum
Phlegmasia alba dolens (puerperal)
Use additional code to identify the deep vein thrombosis
(453.40-453.42, 453.50-453.52, 453.72-453.79, 453.82-453.89)
Use additional code for long term (current) use of anticoagulants, if applicable (V58.61)
671.5 Other phlebitis and thrombosis
[0–4] Cerebral venous thrombosis
Thrombosis of intracranial venous sinus
671.8 Other venous complications
[0–4] Hemorrhoids
671.9 Unspecified venous complication
[0–4]

672 Pyrexia of unknown origin during the puerperium
[0,2,4] Postpartum fever NOS
Puerperal fever NOS
Puerperal pyrexia NOS
Requires fifth digit; valid digits are in [brackets] under each code. See beginning of section 670–676 for definitions. Use 0 as fourth digit for category 672.

673 Obstetrical pulmonary embolism
Requires fifth digit; valid digits are in [brackets] under each code. See beginning of section 670–676 for definitions.
Includes: pulmonary emboli in pregnancy, childbirth, or the puerperium, or specified as puerperal
Excludes: embolism following abortion (639.6)
673.0 Obstetrical air embolism
[0–4]
673.1 Amniotic fluid embolism
[0–4]
673.2 Obstetrical blood-clot embolism
[0–4] Puerperal pulmonary embolism NOS
673.3 Obstetrical pyemic and septic embolism
[0–4]
673.8 Other pulmonary embolism
[0–4] Fat embolism

674 Other and unspecified complications of the puerperium, not elsewhere classified
Requires fifth digit; valid digits are in [brackets] under each code. See beginning of section 670–676 for definitions.
674.0 Cerebrovascular disorders in the puerperium
[0–4] **Excludes:** intracranial venous sinus thrombosis (671.5)
674.1 Disruption of cesarean wound
[0,2,4] Dehiscence or disruption of uterine wound
Excludes: uterine rupture before onset of labor (665.0)
uterine rupture during labor (665.1)
674.2 Disruption of perineal wound
[0,2,4] Breakdown of perineum
Disruption of wound of:
episiotomy
perineal laceration
secondary perineal tear
674.3 Other complications of obstetrical surgical wounds
[0,2,4] Hematoma of cesarean section or perineal wound
Hemorrhage of cesarean section or perineal wound
Infection of cesarean section or perineal wound

Excludes: damage from instruments in delivery (664.0–665.9)

674.4 Placental polyp
[0,2,4]

674.5 Peripartum cardiomyopathy
[0–4] Postpartum cardiomyopathy

674.8 Other
[0,2,4] Hepatorenal syndrome, following delivery
Postpartum:
subinvolution of uterus
uterine hypertrophy

674.9 Unspecified
[0,2,4] Sudden death of unknown cause during the puerperium

675 **Infections of the breast and nipple associated with childbirth**
Requires fifth digit; valid digits are in [brackets] under each code. See beginning of section 670–676 for definitions.
Includes: the listed conditions during pregnancy, childbirth, or the
puerperium

675.0 Infections of nipple
[0–4] Abscess of nipple

675.1 Abscess of breast
[0–4] Abscess:
mammary
subareolar
submammary
Mastitis:
purulent
retromammary
submammary

675.2 Nonpurulent mastitis
[0–4] Lymphangitis of breast
Mastitis:
NOS
interstitial
parenchymatous

675.8 Other specified infections of the breast and nipple
[0–4]

675.9 Unspecified infection of the breast and nipple
[0–4]

676 **Other disorders of the breast associated with childbirth and disorders**
of lactation
Requires fifth digit; valid digits are in [brackets] under each code. See beginning of section 670–676 for definitions.
Includes: the listed conditions during pregnancy, the puerperium, or
lactation

676.0 Retracted nipple
[0–4]
676.1 Cracked nipple
[0–4] Fissure of nipple
676.2 Engorgement of breasts
[0–4]
676.3 Other and unspecified disorder of breast
[0–4]
676.4 Failure of lactation
[0–4] Agalactia
676.5 Suppressed lactation
[0–4]
676.6 Galactorrhea
[0–4] **Excludes:** galactorrhea not associated with childbirth
(611.6)
676.8 Other disorders of lactation
[0–4] Galactocele
676.9 Unspecified disorder of lactation
[0–4]

677 **Late effect of complication of pregnancy, childbirth, and the puerperium**
This category is to be used to indicate conditions in 632–648.9 and 651–676.9 as the cause of the late effect, themselves classifiable elsewhere. The "late effects" include conditions specified as such, or as sequelae, which may occur at any time after the puerperium. Code first any sequelae.

OTHER MATERNAL AND FETAL COMPLICATIONS (678-679)

The following fifth-digit subclassification is for use with categories 678–679 to denote the current episode of care:
0 unspecified as to episode of care or not applicable
1 delivered, with or without mention of antepartum condition
2 delivered, with mention of postpartum complication
3 antepartum condition or complication
4 postpartum condition or complication

678 **Other fetal conditions**
Requires fifth digit; valid digits are in [brackets] under each code.
See beginning of section 678–679 for definitions.
678.0 Fetal hematologic conditions
[0,1,3] Fetal anemia
Fetal thrombocytopenia
Fetal twin to twin transfusion
Excludes: fetal-maternal hemorrhage (656.00–656.03)
isoimmunization incompatibility (656.10–656.13,
656.20–656.23)

678.1   Fetal conjoined twins
[0,1,3]

679 Complications of in utero procedures
Requires fifth digit; valid digits are in [brackets] under each code.
See beginning of section 678–679 for definitions.

679.0 Maternal complications from in utero procedure
[0–4] **Excludes:** maternal history of in utero procedure during previous
        pregnancy (V23.86)

679.1 Fetal complications from in utero procedure
[0–4] Fetal complications from amniocentesis

DISEASES OF THE SKIN AND SUBCUTANEOUS TISSUE (680–709)

INFECTIONS OF SKIN AND SUBCUTANEOUS TISSUE

Excludes: certain infections of skin classified under "Infectious and Parasitic
        Diseases," such as:
          herpes:
            simplex (054.1)
            zoster (053.7–053.9)
          molluscum contagiosum (078.0)
          viral warts (078.10-078.19)

680 Carbuncle and furuncle
Includes: boil
          furunculosis

680.2 Trunk
        Abdominal wall
        Back (any part, except buttocks)
        Breast
        Chest wall
        Flank
        Groin
        Pectoral region
        Perineum
        Umbilicus
        Excludes: buttocks (680.5)
                external genital organs (616.4)

680.3 Upper arm and forearm
        Arm (any part, except hand)
        Axilla
        Shoulder

680.5 Buttock
        Anus
        Gluteal region

680.8 Other specified sites
    Head (any part, except face)
    Scalp
    Excludes: external genital organs (616.4)
680.9 Unspecified site
    Boil NOS
    Carbuncle NOS
    Furuncle NOS

682 Other cellulitis and abscess
  Includes: abscess (acute) (with lymphangitis) except of finger or toe
        cellulitis (diffuse) (with lymphangitis) except of finger or toe
        lymphangitis, acute (with lymphangitis) except of finger or toe
  Use additional code to identify organism, such as Staphylococcus (041.1)
682.2 Trunk
    Abdominal wall
    Back (any part, except buttock)
    Chest wall
    Flank
    Groin
    Pectoral region
    Perineum
    Umbilicus, except newborn
    Excludes: anal and rectal regions (566)
          breast:
              NOS (611.0)
              puerperal (675.1)
          external genital organs (616.3–616.4)
682.5 Buttock
    Gluteal region
    Excludes: anal and rectal regions (566)

683 Acute lymphadenitis
  Abscess (acute) lymph gland or node, except mesenteric
  Adenitis, acute lymph gland or node, except mesenteric
  Lymphadenitis, acute lymph gland or node, except mesenteric
  Use additional code to identify organism such as Staphylococcus (041.1)
  Excludes: enlarged glands NOS (785.6)
         lymphadenitis, unspecified (289.3)

685 Pilonidal cyst
  Includes: fistula, coccygeal or pilonidal
        sinus, coccygeal or pilonidal
685.0 With abscess
685.1 Without mention of abscess

OTHER INFLAMMATORY CONDITIONS OF SKIN AND SUBCUTANEOUS TISSUE

691 Atopic dermatitis and related conditions
  691.8 Other atopic dermatitis and related conditions
692 Contact dermatitis and other eczema
  692.3 Due to drugs and medicine in contact with skin
  692.6 Due to plants (except food)
  692.7 Due to solar radiation
    692.71 Sunburn
    692.72 Acute dermatitis due to solar radiation
    692.73 Actinic reticuloid and actinic granuloma
    692.74 Other chronic dermatitis due to solar radiation
    692.75 Disseminated superficial actinic porokeratosis (DSAP)
    692.76 Sunburn of second degree
    692.77 Sunburn of third degree
    692.79 Other dermatitis due to solar radiation
  692.8 Due to other specified agents
    692.82 Dermatitis due to other radiation
    692.83 Dermatitis due to metals
    692.89 Other
  692.9 Unspecified cause

695 Erythematous conditions
  695.1 Erythema multiforme
  695.2 Erythema nodosum
  695.3 Rosacea
    Acne:
      erythematosa
      rosacea
    Perioral dermatitis
    Rhinophyma
  695.4 Lupus erythematosus
    Lupus:
      erythematodes (discoid)
      erythematosus (discoid), not disseminated
    Excludes: systemic (disseminated) lupus erythematosus (710.0)

696 Psoriasis and similar disorders
  696.0 Psoriatic arthropathy
  696.1 Other psoriasis
  696.2 Parapsoriasis
  696.3 Pityriasis rosea
  696.4 Pityriasis rubra pilaris
  696.5 Other and unspecified pityriasis

698 **Pruritus and related conditions**
  698.0 Pruritus ani
        Perianal itch
  698.1 Pruritus of genital organs
  698.2 Prurigo
        Lichen urticatus
        Prurigo:
          NOS
          Hebra's
          mitis
          simplex
        Urticaria papulosa (Hebra)
  698.8 Other specified pruritic conditions
        Pruritus:
          hiemalis
          senilis
        Winter itch
  698.9 Unspecified pruritic disorder
        Itch NOS
        Pruritus NOS

OTHER DISEASES OF SKIN AND SUBCUTANEOUS TISSUE
Excludes: congenital conditions of skin, hair, and nails (757.3–757.9)

701 **Other hypertrophic and atrophic conditions of skin**
  Excludes: scleroderma (generalized) (710.1)
  701.0 Circumscribed scleroderma
        Addison's keloid
        Dermatosclerosis, localized
        Lichen sclerosus et atrophicus
        Morphea
        Scleroderma, circumscribed or localized
  701.2 Acquired acanthosis nigricans
        Keratosis nigricans
  701.3 Striae atrophicae
        Atrophic spots of skin
        Atrophoderma maculatum
        Atrophy blanche (of Milian)
        Degenerative colloid atrophy
        Senile degenerative atrophy
        Striae distensae
  701.4 Keloid scar
        Cheloid
        Hypertrophic scar
        Keloid

701.5 Other abnormal granulation tissue
Excessive granulation
701.8 Other specified hypertrophic and atrophic conditions of skin
Acrodermatitis atrophicans chronica
Atrophia cutis senilis
Atrophoderma neuriticum
Confluent and reticulate papillomatosis
Cutis laxa senilis
Elastosis senilis
Folliculitis ulerythematosa reticulata
Gougerot–Carteaud syndrome or disease
701.9 Unspecified hypertrophic and atrophic conditions of skin
Atrophoderma

702 Other dermatoses
Excludes: carcinoma in situ (232.0–232.9)
702.0 Actinic keratosis
702.1 Seborrheic keratosis
702.11 Inflamed seborrheic keratosis
702.19 Other seborrheic keratosis
Seborrheic keratosis NOS
Other specified dermatoses

704 Diseases of hair and hair follicles
Excludes: congenital anomalies (757.4)
704.0 Alopecia
Excludes: Syphilitic alopecia (091.82)
704.00 Alopecia, unspecified
704.02 Telogen effluvium
704.09 Other
Folliculitis decalvans
Hypotrichosis:
NOS
Postinfectional
Pseudopelade
704.1 Hirsutism
Hypertrichosis: Polytrichia
NOS
Lanuginose, acquired

705 Disorders of sweat glands
705.8 Other specified disorders of sweat glands
705.82 Fox–Fordyce disease
705.83 Hidradenitis
Hidradenitis suppurativa

706 **Diseases of sebaceous glands**
706.1 Other acne
Acne:
NOS
conglobata
cystic
pustular
vulgaris
Blackhead
Comedo
Excludes: acne rosacea (695.3)
706.2 Sebaceous cyst
Atheroma, skin
Keratin cyst
Wen
706.3 Seborrhea
Excludes: seborrheic keratosis (702.11–702.19)
706.8 Other specified diseases of sebaceous glands
Asteatosis (cutis)
Xerosis cutis
706.9 Unspecified disease of sebaceous glands

707 **Chronic ulcer of skin**
Includes: noninfected sinus of skin
nonhealing ulcer
Excludes: varicose ulcer (454.0, 454.2)
707.0 Pressure ulcer
Bed sore
Decubitus ulcer
Plaster ulcer
707.00 Unspecified site

708 **Urticaria**
Excludes: edema, angioneurotic (995.1)
urticaria:
giant (995.1)
papulosa (Hebra) (698.2)
708.0 Allergic urticaria
708.1 Idiopathic urticaria
708.2 Urticaria due to cold and heat
Thermal urticaria
708.3 Dermatographic urticaria
Dermatographia
Factitial urticaria

708.4 Vibratory urticaria
708.5 Cholinergic urticaria
708.8 Other specified urticaria
Nettle rash
Urticaria:
chronic
recurrent periodic
708.9 Urticaria, unspecified
Hives NOS

709 Other disorders of skin and subcutaneous tissue
709.0 Dyschromia
Excludes: pigmented nevus (216.5–216.8)
709.00 Dyschromia, unspecified
709.01 Vitiligo
709.09 Other
709.1 Vascular disorders of skin
Angioma serpiginosum
Purpura (primary) annularis telangiectodes
709.2 Scar conditions and fibrosis of skin
Adherent scar (skin)
Cicatrix
Disfigurement (due to scar)
Fibrosis, skin NOS
Scar NOS
Excludes: keloid scar (701.4)
709.3 Degenerative skin disorders
Calcinosis:
circumscripta
cutis
Colloid milium
Degeneration, skin
Deposits, skin
Senile dermatosis NOS
Subcutaneous calcification
709.4 Foreign body granuloma of skin and subcutaneous tissue
Excludes: residual foreign body without granuloma of skin and sub-
cutaneous tissue (729.6)
709.8 Other specified disorders of skin
Epithelial hyperplasia
Menstrual dermatosis
Vesicular eruption
709.9 Unspecified disorder of skin and subcutaneous tissue
Dermatosis NOS

DISEASES OF THE MUSCULOSKELETAL SYSTEM AND CONNECTIVE TISSUE (710–739)

ARTHROPATHIES AND RELATED DISORDERS

Excludes: disorders of back (724)

710 Diffuse diseases of connective tissue
Includes: all collagen diseases whose effects are not mainly confined to a single system
Excludes: those affecting mainly the cardiovascular system, ie, polyarteritis nodosa and allied conditions (446.0–446.1)

710.0 Systemic lupus erythematosus
Disseminated lupus erythematosus
Libman-Sacks disease
Use additional code to identify manifestation
Excludes: lupus erythematosus (discoid) NOS (695.4)

710.1 Systemic sclerosis
Acrosclerosis
CRST syndrome
Progressive systemic sclerosis
Scleroderma
Use additional code to identify manifestation
Excludes: circumscribed scleroderma (701.0)

714 Rheumatoid arthritis and other inflammatory polyarthropathies
714.0 Rheumatoid arthritis
Arthritis or polyarthritis:
atrophic
rheumatic (chronic)
Use additional code to identify manifestation

The following fifth-digit subclassification is for use with categories 715–716. Valid digits are in [brackets] under each code.
0   site unspecified
5   pelvic region and thigh
buttock
femur
hip (joint)
8   other specified sites
trunk
9   multiple sites

715 **Osteoarthrosis and allied disorders**
Localized, in the subcategories below, includes bilateral involvement of the same site.
Includes: arthritis or polyarthritis:
  degenerative
  hypertrophic
  degenerative joint disease
  osteoarthritis

715.0 Osteoarthrosis, generalized
[0] Degenerative joint disease, involving multiple joints
  Primary generalized hypertrophic osteoarthrosis
715.1 Osteoarthrosis, localized, primary
[0–8] Localized osteoarthropathy, idiopathic
715.9 Osteoarthrosis, unspecified whether generalized or localized
[0–8]

716 **Other and unspecified arthropathies**
Requires fifth digit. Valid digits are in [brackets] under each code. See list preceding category 715 for definitions.

716.3 Climacteric arthritis
[0–8] Menopausal arthritis
716.9 Arthropathy, unspecified
[0–8] Arthritis, (acute) (chronic) (subacute)
  Arthropathy, (acute) (chronic) (subacute)
  Articular rheumatism, (chronic)
  Inflammation of joint, NOS

724 **Other and unspecified disorders of back**
Excludes: collapsed vertebra (code to cause, eg, osteoporosis,
  733.00–733.09)
724.2 Lumbago
  Low back pain
  Low back syndrome
  Lumbalgia
724.3 Sciatia
724.4 Thoracic or lumbosacral neuritis or radiculitis, unspecified
724.5 Backache, unspecified
  Vertebrogenic (pain) syndrome NOS
724.7 Disorders of coccyx
  724.70 Unspecified disorder of coccyx
  724.71 Hypermobility of coccyx
  724.79 Other

RHEUMATISM, EXCLUDING THE BACK

Includes: disorders of muscles and tendons and their attachments, and of other soft tissues

727 Other disorders of synovium, tendon, and bursa
727.1 Bunion

729 Other disorders of soft tissues
Excludes: carpal tunnel syndrome (354.0)
disorders of the back (724)
729.0 Rheumatism, unspecified and fibrositis
729.1 Myalgia and myositis, unspecified
Fibromyositis NOS
729.2 Neuralgia, neuritis, and radiculitis, unspecified
Excludes: lumbosacral radiculitis (724.4)
mononeuritis (354.0–355.9)
sciatica (724.3)
729.4 Fasciitis, unspecified
729.5 Pain in limb
729.6 Residual foreign body in soft tissue
Excludes: foreign body granuloma:
skin and subcutaneous tissue (709.4)
729.8 Other musculoskeletal symptoms referable to limbs
729.81 Swelling of limb
729.89 Other
729.9 Other and unspecified disorders of soft tissue
729.90 Disorders of soft tissue, unspecified
729.91 Post-traumatic seroma
Excludes: seroma complicating a procedure (998.13)
729.92 Nontraumatic hematoma of soft tissue
Nontraumatic hematoma of muscle
729.99 Other disorders of soft tissue
Polyalgia

OSTEOPATHIES, CHONDROPATHIES, AND ACQUIRED MUSCULOSKELETAL DEFORMITIES

733 Other disorders of bone and cartilage
733.0 Osteoporosis
733.00 Osteoporosis, unspecified
Wedging of vertebra NOS
733.01 Senile osteoporosis
Postmenopausal osteoporosis
733.02 Idiopathic osteoporosis
733.03 Disuse osteoporosis

TABULAR LIST: DISEASES OF THE MUSCULOSKELETAL SYSTEM AND CONNECTIVE TISSUE (710–739)

733.09 Other
Drug-induced osteoporosis
Use additional E code to identify drug
733.9 Other and unspecified disorders of bone and cartilage
733.90 Disorders of bone and cartilage, unspecified
Osteopenia

738 Other acquired deformity
Excludes: congenital (758)
738.6 Acquired deformity of pelvis
Pelvic obliquity
Excludes: that in relation to labor and delivery (653.0–653.4,
653.8–653.9)

739 Nonallopathic lesions, not elsewhere classified
Includes: segmental dysfunction
somatic dysfunction
739.5 Pelvic region
Hip region
Pubic region
739.9 Abdomen and other

CONGENITAL ANOMALIES (740–759)

752 Congenital anomalies of genital organs
Excludes: syndromes associated with anomalies in the number and form of
chromosomes (758.0–758.9)
Code descriptions include terminology from American Society for
Reproductive Medicine (ASRM) Classification of Müllerian Anomalies
when appropriate. If anomaly is DES drug related (eg, ASRM Class VII
Müllerian Anomaly), report also code 760.76
752.0 Anomalies of ovaries
Absence, congenital, of ovary
Accessory ovary
Ectopic ovary
Streak of ovary
752.1 Anomalies of fallopian tubes and broad ligaments
752.10 Unspecified anomaly of fallopian tubes and broad ligaments
752.11 Embryonic cyst of fallopian tubes and broad ligaments
Cyst:
epoophoron
fimbrial
parovarian

752.19 Other
          Absence of fallopian tube or broad ligament
          Accessory fallopian tube or broad ligament
          Atresia of fallopian tube or broad ligament
752.2 Doubling of uterus
        Didelphus uterus (ASRM Class III Müllerian Anomaly)
        Doubling of uterus (any degree) (associated with doubling of
        cervix and vagina)
        Septate uterus (ASRM Class V Müllerian Anomaly)
752.3 Other anomalies of uterus
        Absence, congenital, of uterus
        Acurate (ASRM Class VI Müllerian Anomaly)
        Agenesis of uterus
        Aplasia or hypoplasia of uterus (ASRM Class I Müllerian Anomaly)
        Bicornuate uterus (complete or partial) (ASRM Class IV Müllerian
        Anomaly)
        Hypoplasia (ASRM Class I Müllerian Anomaly)
        Unicornuate uterus (ASRM Class II Müllerian Anomaly)
        Uterus with only one functioning horn
752.4 Anomalies of cervix, vagina, and external female genitalia
        752.40 Unspecified anomaly of cervix, vagina, and external
                 genitalia
        752.41 Embryonic cyst of cervix, vagina, and external female
                 genitalia
                 Cyst of:
                     Gartner's duct
                     canal of Nuck, congenital
                     vagina, embryonal
                     vulva, congenital
        752.42 Imperforate hymen
        752.49 Other anomalies of cervix, vagina, and external female
                 genitalia
                 Absence of cervix, clitoris, vagina, or vulva
                 Agenesis of cervix, clitoris, vagina, or vulva (ASRM Class I
                 Müllerian Anomaly)
                 Congenital stenosis or stricture of:
                     cervical canal
                     vagina
                 Hypoplasia (ASRM Class I Müllerian Anomaly)
                 Excludes: double vagina associated with total
                              duplication (752.2)

752.7 Indeterminate sex and pseudohermaphroditism
Gynandrism
Hermaphroditism
Ovotestis
Pseudohermaphroditism (male) (female)
Pure gonadal dysgenesis
Excludes: pseudohermaphroditism:
with specified chromosomal anomaly (758.0–758.9)
752.9 Unspecified anomaly of genital organs
Congenital:
anomaly NOS of genital organ, NEC
deformity NOS of genital organ, NEC

753 Congenital anomalies of urinary system
753.1 Cystic kidney disease
753.12 Polycystic kidney, unspecified type
753.2 Obstructive defects of renal pelvis and ureter
753.20 Unspecified obstructive defect of renal pelvis and ureter
753.21 Congenital obstruction of ureteropelvic junction
753.22 Congenital obstruction of ureterovesical junction
Adynamic ureter
Congenital hydroureter
753.23 Congenital ureterocele
753.29 Other
753.4 Other specified anomalies of ureter
Absent ureter
Accessory ureter
Deviation of ureter
Displaced ureteric orifice
Double ureter
Ectopic ureter
Implantation, anomalous, of ureter
753.6 Atresia and stenosis of urethra and bladder neck
Congenital obstruction:
bladder neck
urethra
Congenital stricture of:
urethra (valvular)
urinary meatus
vesicourethral orifice
Imperforate urinary meatus
Impervious urethra
Urethral valve formation

753.8 Other specified anomalies of bladder and urethra
Absence, congenital of:
bladder
urethra
Accessory:
bladder
urethra
Congenital:
diverticulum of bladder
hernia of bladder
Congenital urethrorectal fistula
Congenital prolapse of:
bladder (mucosa)
urethra
Double:
urethra
urinary meatus

753.9 Unspecified anomaly of urinary system
Congenital:
anomaly NOS of urinary system (any part, except urachus)
deformity NOS of urinary system (any part, except urachus)

757 **Congenital anomalies of the integument**
Includes: anomalies of skin, subcutaneous tissue, hair, nails, and breast
Excludes: pigmented nevus (216.5–216.8)

757.3 Other specified anomalies of skin
757.32 Vascular hamartomas
Birthmarks
Port-wine stain
Strawberry nevus

757.6 Specified congenital anomalies of breast
Congenital absent breast or nipple
Accessory breast or nipple
Supernumerary breast or nipple
Excludes: hypoplasia of breast (611.82)
micromastia (611.82)

757.9 Unspecified anomaly of the integument
Breast

758 Chromosomal anomalies
Includes: syndromes associated with anomalies in the number and
form of chromosomes
Use additional codes for conditions associated with chromosomal anomalies.
758.0 Down's syndrome
Mongolism
Translocation Down's syndrome
Trisomy:
21 or 22
G
758.1 Patau's syndrome
Trisomy:
13
D1
758.2 Edward's syndrome
Trisomy:
18
E3
758.3 Autosomal deletion syndromes
758.33 Other microdeletions
758.39 Other autosomal deletions
758.4 Balanced autosomal translocation in normal individual
Robertsonian translocation in normal individual
758.5 Other conditions due to autosomal anomalies
Accessory autosomes NEC
758.6 Gonadal dysgenesis
Ovarian dysgenesis
Turner's syndrome
XO syndrome
Excludes: pure gonadal dysgenesis (752.7)
758.7 Klinefelter's syndrome
XXY syndrome
758.8 Other conditions due to chromosome anomalies
758.81 Other conditions due to sex chromosome anomalies
758.89 Other
758.9 Conditions due to anomaly of unspecified chromosome

CERTAIN CONDITIONS ORIGINATING IN THE PERINATAL PERIOD (760–779)

Includes: conditions which have their origin in the perinatal period before birth through the first 28 days after birth even though death or morbidity occurs later. Use additional code(s) to further specify condition.

MATERNAL CAUSES OF PERINATAL MORBIDITY AND MORTALITY

760 **Fetus or newborn affected by maternal conditions which may be unrelated to present pregnancy**

760.7 Noxious influences affecting fetus or newborn via placenta or breast milk
Fetus or newborn affected by noxious substance transmitted via placenta or breast milk
760.76 Diethylstilbestrol (DES)

SYMPTOMS, SIGNS, AND ILL-DEFINED CONDITIONS (780–799)

780 **General symptoms**

780.2 Syncope and collapse
Blackout
Fainting
(Near) (Pre)syncope
Vasovagal attack
Excludes: shock NOS (785.50)

780.3 Convulsions
780.39 Other convulsions
Eclamptic delirium
Seizures NOS

780.4 Dizziness and giddiness
Light-headedness
Vertigo NOS

780.5 Sleep disturbances
780.50 Sleep disturbance, unspecified
780.51 Insomnia with sleep apnea, unspecified
780.52 Insomnia, unspecified
780.53 Hypersomnia with sleep apnea, unspecified
780.54 Hypersomnia, unspecified
780.55 Disruptions of 24 hour sleep wake cycle, unspecified
780.59 Other

780.6 Fever and other physiologic disturbances of temperature regulation
    780.60 Fever, unspecified
        Chills with fever
        Fever NOS
        Fever of unknown origin (FUO)
        Hyperpyrexia NOS
        Pyrexia NOS
        Pyrexia of unkown origin
        Excludes: chills without fever (780.64)
                  pyrexia of unkown origin (during):
                  labor (659.2)
                  the puerperium (672)
    780.61 Fever presenting with conditions classified elsewhere
        Code first underlying condition when associated fever is present, such as with:
        sickle-cell disease (282.60–282.69)
    780.62 Postprocedural fever
        Excludes: postvaccination fever (780.63)
    780.63 Postvaccination fever
        Postimmunization fever
    780.64 Chills (without fever)
        Chills NOS
        Excludes: chills with fever (780.66)
    780.65 Hypothermia not associated with low environmental temperature
        Excludes: hypothermia:
                due to anesthesia (995.89)
780.7 Malaise and fatigue
    Excludes: fatigue (during):
            combat (308.0–308.9)
            heat (992.6)
            pregnancy (646.8)
        neurasthenia (300.5)
        senile asthenia (797)
    780.71 Chronic fatigue syndrome
        Functional quadriplegia
        Complete immobility due to severe physical disability or frailty
        Excludes: hysterical paralysis (300.11)
    780.79 Other malaise and fatigue
        Asthenia NOS
        Lethargy
        Postviral (asthenic) syndrome
        Tiredness

780.8 Generalized hyperhidrosis
Diaphoresis
Excessive sweating
Secondary hyperhidrosis

781 Symptoms involving nervous and musculoskeletal systems
781.9 Other symptoms involving nervous and musculoskeletal systems
781.91 Loss of height

782 Symptoms involving skin and other integumentary tissue
Excludes: symptoms relating to breast (611.71–611.79)
782.0 Disturbance of skin sensation
Anesthesia of skin
Burning or prickling sensation
Hyperesthesia
Hypoesthesia
Numbness
Paresthesia
Tingling
782.1 Rash and other nonspecific skin eruption
Exanthem
Excludes: vesicular eruption (709.8)
782.2 Localized superficial swelling, mass, or lump
Subcutaneous nodules
Excludes: localized adiposity (278.1)
782.3 Edema
Anasarca
Dropsy
Localized edema NOS
Excludes: ascites (789.51–789.59)
edema of pregnancy (642.0–642.9, 646.1)
fluid retention (276.6)
782.6 Pallor and flushing
782.61 Pallor
782.62 Flushing
Excessive blushing
782.7 Spontaneous ecchymoses
Petechiae
Excludes: purpura (287.2–287.5)
782.8 Changes in skin texture
Induration of skin
Thickening of skin
782.9 Other symptoms involving skin and integumentary tissues

783 Symptoms concerning nutrition, metabolism, and development
783.0 Anorexia
Loss of appetite
Excludes: anorexia nervosa (307.1)
loss of appetite of nonorganic origin (307.59)
783.1 Abnormal weight gain
Excludes: excessive weight gain in pregnancy (646.1)
obesity (278.00)
morbid (278.01)
783.2 Abnormal loss of weight and underweight
Use additional code to identify Body Mass Index (BMI), if known
(V85.0–V85.54)
783.21 Loss of weight
783.22 Underweight
783.5 Polydipsia
Excessive thirst
783.6 Polyphagia
Excessive eating
Hyperalimentation NOS
Excludes: disorders of eating of nonorganic origin (307.50–307.59)
783.7 Adult failure to thrive
783.9 Other symptoms concerning nutrition, metabolism, and development
Hypometabolism
Excludes: abnormal basal metabolic rate (794.7)
dehydration (276.51)
other disorders of fluid, electrolyte, and acid-
base balance (276.0–276.9)

784 Symptoms involving head and neck
784.0 Headache
Facial pain
Pain in head NOS
Excludes: migraine (346.0–346.9)
784.1 Throat pain
Excludes: dysphagia (787.20–787.29)
sore throat (462)
chronic (472.1)
784.7 Epistaxis
Hemorrhage from nose
Nosebleed

785 Symptoms involving cardiovascular system
785.0 Tachycardia, unspecified
Rapid heart beat
Excludes: paroxysmal tachycardia (427.0–427.2)

785.1 Palpitations
       Awareness of heart beat
       Excludes: specified dysrhythmias (427.0–427.9)
785.2 Undiagnosed cardiac murmurs
       Heart murmur NOS
785.5 Shock without mention of trauma
       785.50 Shock, unspecified
               Failure of peripheral circulation
       785.51 Cardiogenic shock
       785.52 Septic shock
               endotoxic
               gram-negative
               Code first systemic inflammatory response syndrome due to
               noninfectious process with organ dysfunction
               (995.94)
       785.59 Other
               Shock:
                   hypovolemic
               Excludes: shock (due to):
                                   anesthetic (995.4)
                                   anaphylactic (995.0)
                                   due to serum (999.4)
                                   following abortion (639.5)
                                   obstetrical (669.1)
                                   postoperative (998.0)
                                   traumatic (958.4)
785.6 Enlargement of lymph nodes
       Lymphadenopathy
       "Swollen glands"
       Excludes: acute (683)

786 **Symptoms involving respiratory system and other chest symptoms**
786.0 Dyspnea and respiratory abnormalities
       786.00 Respiratory abnormality, unspecified
       786.01 Hyperventilation
       786.02 Orthopnea
       786.03 Apnea
               Excludes: sleep apnea (780.51, 780.53, 780.57)
       786.04 Cheyne–Stokes respiration
       786.05 Shortness of breath
       786.06 Tachypnea
       786.07 Wheezing
       786.09 Other
               Respiratory distress or insufficiency

786.2 Cough
    Excludes: cough:
        smokers' (491.0)
        with hemorrhage (786.3)
786.3 Hemoptysis
    Cough with hemorrhage
    Pulmonary hemorrhage NOS
786.4 Abnormal sputum
    Abnormal amount, color or odor of sputum
786.5 Chest pain
    786.50 Chest pain, unspecified
    786.51 Precordial pain
    786.52 Painful respiration
        Pain:
            anterior chest wall
            pleuritic
        Pleurodynia
    786.59 Other
        Discomfort in chest
        Pressure in chest
        Tightness in chest
        Excludes: pain in breast (611.71)
786.7 Abnormal chest sounds
    Abnormal percussion, chest
    Friction sounds, chest
    Rales
    Tympany, chest
    Excludes: wheezing (786.07)
786.8 Hiccough
786.9 Other symptoms involving respiratory system and chest
    Breath-holding spell
787 Symptoms involving digestive system
Excludes: constipation (564.0–564.9)
787.0 Nausea and vomiting
    Emesis
    Excludes: hematemesis NOS (578.0)
        vomiting:
            associated with migraine (346.2)
            excessive, in pregnancy (643.0–643.9)
            psychogenic NOS (307.54)
    787.01 Nausea with vomiting
    787.02 Nausea alone
    787.03 Vomiting alone
    787.04 Billious emesis
        Billious vomiting

787.1 Heartburn
Pyrosis
Waterbrash

787.2 Dysphagia
787.20 Dysphagia, unspecified
787.29 Other dysphagia

787.3 Flatulence, eructation, and gas pain
Abdominal distention (gaseous)
Bloating
Tympanites (abdominal) (intestinal)

787.5 Abnormal bowel sounds
Absent bowel sounds
Hyperactive bowel sounds

787.6 Incontinence of feces
Encopresis NOS
Incontinence of sphincter ani

787.7 Abnormal feces
Bulky stools
Excludes: abnormal stool content (792.1)
Melena NOS (578.1)

787.9 Other symptoms involving digestive system
Excludes: gastrointestinal hemorrhage (578.0–578.9)
specific functional digestive disorders, those not
elsewhere classified (564.0–564.9)
787.91 Diarrhea
Diarrhea NOS
787.99 Other
Change in bowel habits
Tenesmus (rectal)

788 Symptoms involving urinary system
Excludes: hematuria (599.70–599.72)
nonspecific findings on examination of the urine
(791.0–791.9)

788.0 Renal colic
Colic (recurrent) of:
kidney
ureter

788.1 Dysuria
Painful urination
Strangury

788.2 Retention of urine
788.20 Retention of urine, unspecified
788.21 Incomplete bladder emptying
788.29 Other specified retention of urine

788.3 Urinary incontinence
Code, if applicable, any causal condition first, such as:
genital prolapse (618.00–618.9)
Excludes: functional urinary incontinence (788.91)
urinary incontinence associated with cognitive impairment
(788.91)
    788.30 Urinary incontinence, unspecified
Enuresis NOS
    788.31 Urge incontinence
    788.33 Mixed incontinence
Urge and stress
    788.34 Incontinence without sensory awareness
    788.35 Post-void dribbling
    788.36 Nocturnal enuresis
    788.37 Continuous leakage
    788.38 Overflow incontinence
    788.39 Other urinary incontinence
788.4 Frequency of urination and polyuria
    788.41 Urinary frequency
Frequency of micturition
    788.42 Polyuria
    788.43 Nocturia
788.5 Oliguria and anuria
Deficient secretion of urine
Suppression of urinary secretion
Excludes: that complicating:
abortion (634–638 with .3, 639.3)
ectopic or molar pregnancy (639.3)
pregnancy, childbirth, or the puerperium
(642.0–642.9, 646.2)
788.6 Other abnormality of urination
    788.61 Splitting of urinary stream
Intermittent urinary stream
    788.62 Slowing of urinary stream
Weak stream
    788.63 Urgency of urination
Excludes: urge incontinence (788.31, 788.33)
    788.64 Urinary hesitancy
    788.65 Straining on urination
    788.69 Other
788.7 Urethral discharge
Urethrorrhea
788.8 Extravasation of urine

788.9 Other symptoms involving urinary system
    788.91 Functional urinary incontinence
        Urinary incontinence due to cognitive impairment, or severe
        physical disability or immobility
        Excludes: urinary incontinence due to physiologic condition
        (788.30–788.39)
    788.99 Other symptoms involving urinary system
        Extrarenal uremia
        Vesical:
            pain
            tenesmus

789 **Other symptoms involving abdomen and pelvis**

The following fifth-digit subclassification is to be used for codes 789.0, 789.3, 789.4, and 789.6.
0   unspecified site
1   right upper quadrant
2   left upper quadrant
3   right lower quadrant
4   left lower quadrant
5   periumbilic
6   epigastric
7   generalized
9   other specified site
    multiple sites

Excludes: symptoms referable to genital organs:
        female (625.0–625.9)
        psychogenic (302.70–302.79)

789.0 Abdominal pain
[0-7,9]
        Cramps, abdominal
789.3 Abdominal or pelvic swelling, mass, or lump
[0-7,9]   Diffuse or generalized swelling or mass:
        abdominal NOS
        umbilical
    Excludes: abdominal distention (gaseous) (787.3)
        ascites (789.51–789.59)
789.4 Abdominal rigidity
[0-7,9]

789.5   Ascites
    Fluid in peritoneal cavity
    789.51   Malignant ascites
        Code first malignancy, such as:
            malignant neoplasm of ovary (183.0)
            secondary malignant neoplasm of retroperitoneum and
            peritoneum (197.6)
    789.59   Other ascites
789.6   Abdominal tenderness
[0-7,9]   Rebound tenderness
789.9   Other symptoms involving abdomen and pelvis
    Umbilical:
        bleeding
        discharge

NONSPECIFIC ABNORMAL FINDINGS

790   Nonspecific findings on examination of blood
    Excludes: abnormality of platelets (thrombocytes) (287.0–287.9)
    790.0   Abnormality of red blood cells
        Excludes: anemia:
                    other specified types (280.0–285.2)
                    hemoglobin disorders (282.5–282.6)
        790.01   Precipitous drop in hematocrit
            Drop in hematocrit
            Drop in hemoglobin
        790.09   Other abnormality of red blood cells
            Abnormal red cell morphology NOS
            Abnormal red cell volume NOS
            Anisocytosis
            Poikilocytosis
    790.1   Elevated sedimentation rate
    790.2   Abnormal glucose
        Excludes: diabetes mellitus (249.00–249.91, 250.00–250.93)
                    gestational diabetes (648.8)
                    glycosuria (791.5)
                    hypoglycemia (251.2)
                    that complicating pregnancy, childbirth, or the
                    puerperium (648.8)
        790.21   Impaired fasting glucose
            Elevated fasting glucose
        790.22   Impaired glucose tolerance test (oral)
            Elevated glucose tolerance test
        790.29   Other abnormal glucose
            Abnormal glucose NOS
            Abnormal nonfasting glucose

Hyperglycemia NOS
Pre-diabetes NOS

790.3 Excessive blood level of alcohol
Elevated blood-alcohol

790.4 Nonspecific elevation of levels of transaminase or lactic acid dehydrogenase (LDH)

790.5 Other nonspecific abnormal serum enzyme levels
Abnormal serum level of:
acid phosphatase
alkaline phosphatase
amylase
lipase

790.7 Bacteremia
Excludes: septicemia (038)
Use additional code to identify organism (041)

790.8 Viremia, unspecified

790.9 Other nonspecific findings on examination of blood
790.91 Abnormal arterial blood gases
790.92 Abnormal coagulation profile
Abnormal or prolonged:
bleeding time
coagulation time
partial thromboplastin time (PTT)
prothrombin time (PT)
Excludes: coagulation (hemorrhagic) disorders (286.0–286.9)
790.95 Elevated C-reactive protein (CRP)

791 **Nonspecific findings on examination of urine**
Excludes: hematuria NOS (599.70–599.72)

791.0 Proteinuria
Albuminuria
Bence-Jones proteinuria
Excludes: that arising during pregnancy or the puerperium (642.0–642.9, 646.2)

791.1 Chyluria

791.2 Hemoglobinuria

791.3 Myoglobinuria

791.4 Biliuria

791.5 Glycosuria

791.6 Acetonuria
Ketonuria

791.7 Other cells and casts in urine

791.9 Other nonspecific findings on examination of urine
Crystalluria

Elevated urine levels of:
17-ketosteroids
catecholamines
indolacetic acid
vanillylmandelic acid (VMA)
Melanuria

792 Nonspecific abnormal findings in other body substances
Excludes: that in chromosomal analysis (795.2)
792.1 Stool contents
Abnormal stool color
Fat in stool
Mucus in stool
Occult blood
Pus in stool
Excludes: blood in stool (melena) (578.1)
792.2 Semen
792.3 Amniotic fluid
792.9 Other nonspecific abnormal findings in body substances
Peritoneal fluid
Pleural fluid
Synovial fluid
Vaginal fluids

793 Nonspecific (abnormal) findings on radiological and other examination
of body structure
Includes: nonspecific abnormal findings of:
thermography
ultrasound examination (echogram)
X-ray examination
Excludes: abnormal results of function studies and radioisotope
scans (794.5–794.9)
793.4 Gastrointestinal tract
793.5 Genitourinary organs
Filling defect:
bladder
kidney
ureter
793.6 Abdominal area, including retroperitoneum
793.8 Breast
793.80 Abnormal mammogram, unspecified
793.81 Mammographic microcalcification
Excludes: Mammographic calcification (793.89)
Mammographic calculus (793.89)
793.82 Inconclusive mammogram

Dense breasts NOS
Inconclusive mammogram NEC
Inconclusive mammography due to dense breasts
Inconclusive mammography NEC

793.89   Other (abnormal) findings on radiological examination of
breast
Mammographic calcification
Mammographic calculus

793.9 Other
Excludes: abnormal finding by radioisotope localization of
placenta (794.9)

793.91   Image test inconclusive due to excess body fat
Use additional code to identify Body Mass Index (BMI), if
known (V85.0–V85.54)

793.99   Other nonspecific (abnormal) findings on radiological and other
examinations of body structures
Abnormal:
placental findings by X-ray or ultrasound method
radiological findings in skin and subcutaneous tissue

794 Nonspecific abnormal results of function studies
Includes: radioisotope:
scans
uptake studies
scintiphotography

794.5 Thyroid
Abnormal thyroid: scan
Abnormal thyroid: uptake

794.7 Basal metabolism
Abnormal basal metabolic rate (BMR)

794.9 Bladder studies

**795 Other and nonspecific abnormal cytological, histological, immuno-
logical, and DNA test findings**
For additional information concerning reporting of abnormal Pap smears, see
Appendix B.

795.0 Abnormal Papanicolaou smear of cervix and cervical HPV
Abnormal thin preparation smear of cervix
Abnormal cervical cytology
Excludes: Abnormal cytologic smear of vagina and vaginal HPV
(795.10–795.19)
Carcinoma in situ of cervix (233.1)
Cervical intraepithelial neoplasia I (CIN I) (622.11)
Cervical intraepithelial neoplasia II (CIN II) (622.12)

Cervical intraepithelial neoplasia III (CIN III) (233.1)
Dysplasia (histologically confirmed) of cervix
(uteri) NOS (622.10)
Mild cervical dysplasia (histologically confirmed) (622.11)
Moderate cervical dysplasia (histologically confirmed)
(622.12)
Severe cervical dysplasia (histologically confirmed) (233.1)

795.00 Abnormal glandular Papanicolaou smear of cervix
Atypical endocervical cells NOS
Atypical endometrial cells NOS
Atypical cervical glandular cells NOS

795.01 Papanicolaou smear of cervix with atypical squamous cells
of undetermined significance (ASC-US)

795.02 Papanicolaou smear of cervic with atypical squamous cell
changes cannot exclude high grade squamous intraepithelial lesion (ASC-H)

795.03 Papanicolaou smear of cervix with low grade squamous
intraepithelial lesion (LGSIL)

795.04 Papanicolaou smear of cervix with high grade squamous
intraepithelial lesion (HGSIL)

795.05 Cervical high risk human papillomavirus (HPV) DNA test
positive

795.06 Papanicolaou smear of cervix with cytologic evidence
of malignancy

795.07 Satisfactory cervical smear but lacking transformation zone

795.08 Unsatisfactory cervical cytology smear
Inadequate cervical cytology sample

795.09 Other abnormal Papanicolaou smear of cervix and cervical
HPV
Cervical low risk human papillomavirus (HPV) DNA test positive
Use additional code for associated human papillomavirus
(079.4)
Excludes: encounter for Papanicolaou cervical
smear to confirm findings of recent
normal smear following initial abnormal
smear (V72.32)

795.1 Abnormal Papanicolaou smear of vagina and vaginal HPV
Abnormal thin preparation smear of vagina NOS
Abnormal vaginal cytology NOS
Use additional code to identify acquired absence of uterus and cervix,
if applicable (V88.01–V88.03)

Excludes: abnormal cytology smear of cervix and cervical HPV (795.00–795.09)
carcinoma in situ of vagina (233.31)
carcinoma in situ of vulva (233.32)
dysplasia (histologically confirmed) of vagina NOS (623.0, 233.31)
dysplasia (histologically confirmed) of vulva NOS (624.01, 624.02, 233.32)
mild vaginal dysplasia (histologically confirmed) (623.0)
mild vulvar dysplasia (histologically confirmed) (624.01)
moderate vaginal dysplasia (histologically confirmed) (623.0)
moderate vulvar dysplasia (histologically confirmed) (624.02)
severe vaginal dysplasia (histologically confirmed) (233.31)
severe vulvar dysplasia (histologically confirmed) (233.32)
vaginal intraepithelial neoplasia I (VAIN I) (623.0)
vaginal intraepithelial neoplasia II (VAIN II) (623.0)
vaginal intraepithelial neoplasia III (VAIN III) (233.31)
vulvar intraepithelial neoplasia I (VIN I) (624.01)
vulvar intraepithelial neoplasia II (VIN II) (624.02)
vulvar intraepithelial neoplasia III (VIN III) (233.32)

795.10 Abnormal glandular Papanicolaou smear of vagina
Atypical vaginal glandular cells NOS

795.11 Papanicolaou smear of vagina with atypical squamous cells of undetermined significance (ASC-US)

795.12 Papanicolaou smear of vagina with atypical squamous cells cannot exclude high grade squamous intraepithelial lesion (ASC-H)

795.13 Papanicolaou smear of vagina with low grade squamous intraepithelial lesion (LGSIL)

795.14 Papanicolaou smear of vagina with high grade squamous intraepithelial lesion (HGSIL)

795.15 Vaginal high risk human papillomavirus (HPV) DNA test positive
Excludes: condyloma acuminatum (078.11)
genital warts (078.11)

795.16 Papanicolaou smear of vagina with cytologic evidence of malignancy

795.18 Unsatisfactory vaginal cytology smear
Inadequate vaginal cytology sample

795.19 Other abnormal Papanicolaou smear of vagina and vaginal HPV
Vaginal low risk human papillomavirus (HPV) DNA test positive
Use additional code for associated human papillomavirus (079.4)

TABULAR LIST: SYMPTOMS, SIGNS, AND ILL-DEFINED CONDITIONS (780–799)

795.2   Nonspecific abnormal findings on chromosomal analysis
Abnormal karyotype

795.3   Nonspecific positive culture findings
Positive culture findings in:
nose
sputum
throat
wound
Excludes: that of:
blood (790.7–790.8)
urine (791.9)

    795.39   Other nonspecific positive culture findings
        Excludes: colonization status (V02.5-V02.9)

795.4   Other nonspecific abnormal histological findings

795.5   Nonspecific reaction to tuberculin skin test without active tuberculosis
Abnormal result of Mantoux test
PPD positive
Tuberculin (skin test):
positive
reactor

795.6   False positive serological test for syphilis
False positive Wassermann reaction

795.7   Other nonspecific immunological findings
Excludes: Abnormal tumor markers (795.81–795.89)
isoimmunization, in pregnancy (656.1–656.2)

    795.71   Nonspecific serologic evidence of human immunodeficiency virus (HIV)
Inconclusive (HIV) test (adult) (infant)
Note: This code is only to be used when a test finding is reported as nonspecific. Asymptomatic positive findings are coded to V08. If any HIV infection symptom or condition is present, see code 042. Negative findings are not coded.
Excludes: acquired immunodeficiency syndrome (AIDS) (042)
asymptomatic HIV infection status (V08)
HIV infection, symptomatic (042)
HIV disease (042)
positive (status) NOS (V08)

    795.79   Other and unspecified nonspecific immunological findings
Raised antibody titer
Raised level of immunoglobulins

795.8   Abnormal tumor markers

    795.81   Elevated carcinoembryonic antigen (CEA)
    795.82   Elevated cancer antigen 125 (CA 125)
    795.89   Other abnormal tumor markers

796 Other nonspecific abnormal findings

796.0 Nonspecific abnormal toxicological findings
Abnormal levels of heavy metals or drugs in blood, urine, or other tissue
Excludes: excessive blood level of alcohol (790.3)

796.2 Elevated blood pressure reading without diagnosis of hypertension
Note: This category is to be used to record an episode of elevated blood pressure in a patient in whom no formal diagnosis of hypertension has been made, or as an incidental finding.

796.3 Nonspecific low blood pressure reading

796.4 Other abnormal clinical findings

796.5 Abnormal finding on antenatal screening

796.7 Abnormal cytologic smear of anus and anal HPV
Excludes: abnormal cytologic smear of cervix and cervical HPV (795.00–795.09)
abnormal cytologic smear of vagina and vaginal HPV (795.10-795.19)
anal intraepithelial neoplasia I (AIN I) (569.44)
anal intraepithelial neoplasia II (AIN II) (569.44)
anal intraepithelial neoplasia III (AIN III) (230.5, 230.6)
carcinoma in situ of anus (230.5, 230.6)
dysplasia (histologically confirmed) of anus NOS (569.44)
mild anal dysplasia (histologically confirmed) (569.44)
moderate anal dysplasia (histologically confirmed) (569.44)
severe anal dysplasia (histologically confirmed) (230.5, 230.6)

796.70 Abnormal glandular Papanicolaou smear of anus
Atypical anal glandular cells NOS

796.71 Papanicolaou smear of anus with atypical squamous cells of undetermined significance (ASC-US)

796.72 Papanicolaou smear of anus with atypical squamous cells cannot exclude high grade squamous intraepithelial lesion (ASC-H)

796.73 Papanicolaou smear of anus with low grade squamous intraepithelial lesion (LGSIL)

796.74 Papanicolaou smear of anus with high grade squamous intraepithelial lesion (HGSIL)

796.75 Anal high risk human papillomavirus (HPV) DNA test positive

796.76 Papanicolaou smear of anus with cytologic evidence of malignancy

796.77 Satisfactory anal smear but lacking transformation zone

796.78 Unsatisfactory anal cytology smear
Inadequate anal cytology sample

796.79 Other abnormal Papanicolaou smear of anus and anal HPV
Anal low risk human papillomavirus (HPV)
DNA test positive
Use additional code for associated human papillomavirus
(079.4)
796.9 Other

ILL-DEFINED AND UNKNOWN CAUSES OF MORBIDITY AND MORTALITY

799 **Other ill-defined and unknown causes of morbidity and mortality**
799.2 Signs and symptoms involving emotional state
Excludes: anxiety (300.00-300.09)
depression (311)
799.21 Nervousness
Nervous
799.22 Irritability
Irritable
799.23 Impulsiveness
Impulsive
Excludes: impulsive neurosis (300.3)
799.24 Emotional lability
799.25 Demoralization and apathy
Apathetic
799.29 Other signs and symptoms involving emotional state
799.8 Other ill-defined conditions
799.81 Decreased libido
Decreased sexual desire
Excludes: psychosexual dysfunction with inhibited sexual
desire (302.71)
799.89 Other ill-defined conditions

INJURY AND POISONING (800–999)

INTERNAL INJURY OF THORAX, ABDOMEN, AND PELVIS

Includes: blunt trauma of internal organs
bruise of internal organs
concussion injuries (except cerebral) of internal organs
crushing of internal organs
hematoma of internal organs
laceration of internal organs
puncture of internal organs
tear of internal organs
traumatic rupture of internal organs
Note: The description "with open wound," used in the fourth-digit
subdivisions, includes those with mention of infection or foreign body.

863   **Injury to gastrointestinal tract**
      Excludes: anal sphincter laceration during delivery (664.2)
      863.4   Colon or rectum, without mention of open wound into cavity
              863.45   Rectum
              863.46   Multiple sites in colon and rectun
              863.49   Other
      863.5   Colon or rectum, with open wound into cavity
              863.55   Rectum
              863.56   Multiple sites in colon and rectum
              863.59   Other
      863.8   Other and unspecified gastrointestinal sites, without mention of
              open wound into cavity
              863.85   Appendix
      863.9   Other and unspecified gastrointestinal sites, with open wound into
              cavity
              863.95   Appendix

867   **Injury to pelvic organs**
      Excludes: injury during delivery (664.0–665.9)
      867.0   Bladder and urethra, without mention of open wound into cavity
      867.1   Bladder and urethra, with open wound into cavity
      867.2   Ureter, without mention of open wound into cavity
      867.3   Ureter, with open wound into cavity
      867.4   Uterus, without mention of open wound into cavity
      867.5   Uterus, with open wound into cavity
      867.6   Other specified pelvic organs, without mention of open wound
              into cavity
              Fallopian tube
              Ovary
      867.7   Other specified pelvic organs, with open wound into cavity
      867.8   Unspecified pelvic organ, without mention of open wound into cavity
      867.9   Unspecified pelvic organ, with open wound into cavity

OPEN WOUND OF HEAD, NECK, AND TRUNK
877   **Open wound of buttock**
      Includes: sacroiliac region
      877.0   Without mention of complication
      877.1   Complicated

878   **Open wound of genital organs (external), including traumatic amputation**
      Excludes: injury during delivery (664.0–665.9)
                       internal genital organs (867.0–867.9)
      878.4   Vulva, without mention of complication
              Labium (majus) (minus)
      878.5   Vulva, complicated

878.6 Vagina, without mention of complication
878.7 Vagina, complicated
878.8 Other and unspecified parts, without mention of complication
878.9 Other and unspecified parts, complicated

879 Open wound of other and unspecified sites, except limbs
879.0 Breast, without mention of complication
879.1 Breast, complicated
879.2 Abdominal wall, anterior, without mention of complication
Abdominal wall NOS
Epigastric region
Hypogastric region
Pubic region
Umbilical region
879.3 Abdominal wall, anterior, complicated
879.4 Abdominal wall, lateral, without mention of complication
Flank
Groin
Hypochondrium
Iliac (region)
Inguinal region
879.5 Abdominal wall, lateral, complicated
879.6 Other and unspecified parts of trunk, without mention of compli-
cation
Pelvic region
Perineum
Trunk NOS
879.7 Other and unspecified parts of trunk, complicated
879.8 Open wound(s) (multiple) of unspecified site(s) without mention
of complication
Multiple open wounds NOS
Open wound NOS
Open wound(s) (multiple) of unspecified site(s), complicated

INJURY TO BLOOD VESSELS

Includes: arterial hematoma of blood vessel, secondary to other injuries
avulsion of blood vessel, secondary to other injuries
laceration of blood vessel, secondary to other injuries
rupture of blood vessel, secondary to other injuries
traumatic aneurysm or fistula (arteriovenous) of blood vessel,
secondary to other injuries
Excludes: accidental puncture or laceration during medical procedure (998.2)
902 Injury to blood vessels of abdomen and pelvis
902.5 Iliac blood vessels
902.55 Uterine artery

902.56   Uterine vein
902.59   Other
902.8   Other specified blood vessels of abdomen and pelvis
902.81   Ovarian artery
902.82   Ovarian vein
902.87   Multiple blood vessels of abdomen and pelvis
902.89   Other
Unspecified blood vessel of abdomen and pelvis

LATE EFFECTS OF INJURIES, POISONINGS, TOXIC EFFECTS, AND OTHER EXTERNAL CAUSES

These categories are to be used to indicate conditions classifiable to 800–999 as the cause of late effects, which are themselves classified elsewhere. The "late effects" include those specified as such, or as sequelae, which may occur at any time after the acute injury.

908   Late effects of other and unspecified injuries
908.1   Late effect of internal injury to intra-abdominal organs
908.2   Late effect of internal injury to other internal organs
908.4   Late effect of injury to blood vessel of thorax, abdomen, and pelvis
908.5   Late effect of foreign body in orifice

909   Late effects of other and unspecified external causes
909.2   Late effect of radiation
Late effect of conditions classifiable to 990
909.3   Late effect of complications of surgical and medical care
Late effect of conditions classifiable to 996–999

SUPERFICIAL INJURY

911   Superficial injury of trunk
Includes: abdominal wall
anus
breast
buttock
labium (majus) (minus)
perineum
vagina
vulva
911.8   Other and unspecified superficial injury of trunk, without mention of infection
911.9   Other and unspecified superficial injury of trunk, infected

919   Superficial injury of other, multiple, and unspecified sites
919.8   Other and unspecified superficial injury of trunk, without mention of infection

919.9   Other and unspecified superficial injury of trunk, infected

CONTUSION WITH INTACT SKIN SURFACE

Includes: bruise without fracture or open wound
            hematoma without fracture or open wound
Excludes: internal organs (863–867)
            open wound (877)

921   Contusion of eye and adnexa
921.0   Black eye, NOS

922   Contusion of trunk
922.0   Breast
922.2   Abdominal wall
        Flank
        Groin
922.3   Back
        922.31   Back
        922.32   Buttock
922.4   Genital organs
        Labium (majus) (minus)
        Perineum
        Vagina
        Vulva
922.8   Multiple sites of trunk
922.9   Unspecified part
        Trunk NOS

CRUSHING INJURY

Use additional code to identify any associated injuries, such as:
internal injuries (863–867)

926   Crushing injury of trunk
926.0   External genitalia
        Labium (majus) (minus)
        Vulva
926.1   Other specified sites
        926.19   Other
                 Breast
926.8   Multiple sites of trunk
926.9   Unspecified site
        Trunk NOS

929   Crushing injury of multiple and unspecified sites
929.0   Multiple sites, not elsewhere classified
929.9   Unspecified site

EFFECTS OF FOREIGN BODY ENTERING THROUGH ORIFICE

Excludes: foreign body:
  inadvertently left in operative wound (998.4, 998.7)
  in open wound (800–839, 851–897)
  residual, in soft tissues (729.6)

937 Foreign body in anus and rectum
Rectosigmoid (junction)

939 Foreign body in genitourinary tract
939.0 Bladder and urethra
939.1 Uterus, any part
       Excludes: intrauterine contraceptive device:
                 complications from (996.32, 996.65)
                 presence of (V45.51)
939.2 Vulva and vagina
939.9 Unspecified site

BURNS

Includes: burns from:
  electrical heating appliance
  electricity
  flame
  hot object
  lightning
  radiation
  chemical burns (external) (internal)
       scalds
Excludes: sunburn (692.71, 692.76–692.77)

942 Burn of trunk
The following fifth-digit subclassification is for use with category 942:
0   trunk, unspecified site
1   breast
2   chest wall, excluding breast and nipple
3   abdominal wall
     Flank
5   genitalia
     Labium (majus) (minus)
     Perineum
     Vulva
9   other and multiple sites of trunk

942.0 Unspecified degree
942.1 Erythema (first degree)

942.2 Blisters, epidermal loss (second degree)
942.3 Full-thickness skin loss (third degree NOS)
942.4 Deep necrosis of underlying tissues (deep third degree) without mention of loss of a body part
942.5 Deep necrosis of underlying tissues (deep third degree) with loss of a body part

947 Burn of internal organs
Includes: burns from chemical agents (ingested)
947.4 Vagina and uterus
947.8 Other specified sites
947.9 Unspecified site

CERTAIN TRAUMATIC COMPLICATIONS AND UNSPECIFIED INJURIES

958 Certain early complications of trauma
Excludes: post-traumatic seroma (729.91)
  that occurring during or following medical procedures (996.0–999.9)
958.1 Fat embolism
  Excludes: that complicating:
    abortion (634–638 with .6, 639.6)
    pregnancy, childbirth, or the puerperium (673.8)
958.2 Secondary and recurrent hemorrhage
958.3 Posttraumatic wound infection, not elsewhere classified
  Excludes: infected open wounds—code to complicated open wound of site
958.4 Traumatic shock
  Shock (immediate) (delayed) following injury
  Excludes: shock:
    anaphylactic (995.0)
      due to serum (999.4)
    anesthetic (995.4)
    electric (994.8)
    following abortion (639.5)
    lightning (994.0)
    nontraumatic NOS (785.50)
    obstetric (669.1)
    postoperative (998.0)
958.5 Traumatic anuria
  Crush syndrome
  Renal failure following crushing
  Excludes: that due to a medical procedure (997.5)
958.8 Other early complications of trauma

959 Injury, other and unspecified
Includes: injury NOS
Excludes: injury NOS of:
blood vessels (902)
eye (921.0)
internal organs (863-867)
959.1 Trunk
959.12 Other injury of abdomen
959.14 Other injury of external genitals
959.19 Other injury of other sites of trunk
Injury of trunk NOS
959.8 Other specified sites, including multiple
Excludes: multiple sites classifiable to the same four-digit
category (959.0–959.7)

962 Poisoning by hormones and synthetic substitutes
962.2 Ovarian hormones and synthetic substitutes
Contraceptives, oral
Estrogens
Estrogens and progestogens, combined
Progestogens
962.3 Insulins and antidiabetic agents
Acetohexamide
Biguanide derivatives, oral
Chlorpropamide
Glucagon
Insulin
Phenformin
Sulfonylurea derivatives, oral
Tolbutamide
962.4 Anterior pituitary hormones
Corticotropin
Gonadotropin

968 Poisoning by other central nervous system depressants and anesthetics
968.4 Other and unspecified general anesthetics

OTHER AND UNSPECIFIED EFFECTS OF EXTERNAL CAUSES

990 Effects of radiation, unspecified
Complication of:
phototherapy
radiation therapy
Radiation sickness

Excludes: specified adverse effects of radiation. Such conditions are to be classified according to the nature of the adverse effect, as:
    burns (942–947)
    dermatitis (692.7–692.8)
    sunburn (692.71, 692.76–692.77)

995 Certain adverse effects not elsewhere classified
Excludes: complications of surgical and medical care (996.0–999.9)
995.0 Other anaphylactic shock
    Allergic shock NOS or due to adverse effect of correct medicinal substance properly administered
    Anaphylactic reaction NOS or due to adverse effect of correct medicinal substance properly administered
    Anaphylaxis NOS or due to adverse effect of correct medicinal substance properly administered
    Excludes: anaphylactic reaction to serum (999.4)
995.1 Angioneurotic edema
    Giant urticaria
    Excludes: urticaria:
        due to serum (999.5)
        other specified (698.2, 708.0–708.9)
995.2 Other and unspecified adverse effect of drug, medicinal and biological substance (due) to correct medicinal substance properly administered
    Adverse effect to correct medicinal substance properly administered
    Allergic reaction to correct medicinal substance properly administered
    Hypersensitivity to correct medicinal substance properly administered
    Idiosyncrasy due to correct medicinal substance properly administered
    Drug:
        hypersensitivity NOS
        reaction NOS
    995.20 Unspecified adverse effect of unspecified drug, medicinal and biological substance
    995.22 Unspecified adverse effect of anesthesia
    995.23 Unspecified adverse effect of insulin
    995.24 Failed moderate sedation during procedure
        Failed conscious sedation during procedure
    995.27 Other drug allergy
    995.29 Unspecified adverse effect of other drug, medicinal and biological substance
995.3 Allergy, unspecified
    Allergic reaction NOS
    Hypersensitivity NOS
    Idiosyncrasy NOS

Excludes: allergic reaction NOS to correct medicinal substance properly administered (995.22)
specific types of allergic reaction, such as:
dermatitis (691–692)
hayfever (477.0–477.8)

995.4 Shock due to anesthesia
Shock due to anesthesia in which the correct substance was properly
administered
Excludes: complications of anesthesia in labor or delivery
(668.0–668.9)
overdose or wrong substance given (968.4–969.9)
postoperative shock NOS (998.0)
specified adverse effects of anesthesia classified
elsewhere, such as: hepatitis (070.0–070.9), etc.
unspecified adverse effect of anesthesia (995.22)

995.5 Child maltreatment syndrome
Use additional code(s), if applicable, to identify any associated
injuries
Use additional E code to identify:
nature of abuse (E960–E968)
perpetrator (E967.0–E967.9)

995.50 Child abuse, unspecified
995.51 Child emotional/psychological abuse
995.52 Child neglect (nutritional)
Use additional code to identify intent of neglect (E904.0,
E968.4)
995.53 Child sexual abuse
995.54 Child physical abuse
Battered baby or child syndrome
995.59 Other child abuse and neglect
Multiple forms of abuse

995.8 Other specified adverse effects, not elsewhere classified
995.80 Adult maltreatment, unspecified
Abused person NOS
Use additional code to identify:
any associated injury
nature of abuse (E960–E968)
perpetrator (E967.0–E967.9)
995.81 Adult physical abuse
Battered:
person syndrome NEC
spouse
woman

Use additional code to identify:
any associated injury
nature of abuse (E960–E968)
perpetrator (E967.0–E967.9)

995.82 Adult emotional/psychological abuse
Use additional E code to identify perpetrator (E967.0–E967.9)

995.83 Adult sexual abuse
Use additional code to identify:
any associated injury
perpetrator (E967.0–E967.9)

995.84 Adult neglect (nutritional)
Use additional code to identify:
intent of neglect (E904.0–E968.4)
perpetrator (E967.0–E967.9)

995.85 Other adult abuse and neglect
Multiple forms of abuse and neglect
Use additional code to identify:
any associated injury
intent of neglect (E904.0, E968.4)
nature of abuse (E960–E968)
perpetrator (E967.0–E967.9)

995.86 Malignant hyperthermia
Malignant hyperpyrexia due to anesthesia

995.89 Other
Hypothermia due to anesthesia

995.9 Systemic inflammatory response syndrome (SIRS)

995.91 Sepsis
Systemic inflammatory response syndrome due to infectious process without acute organ dysfunction
Code first underlying infection
Excludes: sepsis with acute organ dysfunction (995.92)
sepsis with multiple organ dysfunction (995.92)
severe sepsis (995.92)

995.92 Severe sepsis
Sepsis with acute organ dysfunction
Sepsis with multiple organ dysfunction (MOD)
Systemic inflammatory response syndrome due to infectious process with acute organ dysfunction
Code first underlying infection
Use additional code to specify acute organ dysfunction, such as:
acute kidney failure (584.5-584.9)
disseminated intravascular coagulopathy (DIC) syndrome (286.6)

995.93 Systemic inflammatory response syndrome due to noninfectious process without acute organ dysfunction
Code first underlying conditions, such as:
acute pancreatitis (577.0)
trauma
Excludes: systemic inflammatory response syndrome due to noninfectious process with acute organ dysfunction (995.94)

995.94 Systemic inflammatory response syndrome due to noninfectious process with acute organ dysfunction
Code first underlying condition, such as:
acute pancreatitis (577.0)
trauma
Use additional code to specify acute organ dysfunction, such as:
acute kidney failure (584.5-584.9)
disseminated intravascular coagulopathy (DIC) syndrome (286.6)
Excludes: severe sepsis (995.92)

COMPLICATIONS OF SURGICAL AND MEDICAL CARE, NOT ELSEWHERE CLASSIFIED

Excludes: adverse effects of medicinal agents (010–799.8, 995.0–995.8)
burns from local applications and irradiation (942–947)
complications of:
conditions for which the procedure was performed
surgical procedures during abortion, labor, and delivery (630–676.9)
poisoning and toxic effects of drugs and chemicals (962–968)
postoperative conditions in which no complications are present, such as:
artificial opening status (V44.0–V44.7)
closure of external stoma (V55.0–V55.7)
fitting of prosthetic device (V52.4)
specified complications classified elsewhere:
anesthetic shock (995.4)
electrolyte imbalance (276.0–276.9)
postmastectomy lymphedema syndrome (457.0)
any other condition classified elsewhere in the Alphabetic Index when described as due to a procedure

TABULAR LIST: INJURY AND POISONING (800–999)

996   Complications peculiar to certain specified procedures
Includes: complications, not elsewhere classified, in the use of artificial substitutes (eg, Dacron, metal, Silastic, Teflon) or natural
sources (eg, bone) involving:
anastomosis (internal)
graft (bypass) (patch)
implant
internal device:
catheter
electronic
fixation
prosthetic
reimplant
transplant
Excludes: accidental puncture or laceration during procedure
(998.2)
capsular contracture of breast implant (611.83)
complications of internal anastomosis of:
gastrointestinal tract (997.4)
urinary tract (997.5)
other specified complications classified elsewhere, such as:
serum hepatitis (070.2–070.3)
996.3   Mechanical complication of genitourinary device, implant, and
graft
996.30   Unspecified device, implant, and graft
996.31   Due to urethral (indwelling) catheter
996.32   Due to intrauterine contraceptive device
996.39   Other
Cystostomy catheter
Prosthetic reconstruction of vas deferens
Repair (graft) of ureter without mention of resection
Excludes: complications due to:
external stoma of urinary tract (997.5)
internal anastomosis of urinary tract (997.5)
996.5   Mechanical complications of other specified prosthetic device,
implant, and graft
996.54   Due to breast prosthesis
Breast capsule (prosthesis)
Mammary implant
996.6   Infection and inflammatory reaction due to internal prosthetic
device, implant, and graft
Infection (causing obstruction) or inflammation due to (presence
of) any device, implant, and graft classifiable to 996.3–996.5
Use additional code to identify specified infections

996.64 Due to indwelling urinary catheter
Use additional code to identify specified infections, such as:
Cystitis (595.0–595.9)
Sepsis (038.0–038.9)
996.65 Due to other genitourinary device, implant and graft
Intrauterine contraceptive device
996.69 Due to other internal prosthetic device, implant, and graft
Breast prosthesis
996.7 Other complications of internal (biological) (synthetic) prosthetic device, implant, and graft
Complication NOS due to (presence of) any device, implant, and graft classifiable to 996.3–996.5:
occlusion NOS
Embolism
Fibrosis
Hemorrhage
Pain
Stenosis
Thrombus
Use additional code to identify complication, such as:
Add venous embolism and thrombosis (453.40-453.9)
Excludes: disruption (dehiscence) of internal suture material (998.31)
996.76 Due to genitourinary device, implant, and graft
996.79 Due to other internal prosthetic device, implant, and graft
Breast implant
Genitourinary NEC

997 Complications affecting specified body systems, not elsewhere classified
Use additional code to identify complication
Excludes: the listed conditions when specified as:
causing shock (998.0)
complications of
anesthesia:
adverse effect (010–799, 995)
in labor or delivery (668.0–668.9)
poisoning (968.0–969.9)
implanted device or graft (996.3–996.7)
obstetrical procedures (669.0–669.4)
997.0 Nervous system complications
997.00 Nervous system complication, unspecified
997.01 Central nervous system complication
Anoxic brain damage
Cerebral hypoxia
Excludes: Cerebrovascular hemorrhage or infarction (997.02)

997.02 Iatrogenic cerebrovascular infarction or hemorrhage
Postoperative stroke
997.09 Other nervous system complications
997.1 Cardiac complications
Cardiac:
arrest during or resulting from a procedure
insufficiency during or resulting from a procedure
Cardiorespiratory failure during or resulting from a procedure
Heart failure during or resulting from a procedure
997.2 Peripheral vascular complications
Phlebitis or thrombophlebitis during or resulting from a procedure
Excludes: the listed conditions due to:
infusion, perfusion, or transfusion (999.2)
997.3 Respiratory complications
Excludes: Mendelson's syndrome in labor and delivery (668.0)
specified complications classified elsewhere
997.31 Ventilator associated pneumonia
Ventilator associated pneumonitis
Use additional code to identify organism
997.39 Other respiratory complications
Mendelson's syndrome resulting from a procedure
Pneumonia (aspiration) resulting from a procedure
997.4 Digestive system complications
Complications of:
intestinal (internal) anastomosis and bypass, not elsewhere
classified, except that involving urinary tract
Hepatic failure specified as due to a procedure
Hepatorenal syndrome specified as due to a procedure
Intestinal obstruction NOS specified as due to a procedure
Excludes: specified gastrointestinal complications classified
elsewhere, such as:
colostomy or enterostomy complications (569.60–
569.69)
infection of external stoma (569.61)
pelvic peritoneal adhesions, female (614.6)
peritoneal adhesions (568.0)
997.5 Urinary complications
Complications of:
external stoma of urinary tract
internal anastomosis and bypass of urinary tract, including
that involving intestinal tract
Oliguria or anuria specified as due to procedure
Renal (kidney):
failure (acute) specified as due to procedure
insufficiency (acute) specified as due to procedure

Tubular necrosis (acute) specified as due to procedure
Excludes: specified complications classified elsewhere, such as:
postoperative stricture of ureter (593.3)
997.9 Complications affecting other specified body systems, not elsewhere classified
Excludes: specified complications classified elsewhere, such as:
broad ligament laceration syndrome (620.6)
postartificial menopause syndrome (627.4)
postoperative stricture of vagina (623.2)
997.91 Hypertension
Excludes: Essential hypertension (401.0–401.9)

998 Other complications of procedures, NEC
998.0 Postoperative shock
Collapse NOS during or resulting from a surgical procedure
Shock (endotoxic) (hypovolemic) (septic) during or resulting from a surgical procedure
Excludes: shock:
anaphylactic due to serum (999.4)
anesthetic (995.4)
following abortion (639.5)
obstetric (669.1)
traumatic (958.4)
998.1 Hemorrhage or hematoma or seroma complicating a procedure
Excludes: hemorrhage, hematoma or seroma:
complicating cesarean section or puerperal perineal wound (674.3)
due to implanted device or graft (996.76–996.79)
998.11 Hemorrhage complicating a procedure
998.12 Hematoma complicating a procedure
998.13 Seroma complicating a procedure
998.2 Accidental puncture or laceration during a procedure
Accidental perforation by catheter or other instrument during a procedure on:
blood vessel
nerve
organ
Excludes: puncture or laceration caused by implanted device intentionally left in operation wound (996.3–996.5)
specified complications classified elsewhere, such as:
broad ligament laceration syndrome (620.6)
trauma from instruments during delivery (664.0–665.9)

998.3 Disruption of wound
Dehiscence of operation wound
Rupture of operation wound
Excludes: disruption of:
    cesarean wound (674.1)
    perineal wound, puerperal (674.2)
  998.30 Disruption of wound, unspecified
    Disruption of wound NOS
  998.31 Disruption or internal operation (surgical) wound
    Deep disruption of dehiscence of operation wound NOS
    Excludes: complications of internal anastomosis of:
        gastrointestinal tract (997.4)
        urinary tract (997.5)
  998.32 Disruption of external operation (surgical) wound
    Disruption of operation wound NOS
    Full-thickness skin disruption or dehiscence
    Superficial disruption or dehiscence of operation wound
  998.33 Disruption of traumatic injury wound repair
    Disruption or dehiscence of closure of traumatic laceration
    (external) (internal)
998.4 Foreign body accidentally left during a procedure
Adhesions due to foreign body accidentally left in operative wound
or body cavity during a procedure
Obstruction due to foreign body accidentally left in operative wound
or body cavity during a procedure
Perforation due to foreign body accidentally left in operative wound or
body cavity during a procedure
Excludes: obstruction or perforation caused by implanted device
    intentionally left in body (996.3–996.5)
998.5 Postoperative infection
Excludes: infection due to:
    implanted device (996.63–996.69)
    infusion, perfusion, or transfusion (999.31–999.39)
    postoperative obstetrical wound infection (674.3)
  998.51 Infected postoperative seroma
    Use additional code to identify organism
  998.59 Other postoperative infection
    Abscess: postoperative
        intra-abdominal postoperative
        stitch postoperative
        subphrenic postoperative
        wound postoperative
    Septicemia postoperative
    Use additional code to identify infection

998.6 Persistent postoperative fistula
998.7 Acute reaction to foreign substance accidentally left during a
procedure
Peritonitis:
aseptic
chemical
998.8 Other specified complications of procedures, not elsewhere classified
  998.81 Emphysema (subcutaneous) (surgical) resulting from a
  procedure
  998.83 Nonhealing surgical wound
  998.89 Other specified complications
998.9 Unspecified complication of procedure, not elsewhere classified
Postoperative complication NOS
Excludes: complication NOS of obstetrical surgery or procedure
(669.4)

999 Complications of medical care, not elsewhere classified
Includes: complications, not elsewhere classified, of:
immunization
infusion
injection
inoculation
perfusion
transfusion
vaccination
Use additional code, where applicable, to identify specific
complication
Excludes: specified complications classified elsewhere such as:
complications of implanted device (996.3–996.7)
contact dermatitis due to drugs (692.3)
transient (293.9)
dialysis disequilibrium syndrome (276.0–276.9)
poisoning and toxic effects of drugs and chemicals (962–968)
water and electrolyte imbalance (276.0–276.9)
999.0 Generalized vaccinia
999.1 Air embolism
Air embolism to any site following infusion, perfusion, or transfusion
Excludes: embolism specified as:
complicating:
abortion (634–638 with .6, 639.6)
ectopic or molar pregnancy (639.6)
pregnancy, childbirth, or the puerperium
(673.0)
due to implanted device (996.7)

999.2 Other vascular complications
Phlebitis following infusion, perfusion, or transfusion
Thromboembolism following infusion, perfusion, or transfusion
Thrombophlebitis following infusion, perfusion, or transfusion
Excludes: extravasation of vesicant drugs (999.81, 999.82)
the listed conditions when specified as:
postoperative NOS (997.2)

999.3 Other infection
Infection following infusion, injection, transfusion, or vaccination
Sepsis following infusion, injection, transfusion, or vaccination
Septicemia following infusion, injection, transfusion, or vaccination
Excludes: the listed conditions when specified as:
due to implanted device (996.64)
postoperative NOS (998.51–998.59)
Use additional code to identify specified infection, such as:
septicemia

999.31 Infection due to central venous catheter

999.39 Infection following other infusion, injection, transfusion, or
vaccination

999.4 Anaphylactic shock due to serum
Excludes: shock:
allergic NOS (995.0)
anaphylactic:
NOS (995.0)
due to drugs and chemicals (995.0)

999.5 Other serum reaction
Intoxication by serum
Protein sickness
Serum rash
Serum sickness
Urticaria due to serum
Excludes: serum hepatitis (070.2–070.3)

999.6 ABO incompatibility reaction
Incompatible blood transfusion
Reaction to blood group incompatibility in infusion or transfusion
Excludes: minor blood group antigens reactions (Duffy) (E)
(K(ell)) (Kidd) (Lewis) (M) (N) (P) (S) (999.89)

999.7 Rh incompatibility reaction
Reactions due to Rh factor in infusion or transfusion

999.8 Other infusion and transfusion reaction
Septic shock due to transfusion
Transfusion reaction NOS
Excludes: postoperative shock (998.0)

999.81 Extravasation of vesicant chemotherapy
　　　　Infiltration of vesicant chemotherapy
999.82 Extravasation of other vesicant agent
　　　　Infiltration of other vesicant agent
999.88 Other infusion reaction
999.89 Other transfusion reaction
　　　　Transfusion reaction NOS
999.9 Other and unspecified complications of medical care, not elsewhere classified
　　　　Complications, not elsewhere classified, of:
　　　　　　ultrasound therapy
　　　　Unspecified misadventure of medical care
　　　　Excludes:　unspecified complication of:
　　　　　　　　　　phototherapy (990)
　　　　　　　　　　radiation therapy (990)
　　　　　　　　　　ventilator associated pneumonia (997.31)

4

SUPPLEMENTARY CLASSIFICATIONS

FACTORS INFLUENCING HEALTH STATUS AND CONTACT WITH HEALTH SERVICES (V01–V89)

V codes are located in a separate section of the Tabular List. These codes are used to report:

▓ An encounter with a patient who is not currently sick, but who is being seen for some specific purpose. Some examples are: Group B streptococcus screening for a pregnant patient (code V28.6), well-woman examination (code V72.31), screening due to family history of malignant neoplasm (code from the category V16).

▓ An encounter with a patient in whom a disease or injury has been previously diagnosed and is being seen now for a specific treatment. An example is chemotherapy (code V58.1).

▓ A situation or problem that influences the patient's health status, but which is not in itself a current illness or injury. An example is family history of breast cancer (code V16.3) as a secondary diagnosis during a preventive visit (code V72.31).

Many payers recognize and process claims with V codes, depending on the patient's coverage. If the reason the patient was seen is best described by a V code, then the V code is reported even if this means the visit will not be covered by her third-party payer.

PERSONS WITH POTENTIAL HEALTH HAZARDS RELATED TO COMMUNICABLE DISEASES

Excludes: personal history of infectious and parasitic diseases (V12.0)

V01 Contact with or exposure to communicable diseases
V01.1 Tuberculosis
Conditions classifiable to 010–018
V01.4 Rubella
Conditions classifiable to 056
V01.6 Venereal diseases
Conditions classifiable to 090–099

V01.7 Other viral diseases
    Conditions classifiable to 042–078, and V08, except as above
    V01.71 Varicella
    V01.79 Other viral diseases
V01.8 Other communicable diseases
    Conditions classifiable to 010–136, except as above
    V01.81 Anthrax
    V01.82 Exposure to SARS-associated coronavirus
    V01.83 *Escherichia coli (E. coli)*
    V01.84 Meningococcus
V01.9 Unspecified communicable disease

V02 Carrier or suspected carrier of infectious diseases
Includes: Colonization status
V02.5 Other specified bacterial diseases
    V02.51 Group B streptococcus
    V02.52 Other streptococcus
    V02.53 Methicillin susceptible Staphylococcus aureus
        MSSA colonization
    V02.54 Methicillin resistant Staphylococcus aureus
        MRSA colonization
    V02.59 Other specified bacterial diseases
        Meningococcal
        Staphylococcal
V02.6 Viral hepatitis
    V02.60 Viral hepatitis carrier, unspecified
    V02.61 Hepatitis B carrier
    V02.62 Hepatitis C carrier
    V02.69 Other viral hepatitis carrier
V02.7 Gonorrhea
V02.8 Other venereal diseases
V02.9 Other specified infectious organism

V03 Need for prophylactic vaccination and inoculation against bacterial diseases
Excludes: vaccination not carried out (V64.00–V64.09)
          vaccines against combinations of diseases (V06.4–V06.8)
V03.2 Tuberculosis (BCG)
V03.7 Tetanus toxoid alone
V03.8 Other specified vaccinations against single bacterial diseases
    V03.81 Hemophilus influenza, type B (Hib)
    V03.82 *Streptococcus pneumoniae* (pneumococcus)
    V03.89 Other specified vaccination
V03.9 Unspecified single bacterial disease

V04 **Need for prophylactic vaccination and inoculation against certain diseases**
　　Excludes: vaccines against combinations of diseases (V06.4–V06.8)
　　　　V04.0　Poliomyelitis
　　　　V04.2　Measles alone
　　V04.3　Rubella alone
　　V04.5　Rabies
　　V04.6　Mumps alone
　　V04.7　Common cold
　　V04.8　Other viral diseases
　　　　V04.81　Influenza
　　　　V04.82　Respiratory syncytial virus (RSV)
　　　　V04.89　Other viral diseases

V05 **Need for prophylactic vaccination and inoculation against single diseases**
　　Excludes: vaccines against combinations of diseases (V06.4–V06.8)
　　V05.3　Viral hepatitis
　　V05.4　Varicella
　　　　Chicken pox
　　V05.8　Other specified disease
　　V05.9　Unspecified single disease

V06 **Need for prophylactic vaccination and inoculation against combinations of diseases**
　　Note:　Use additional single vaccination codes from categories V03–V05 to identify any vaccinations not included in a combination code.
　　V06.4　Measles-mumps-rubella (MMR)
　　V06.6　*Streptococcus pneumoniae* (pneumococcus) and influenza
　　V06.8　Other combinations
　　　　Excludes: multiple single vaccination codes (V03–V05)

Persons With Need for Isolation, Other Potential Health Hazards, and Prophylactic Measures

V07 **Need for isolation and other prophylactic measures**
　　Excludes: prophylactic organ removal (V50.41–V50.49)
　　V07.1　Desensitization to allergens
　　V07.2　Prophylactic immunotherapy
　　　　Administration of:
　　　　　　immune sera (gamma globulin)
　　　　　　RhoGAM
　　V07.3　Other prophylactic chemotherapy
　　　　V07.39　Other prophylactic chemotherapy
　　　　　　Excludes: maintenance chemotherapy following disease (V58.11)

V07.4 Hormone replacement therapy (postmenopausal)
V07.5 Prophylactic use of agents affecting estrogen receptors and
estrogen levels
Code first, if applicable:
malignant neoplasm of breast (174.0–174.9, 175.0–175.9)
malignant neoplasm of prostate (185)
Use additional code, if applicable to identify:
estrogen receptor positive status (V86.0)
family history of breast cancer (V16.3)
genetic susceptibility to cancer (V84.01–V84.09)
personal history of breast cancer (V10.3)
postmenopausal status (V49.81)
Excludes: hormone replacement thrapy (potmenopausal) (V07.4)
V07.51 Prophylactic use of selective estrogen receptor
modulators (SERMs)
Prophylactic use of:
raloxifene (Evista)
tamoxifen (Nolvadex)
toremifene (Fareston)
V07.52 Prophylactic use of aromatase inhibitors
Prophylactic use of:
anastrozole (Arimidex)
exemestane (Aromasin)
letrozole (Femara)
V07.59 Prophylactic use of other agents affecting estrogen receptors
and estrogen levels
Prophylactic use of:
estrogen receptor downregulators
fulvestrant (Faslodex)
gonadotropin-releasing hormone (GnRH) agonist
goserelin acetate (Zoladex)
leuprolide acetate (leuprorelin) (Lupron)
megestrol acetate (Megace)
V07.8 Other specified prophylactic measure

V08 Asymptomatic human immunodeficiency virus (HIV) infection status
HIV positive NOS
This code is only to be used when no HIV infection symptoms or
conditions are present. If any HIV infection symptoms or conditions are
present, see code 042.
Excludes: AIDS (042)
human immunodeficiency virus (HIV) disease (042)
exposure to HIV (V01.79)
nonspecific serologic evidence of HIV (795.71)
symptomatic human immunodeficiency virus (HIV) infection (042)

PERSONS WITH POTENTIAL HEALTH HAZARDS RELATED TO PERSONAL AND FAMILY HISTORY

Excludes: obstetric patients where the possibility that the fetus might be affected is the reason for observation or management during pregnancy (655.0–655.9)

V10 Personal history of malignant neoplasm
V10.0 Gastrointestinal tract
 V10.05 Large intestine
 V10.06 Rectum, rectosigmoid junction, and anus
 V10.07 Liver
V10.1 Trachea, bronchus, and lung
 V10.11 Bronchus and lung
 V10.12 Trachea
V10.3 Breast
 History of conditions classifiable to 174
V10.4 Genital organs
 History of conditions classifiable to 179–184
 V10.40 Female genital organ, unspecified
 V10.41 Cervix uteri
 V10.42 Other parts of uterus
 V10.43 Ovary
 V10.44 Other genital organs
V10.5 Urinary organs
 V10.50 Urinary organ, unspecified
 V10.51 Bladder
 V10.52 Kidney
  Excludes: renal pelvis (V10.53)
 V10.53 Renal pelvis
 V10.59 Other
V10.6 Leukemia
 V10.60 Leukemia, unspecified
 V10.61 Lymphoid leukemia
 V10.62 Myeloid leukemia
 V10.63 Monocytic leukemia
 V10.69 Other
V10.7 Other lymphatic and hematopoietic neoplasms
 Conditions classifiable to 200
 Excludes: listed conditions in 200 in remission
 V10.71 Lymphosarcoma and reticulosarcoma
 V10.72 Hodgkin's disease
 V10.79 Other
V10.8 Personal history of malignant neoplasm of other sites
 History of conditions classifiable to 171–173, 195
 V10.81 Bone
 V10.82 Malignant melanoma of skin

V10.83 Other malignant neoplasm of skin
V10.89 Other
   Perineum/retroperineum
V10.9 Other and unspecified personal history of malignant
   neoplasm
V10.90 Personal history of unspecified malignant
   neoplasm
      Personal history of malignant neoplasm
      NOS

V11 Personal history of mental disorder
V11.0 Schizophrenia
V11.1 Affective disorders
   Personal history of manic-depressive psychosis
   Excludes: that in remission (296.0–296.6 with fifth-digit 5, 6)
V11.2 Neurosis
V11.3 Alcoholism
V11.8 Other mental disorders

V12 Personal history of certain other diseases
V12.0 Infectious and parasitic diseases
   Excludes: personal history of infectious diseases specific to a body
      system
   V12.00 Unspecified infectious and parasitic disease
   V12.01 Tuberculosis
   V12.02 Poliomyelitis
   V12.03 Malaria
   V12.04 Methicillin resistant Staphylococcus aureus
      MRSA
   V12.09 Other
V12.1 Nutritional deficiency
V12.2 Endocrine, metabolic, and immunity disorders
   Excludes: history of allergy (V14.0–V14.8)
V12.5 Diseases of circulatory system
   V12.51 Venous thrombosis and embolism
      Pulmonary embolism
   V12.52 Thrombophlebitis
   V12.53 Sudden cardiac arrest
   V12.54 Transient ischemic attack (TIA) and cerebral infarction with-
      out residual deficits
V12.7 Diseases of digestive system
   V12.71 Peptic ulcer disease
   V12.72 Colonic polyps

V13 Personal history of other diseases
V13.0 Disorders of urinary system
  V13.00 Unspecified urinary disorder
  V13.01 Urinary calculi
  V13.02 Urinary (tract) infection
  V13.03 nephrotic syndrome
  V13.09 Other
V13.1 Trophoblastic disease
  Excludes: supervision during a current pregnancy (V23.1)
V13.2 Other genital system and obstetric disorders
  Excludes: supervision during a current pregnancy of a woman
       with poor obstetric history (V23.0–V23.9)
       habitual aborter (646.3)
           without current pregnancy (629.81)
  V13.21 Personal history of pre-term labor
    Excludes: current pregnancy with history of preterm labor
         (V23.41)
  V13.22 Personal history of cervical dysplasia
    Excludes: personal history of malignant neoplasia of cervix
         uteri (V10.41)
  V13.29 Other genital system and obstetric disorders
V13.3 Diseases of skin and subcutaneous tissue
V13.4 Arthritis

V14 Personal history of allergy to medicinal agents
V14.0 Penicillin
V14.1 Other antibiotic agent
V14.2 Sulfonamides
V14.3 Other anti-infective agent
V14.4 Anesthetic agent
V14.5 Narcotic agent
V14.6 Analgesic agent
V14.7 Serum or vaccine
V14.8 Other specified medicinal agents

V15 Other personal history presenting hazards to health
V15.1 Surgery to heart and great vessels
V15.2 Surgery to other organs
  V15.21 Personal history of undergoing in utero procedure during
       pregnancy
  V15.22 Personal history of undergoing in utero procedure while a
       fetus
  V15.29 Surgery to other organs
V15.3 Irradiation
  Previous exposure to therapeutic or other ionizing radiation

V15.4 Psychological trauma
    Excludes: history of condition classifiable to 293–311 (V11.0–V11.8)
    V15.41 History of physical abuse
        Rape
    V15.42 History of emotional abuse
        Neglect
    V15.49 Other
V15.7 Contraception
    Excludes: current contraceptive management (V25.0–V25.4)
                presence of intrauterine contraceptive device as
                incidental finding (V45.5)
V15.8 Other specified personal history presenting hazards to health
    Excludes: contact with and (suspected) exposure to:
                aromatic compounds and dyes (V87.11–V87.19)
                arsenic and other metals (V87.01–V87.09)
                molds (V87.31)
    V15.81 Noncompliance with medical treatment
    V15.82 History of tobacco use
        Excludes: tobacco dependence (305.1)
    V15.80 History of failed moderate sedation
        History of failed conscious sedation
    V15.83 Underimmunization status
        Delinquent immunization status
        Lapsed immunization schedule status
    V15.88 History of fall at risk for falling
    V15.89 Other
        Medicare high risk patient seen for:
        pelvic examination and clinical breast check
        collection of pap smear specimen
        Excludes: contact with and (suspected) exposure to other
                potentially hazardous chemicals (V87.2)
                contact with and (suspected) exposure
                to other potentially hazardous substances
                (V87.39)
V15.9 Unspecified personal history presenting hazards to health

V16 Family history of malignant neoplasm
V16.0 Gastrointestinal tract
V16.1 Trachea, bronchus, and lung
V16.3 Breast
    Family history of condition classifiable to 174
V16.4 Genital organs
    Family history of condition classifiable to 179–184
    V16.40 Genital organ, unspecified
    V16.41 Ovary

V16.42 Prostate
V16.43 Testis
V16.49 Other
V16.5 Urinary organs
Family history of condition classifiable to 188–189
V16.51 Kidney
V16.59 Other
V16.6 Leukemia

V17 Family history of certain chronic disabling diseases
V17.3 Ischemic heart disease
V17.4 Other cardiovascular diseases
V17.41 Family history of sudden cardiac death (SCD)
Excludes: family history of ischemic heart disease (V17.3)
family history of myocardial infarction (V17.3)
V17.49 Family history of other cardiovascular diseases
V17.8 Other musculoskeletel diseases
V17.81 Osteoporosis
V17.89 Other musculoskeletal diseases

V18 Family history of certain other specific conditions
V18.0 Diabetes mellitus
V18.1 Other endocrine and metabolic diseases
V18.11 Multiple endocrine neoplasia [MEN] syndrome
V18.19 Other endocrine and metabolic diseases
V18.2 Anemia
V18.4 Mental retardation
V18.5 Digestive disorders
V18.51 Colonic polyps
V18.6 Kidney diseases
V18.61 Polycystic kidney
V18.7 Other genitourinary diseases
V18.9 Genetic disease carrier

V19 Family history of other conditions
V19.0 Blindness or visual loss
V19.1 Other eye disorders
V19.2 Deafness or hearing loss
V19.4 Skin conditions

PERSONS ENCOUNTERING HEALTH SERVICES IN CIRCUMSTANCES RELATED TO REPRODUCTION AND DEVELOPMENT

V22 Normal pregnancy
Excludes: pregnancy examination or test, pregnancy unconfirmed (V72.40)
V22.0 Supervision of normal first pregnancy
V22.1 Supervision of other normal pregnancy

V22.2 Pregnant state, incidental
Pregnant state NOS

V23 Supervision of high-risk pregnancy
V23.0 Pregnancy with history of infertility
V23.1 Pregnancy with history of trophoblastic disease
Pregnancy with history of:
hydatidiform mole
vesicular mole
Excludes: that without current pregnancy (V13.1)
V23.2 Pregnancy with history of abortion
Pregnancy with history of conditions classifiable to 634–638
Excludes: habitual aborter:
care during pregnancy (646.3)
that without current pregnancy (629.81)
V23.3 Grand multiparity
Excludes: care in relation to labor and delivery (659.4)
that without current pregnancy (V61.5)
V23.4 Pregnancy with other poor obstetric history
Pregnancy with history of other conditions classifiable to 630–676
V23.41 Pregnancy with history of pre-term labor
V23.49 Pregnancy with other poor obstetric history
V23.5 Pregnancy with other poor reproductive history
Pregnancy with history of stillbirth or neonatal death
V23.7 Insufficient prenatal care
History of little or no prenatal care
V23.8 Other high-risk pregnancy
V23.81 Elderly primigravida
First pregnancy in a woman who will be 35 years of age or
older at expected date of delivery
Excludes: elderly primigravida complicating pregnancy (659.5)
V23.82 Elderly multigravida
Second or more pregnancy in a woman who will be 35
years of age or older at expected date of delivery
Excludes: elderly multigravida complicating pregnancy (659.6)
V23.83 Young primigravida
First pregnancy in a female less than 16 years old at
expected date of delivery
Excludes: young primigravida complicating pregnancy (659.8)
V23.84 Young multigravida
Second or more pregnancy in a female less than 16 years
old at expected date of delivery
Excludes: young multigravida complicating pregnancy
(659.8)
V23.85 Pregnancy resulting from assisted reproductive technology
Pregnancy resulting from in vitro fertilization

V23.86 Pregnancy with history of in utero procedure during previous pregnancy
Excludes: management of pregnancy affected by in utero procedure during current pregnancy (679.0–679.1)
V23.89 Other high-risk pregnancy
V23.9 Unspecified high-risk pregnancy

V24 Postpartum care and examination
V24.0 Immediately after delivery
Care and observation in uncomplicated cases
V24.1 Lactating mother
Supervision of lactation
V24.2 Routine postpartum follow-up

V25 Encounter for contraceptive management
V25.0 General counseling and advice
V25.01 Prescription of oral contraceptives
V25.02 Initiation of other contraceptive measures
Fitting of diaphragm
Prescription of foams, creams, or other agents
V25.03 Encounter for emergency contraceptive counseling and prescription
Encounter for postcoital contraceptive counseling and prescription
V25.04 Counseling and instruction in natural family planning to avoid pregnancy
V25.09 Other
Family planning advice
V25.1 Insertion of intrauterine contraceptive device
V25.2 Sterilization
Admission for interruption of fallopian tubes or vas deferens
V25.3 Menstrual extraction
Menstrual regulation
V25.4 Surveillance of previously prescribed contraceptive methods
Checking, reinsertion, or removal of contraceptive device
Repeat prescription for contraceptive method
Routine examination in connection with contraceptive maintenance
Excludes: presence of intrauterine contraceptive device as incidental finding (V45.5)
V25.40 Contraceptive surveillance, unspecified
V25.41 Contraceptive pill
V25.42 Intrauterine contraceptive device
Checking, reinsertion, or removal of intrauterine device
V25.43 Implantable subdermal contraceptive
V25.49 Other contraceptive method

V25.5 Insertion of implantable subdermal contraceptive
V25.8 Other specified contraceptive management
Postvasectomy sperm count
Excludes: sperm count following sterilization reversal (V26.22)
sperm count for fertility testing (V26.21)
V25.9 Unspecified contraceptive management

V26 Procreative management
V26.0 Tuboplasty or vasoplasty after previous sterilization
V26.1 Artificial insemination
V26.2 Investigation and testing
Excludes: postvasectomy sperm count (V25.8)
V26.21 Fertility testing
Fallopian insufflation
Sperm count for fertility testing
Excludes: genetic counseling and testing (V26.31–V26.39)
V26.22 Aftercare following sterilization reversal
Fallopian insufflation following sterilization reversal
Sperm count following sterilization reversal
V26.29 Other investigation and testing
V26.3 Genetic counseling and testing
Excludes: fertility testing (V26.21)
nonprocreative genetic screening (V82.71, V82.79)
V26.31 Testing of female for genetic disease carrier status
V26.32 Other genetic testing of female
Use additional code to identify habitual aborter
(629.81, 646.3)
V26.33 Genetic counseling
V26.34 Testing of male for genetic disease carrier
V26.35 Encounter for testing of male partner of habitual aborter
V26.39 Other genetic testing of male
V26.4 General counseling and advice
V26.41 Procreative counseling and advice using natural family planning
V26.42 Encounter for fertility preservation counseling
Encounter for fertility preservation counseling prior to
cancer therapy
Encounter for fertility preservation counseling prior to
surgical removal of gonads
V26.49 Other procreative management counseling and advice
V26.5 Sterilization status
V26.51 Tubal ligation status
Excludes: infertility not due to previous tubal ligation
(628.0–628.9)
V26.8 Other specified procreative management
V26.81 Encounter for assisted reproductive fertility procedure cycle
Patient undergoing in vitro fertilization cycle

Use additional code to identify type of infertility
Excludes: precycle diagnosis and testing—code to reason for
encounter
V26.82 Encounter for fertility preservation procedure
Encounter for fertility preservation procedure prior to
cancer therapy
Encounter for fertility preservation procedure prior to
surgical removal of gonads
V26.89 Other specified procreative management
V26.9 Unspecified procreative management

V27 Outcome of delivery
This category is intended for the coding of the outcome of delivery on the
mother's record.
V27.0 Single liveborn
V27.1 Single stillborn
V27.2 Twins, both liveborn
V27.3 Twins, one liveborn and one stillborn
V27.4 Twins, both stillborn
V27.5 Other multiple birth, all liveborn
V27.6 Other multiple birth, some liveborn
V27.7 Other multiple birth, all stillborn
V27.9 Unspecified outcome of delivery

V28 Encounter for antenatal screening of mother
For additional information concerning diagnostic coding for ultrasound pro-
cedures, see Appendix C.
Excludes: abnormal findings on screening—code to findings
routine prenatal care (V22.0–V23.9)
V28.0 Screening for chromosomal abnormalities by amniocentesis
V28.1 Screening for raised alpha-fetoprotein levels in amniotic fluid
V28.2 Other screening based on amniocentesis
V28.3 Encounter for routine screening for malformation using ultrasonics
Encounter for routine fetal ultrasound NOS
Excludes: encounter for fetal anatomic survey (V28.81)
genetic counseling and testing (V26.31–V26.39)
V28.4 Screening for fetal growth retardation using ultrasonics
V28.5 Screening for isoimmunization
V28.6 Screening for Streptococcus B
V28.8 Other specified antenatal screening
V28.81 Encounter for fetal anatomic survey
V28.82 Encounter for screening for risk of pre-term labor
V28.89 Other specified antenatal screening
Chorionic villus sampling
Genomic screening
Nuchal translucency testing

Proteomic screening
V28.9 Unspecified antenatal screening

PERSONS WITH A CONDITION INFLUENCING THEIR HEALTH STATUS

These categories are intended for use when these conditions are recorded as "diagnoses" or "problems."

V40 Mental and behavioral problems
V40.1 Problems with communication (including speech)

V41 Problems with special senses and other special functions
V41.7 Problems with sexual function
Excludes: marital problems (V61.10)
psychosexual disorders (302.7)

V43 Organ or tissue replaced by other means
Includes: organ or tissue assisted by other means
replacement of organ by:
artificial device
mechanical device
prosthesis
Excludes: fitting and adjustment of prosthetic device (V52.4)
renal dialysis status (V45.1)
V43.2 Heart
V43.21 Heart assist device
V43.22 Fully implantable artificial heart
V43.6 Joint
V43.69 Other
V43.8 Other organ or tissue
V43.82 Breast

V44 Artificial opening status
Excludes: artificial openings requiring attention or management
(V55.1–V55.7)
V44.0 Tracheostomy
V44.1 Gastrostomy
V44.2 Ileostomy
V44.3 Colostomy
V44.5 Cystostomy
V44.59 Other cystostomy
V44.7 Artificial vagina

V45 Other postprocedural states
Excludes: aftercare management (V52–V58.8)
malfunction or other complication—code to condition
V45.1 Renal dialysis status

V45.11 Renal dialysis status
    Hemodialysis status
    Patient requiring intermittent renal dialysis
    Peritoneal dialysis status
    Presence of arterial-venous shunt (for dialysis)
  V45.12 Noncompliance with renal dialysis
V45.5 Presence of contraceptive device
  Excludes: checking, reinsertion, or removal of device (V25.42)
       complication from device (996.32)
       insertion of device (V25.1)
  V45.51 Intrauterine contraceptive device
  V45.52 Subdermal contraceptive implant
  V45.59 Other
V45.7 Acquired absence of organ
  V45.71 Acquired absence of breast and nipple
    Excludes: congenital absence of breast and nipple (757.6)
  V45.77 Genital organs
    Excludes: acquired absence of cervix and uterus
       (V88.01–V88.03)
       female genital mutilation status (629.20–629.29)
V45.8 Other postprocedural status
  V45.83 Breast implant removal status
  V45.86 Bariatric surgery status
    Excludes: bariatric surgery status complicating pregnancy,
       childbirth, or puerperium

V49 Other conditions influencing health status
 V49.8 Other specified conditions influencing health status
  V49.81 Asymptomatic postmenopausal status (age-related) (natural)
    Excludes: menopausal and premenopausal disorders
       (627.0–627.9)
       postsurgical menopause (256.2)
       premature menopause (256.31)
       symptomatic menopause (627.0–627.9)

Persons Encountering Health Services for Specific Procedures and Aftercare

Categories V51–V58 are used to indicate a reason for care in patients who may have already been treated for some disease or injury not now present, or who are receiving care to consolidate the treatment, to deal with residual states, or to prevent recurrence.

Excludes: follow-up examination for medical surveillance following treatment
    (V67.0–V67.9)

V50 Elective surgery for purposes other than remedying health states
 V50.1 Other plastic surgery for unacceptable cosmetic appearance
    Breast augmentation or reduction

Face-lift
Excludes: encounter for breast reduction (611.1)
plastic surgery following healed injury or operation
(V51.0–V51.8)
V50.2 Routine or ritual circumcision
Circumcision in the absence of significant medical indication
V50.3 Ear piercing
V50.4 Prophylactic organ removal
Excludes: therapeutic organ removal—code to condition
V50.41 Breast
V50.42 Ovary
V50.49 Other

V51 Aftercare involving the use of plastic surgery
Excludes: plastic surgery as treatment for current condition or injury—
code to condition or injury
V51.0 Encounter for breast reconstruction following mastectomy
Excludes: deformity and disproportion of reconstructed breast
(612.0–612.1)
V51.8 Other aftercare involving the use of plastic surgery

V52 Fitting and adjustment of prosthetic device and implant
Includes: removal of device
Excludes: malfunction or complication of prosthetic device (996.3–996.7)
status only, without need for care (V43.2–V43.8)
V52.4 Breast prosthesis and implant
Elective implant exchange (different material) (different size)
Removal of tissue expander without synchronous insertion of
permanent implant
Excludes: admission for initial breast implant insertion for breast
augmentation (V50.1)
complications of breast implant (996.54, 996.69, 996.79)
encounter for breast reconstruction following mastectomy
(V51.0)

V53 Fitting and adjustment of other device
Includes: removal of device
replacement of device
Excludes: status only, without need for care (V45.1–V45.8)
V53.6 Urinary devices
urinary catheter
Excludes: cystostomy (V55.5)
nephrostomy (V55.6)
ureterostomy (V55.6)
urethrostomy (V55.6)

V55 Attention to artificial openings
Includes: adjustment or repositioning of catheter closure
passage of sounds or bougies
reforming
removal or replacement of catheter
toilet or cleansing
Excludes: complications of external stoma (569.60–569.69, 997.4, 997.5)
status only, without need for care (V44.0–V44.7)
V55.1 Gastrostomy
V55.2 Ileostomy
V55.3 Colostomy
V55.5 Cystostomy
V55.6 Other artificial opening of urinary tract
Nephrostomy
Ureterostomy
Urethrostomy
V55.7 Artificial vagina

V58 Encounter for other and unspecified procedures and aftercare
Excludes: convalescence and palliative care (V66.0–V66.9)
V58.0 Radiotherapy
Encounter or admission for radiotherapy
Excludes: encounter for radioactive implant—code to condition
radioactive iodine therapy—code to condition
V58.1 Chemotherapy
Encounter or admission for chemotherapy
V58.2 Blood transfusion, without reported diagnosis
V58.3 Attention to dressings and sutures
Change or removal of wound packing
Excludes: attention to drains (V58.49)
planned postoperative wound closure (V58.41)
V58.30 Encounter for change or removal of nonsurgical wound
dressing
V58.31 Encounter for change or removal of surgical wound dressing
V58.32 Encounter for removal of sutures or staples
V58.4 Other aftercare following surgery
Note: Codes from this subcategory should be used in conjunction
with other aftercare codes to fully identify the reason for the
aftercare encounter.
Excludes: aftercare following sterilization reversal surgery (V26.22)
attention to artificial openings (V55.1–V55.7)
V58.41 Encounter for planned postoperative wound closure
Excludes: disruption of operative wound (998.31–998.32)
encounter for dressing and suture aftercare
(V58.30–V58.32)
V58.42 Aftercare following surgery for neoplasm

Conditions classifiable to 140–239

V58.43 Aftercare following surgery for injury and trauma
Conditions classifiable to 863–999

V58.49 Other specified aftercare following surgery
Change or removal of drains

V58.6 Long-term (current) drug use
Excludes: drug abuse (305.00–305.93)
drug abuse and dependence complicating pregnancy
(648.3–648.4)
drug dependence (304.00–304.93)
hormone replacement therapy (postmenopausal) (V07.4)
prophylactic use of agents affecting estrogen receptors and
estrogen levels (V07.51–V07.59)

V58.61 Long-term (current) use of anticoagulants
Excludes: long-term (current) use of aspirin (V58.66)

V58.62 Long-term (current) use of antibiotics

V58.63 Long-term (current) use of antiplatelets/antithrombotics
Excludes: long-term (current) use of aspirin (V58.66)

V58.64 Long-term (current) use of nonsteroidal anti-inflammatories
(NSAID)
Excludes: long-term (current) use of aspirin (V58.66)

V58.65 Long-term (current) use of steroids

V58.66 Long-term (current) use of aspirin

V58.67 Long-term (current) use of insulin

V58.69 Long-term (current) use of other medications
Long term current use of methadone
Long term current use of opiate analgesic
Other high-risk medications

V58.7 Aftercare following surgery to specified body systems, not elsewhere
classified
Note: Codes from this subcategory should be used in conjunction
with other aftercare codes to fully identify the reason for the
aftercare encounter.
Excludes: aftercare following surgery for neoplasm (V58.42)

V58.76 Aftercare following surgery of the genitourinary system,
NEC
Conditions classifiable to 584–629
Excludes: aftercare following sterilization reversal (V26.22)

V58.8 Other specified procedures and aftercare

V58.83 Encounter for therapeutic drug monitoring
Use additional code for any associated long-term (current)
drug use (V58.61–V58.69)
Excludes: blood-drug testing for medicolegal
reasons (V70.4)

V59 Donors
  V59.7 Egg (oocyte) (ovum)
    V59.70 Egg (oocyte) (ovum) donor, unspecified
    V59.71 Egg (oocyte) (ovum) donor, under age 35, anonymous
      recipient
      Egg donor, under age 35 NOS
    V59.72 Egg (oocyte) (ovum) donor, under age 35, designated
      recipient
    V59.73 Egg (oocyte) (ovum) donor, age 35 and over, anonymous
      recipient
      Egg donor, age 35 and over NOS
    V59.74 Egg (oocyte) (ovum) donor, age 35 and over, designated
      recipient

PERSONS ENCOUNTERING HEALTH SERVICES IN OTHER CIRCUMSTANCES

V61 Other family circumstances
  Includes: when these circumstances or fear of them, affecting the person
      directly involved or others, are mentioned as the reason, justified
      or not, for seeking or receiving medical advice or care
  V61.0 Family disruption
    V61.01 Family disruption due to family member on military
      deployment
        Individual or family member affected by other family
          member being on deployment
        Excludes: family disruption due to family member on non-
          military extended absence from home (V61.08)
    V61.02 Family disruption due to return of family member from
      military deployment
        Individual or family affected by other family member
        having returned from deployment (current or past
        conflict)
    V61.03 Family disruption due to divorce or legal separation
    V61.04 Family disruption due to parent-child estrangement
      Excludes: other family estrangement (V61.09)
    V61.05 Family disruption due to child in welfare custody
    V61.06 Family disruption due to child in foster care or in care of
      non-parental family member
    V61.06 Other family disruptions
      Family estrangement NOS
    V61.07 Family disruption due to death of family member
    Excludes: bereavement (V62.82)
    V61.08 Family disruption due to other extended absence of family
      member
    Excludes: family disruption due to family member on military deploy
      ment (V61.01)

V61.1 Counseling for marital and partner problems
Excludes: problems related to:
psychosexual disorders (302.7)
sexual function (V41.7)
 V61.10 Counseling for marital and partner problems, unspecified
  Marital conflict
  Partner conflict
 V61.11 Counseling for victim of spousal and partner abuse
  Excludes: encounter for treatment of current injuries due
  to abuse (995.80–995.85)
 V61.12 Counseling for perpetrator of spousal and partner abuse
V61.4 Health problems within family
 V61.41 Alcoholism in family
 V61.42 Substance abuse in family
 V61.49 Other
  Care of sick or handicapped person in family or household
  Presence of sick or handicapped person in family or
  household
V61.5 Multiparity
V61.7 Other unwanted pregnancy
V61.8 Other specified family circumstances
 Problems with family members NEC
V61.9 Unspecified family circumstance

V62 Other psychosocial circumstances
Includes: those circumstances or fear of them, affecting the person
directly involved or others, mentioned as the reason,
justified or not, for seeking or receiving medical advice or
care
Excludes: previous psychological trauma (V15.41–V15.49)
V62.2 Other occupational circumstances or maladjustment
 V62.21 Personal current military deployment status
  Individual (civilian or military) currently deployed in
  theater or in support of military war, peacekeeping and
  humanitarian operations
 V62.22 Personal history of return from military deployment
  Individual (civilian or military) with past history of military
  war, peacekeeping and humanitarian deployment (current
  or past conflict)
 V62.29 Other occupational circumstances or maladjustment
  Career choice problem
  Dissatisfaction with employment
  Occupational problem

V62.6 Refusal of treatment for reasons of religion or conscience
V62.8 Other psychological or physical stress, not elsewhere classified
    V62.81 Interpersonal problems, not elsewhere classified
    V62.82 Bereavement, uncomplicated
        Excludes: bereavement as adjustment reaction (309.0)
    V62.83 Counseling for perpetrator of physical/sexual abuse
        Excludes: counseling for perpetrator of parental
                child abuse (V61.22)
                counseling for perpetrator of spousal and partner
                abuse (V61.12)
    V62.89 Other
        Life circumstance problems
        Phase of life problems
V62.9 Unspecified psychosocial circumstance

V64 Persons encountering health services for specific procedures, not carried out
V64.0 Vaccination not carried out
    V64.00 Vaccination not carried out, unspecified reason
    V64.01 Vaccination not carried out because of acute illness
    V64.02 Vaccination not carried out because of chronic illness or condition
    V64.03 Vaccination not carried out because of immune compromised state
    V64.04 Vaccination not carried out because of allergy to vaccine or component
    V64.05 Vaccination not carried out because of caregiver refusal
        Guardian or parent refusal
        Excludes: vaccination not carried out because of caregiver
                refusal for religious reasons (V64.07)
    V64.06 Vaccination not carried out because of patient refusal
    V64.07 Vaccination not carried out for religious reasons
    V64.08 Vaccination not carried out because patient had disease being vaccinated against
    V64.09 Vaccination not carried out for other reason
V64.1 Surgical or other procedure not carried out because of contra-indication
V64.2 Surgical or other procedure not carried out because of patient's decision
V64.3 Procedure not carried out for other reasons
V64.4 Closed surgical procedure converted to open procedure
    V64.41 Laparoscopic surgical procedure converted to open procedure

V65 Other persons seeking consultation
V65.0 Healthy person accompanying sick person
V65.1 Person consulting on behalf of another person
Advice or treatment for nonattending third party
Excludes: concern (normal) about sick person in family
(V61.41–V61.49)
V65.19 Other person consulting on behalf of another person
V65.2 Person feigning illness
Malingerer
Peregrinating patient
V65.3 Dietary surveillance and counseling
Use additional code to identify Body Mass Index (BMI), if known
(V85.0–V85.54)
Dietary surveillance and counseling (in):
NOS
colitis
diabetes mellitus
food allergies or intolerance
gastritis
hypercholesterolemia
hypoglycemia
obesity
V65.4 Other counseling, not elsewhere classified
Health:
advice
education
instruction
Excludes: counseling (for):
contraception (V25.40–V25.49)
genetic (V26.31–V26.39)
on behalf of third party (V65.19)
procreative management (V26.41–V26.49)
V65.40 Counseling NOS
V65.41 Exercise counseling
V65.42 Counseling on substance use and abuse
V65.43 Counseling on injury prevention
V65.44 Human immunodeficiency virus (HIV) counseling
V65.45 Counseling on other sexually transmitted diseases
V65.49 Other specified counseling
V65.5 Person with feared complaint in whom no diagnosis was made
Feared condition not demonstrated
Problem was normal state
"Worried well"
V65.8 Other reasons for seeking consultation
Excludes: specified symptoms

V65.9 Unspecified reason for consultation

V66 Convalescence and palliative care
V66.0 Following surgery
V66.1 Following radiotherapy
V66.2 Following chemotherapy
V66.5 Following other treatment
V66.6 Following combined treatment
V66.7 Encounter for palliative care
      End-of-life care
      Hospice care
      Terminal care
      Code first underlying disease
V66.9 Unspecified convalescence

V67 Follow-up examination
Includes: surveillance only following completed treatment
Excludes: surveillance of contraception (V25.40–V25.49)
V67.0 Following surgery
    V67.00 Following surgery, unspecified
    V67.01 Follow-up vaginal pap smear
        Vaginal pap smear, status-post hysterectomy for malignant condition
        Use additional code to identify:
            acquired absence of uterus (V88.01–V88.03)
            personal history of malignant neoplasm (V10.40–V10.44)
        Excludes: vaginal pap smear status—post hysterectomy for non-malignant condition (V76.47)
    V67.09 Following other surgery
        Excludes: sperm count following sterilization reversal (V26.22)
                sperm count for fertility testing (V26.21)
V67.1 Following radiotherapy
V67.2 Following chemotherapy
    Cancer chemotherapy follow-up
V67.5 Following other treatment
    V67.51 Following completed treatment with high-risk medication, not elsewhere classified
        Excludes: Long-term (current) drug use (V58.61–V58.69)
    V67.59 Other
V67.6 Following combined treatment
V67.9 Unspecified follow-up examination

V68 Encounters for administrative purposes
V68.0 Issue of medical certificates
    V68.01 Disability examination
        Use additional code(s) to identify:
        specific examination(s), screening, and testing performed
        (V72.0–V82.9)
    V68.09 Other issue of medical certificates
        Excludes: encounter for general medical examination (V70.0–V70.9)
V68.1 Issue of repeat prescriptions
    Issue of repeat prescription for medications
    Excludes: repeat prescription for contraceptives (V25.41–V25.49)
V68.8 Other specified administrative purpose
    V68.81 Referral of patient without examination or treatment
    V68.89 Other
V68.9 Unspecified administrative purpose

V69 Problems related to lifestyle
V69.0 Lack of physical exercise
V69.1 Inappropriate diet and eating habits
    Excludes: anorexia nervosa (307.1)
        bulimia (783.6)
        other and unspecified eating disorders 307.50–307.59)
V69.2 High-risk sexual behavior
V69.4 Lack of adequate sleep
    Sleep deprivation
    Excludes: insomnia (780.52)
V69.8 Other problems related to lifestyle
    Self-damaging behavior
V69.9 Problem related to lifestyle, unspecified

PERSONS WITHOUT REPORTED DIAGNOSES ENCOUNTERED DURING
EXAMINATION AND INVESTIGATION OF INDIVIDUALS AND POPULATIONS
Note: Nonspecific abnormal findings disclosed at the time of these examinations are
    classifiable to categories 790–796.

V70 General medical examination
Use additional code(s) to identify any special screening examination(s)
performed (V73.0–V82.9)
V70.0 Routine general medical examination at a health care facility
    Health checkup
    Excludes: pre-procedural general physical examination (V72.83)
V70.4 Examination for medicolegal reasons
    Blood-alcohol tests

Blood-drug tests
Paternity testing
Excludes: examination and observation following:
accidents (V71.3, V71.4)
assault (V71.6)
rape (V71.5)
V70.8 Other specified general medical examinations
Examination of potential donor of organ or tissue
V70.9 Unspecified general medical examination
V71 **Observation and evaluation for suspected conditions not found**
This category is to be used when persons without a diagnosis are suspected of having an abnormal condition, without signs or symptoms, which requires study, but after examination and observation, is found not to exist. This category is also for use for administrative and legal observation status.
Excludes: suspected maternal and fetal conditions not found (V89.01–V89.09)
V71.1 Observation for suspected malignant neoplasm
V71.2 Observation for suspected tuberculosis
V71.3 Observation following accident at work
V71.4 Observation following other accident
Examination of individual involved in motor vehicle traffic accident
V71.5 Observation following alleged rape or seduction
Examination of victim or culprit
V71.6 Observation following other inflicted injury
Examination of victim or culprit
V71.8 Observation and evaluation for other specified suspected conditions
V71.81 Abuse and neglect
Excludes: adult abuse and neglect (995.80–995.85)
child abuse and neglect (995.50–995.59)
V71.89 Other specified suspected conditions
Hydatidiform mole

V72 **Special investigations and examinations**
Includes: routine examination of specific system
Excludes: general medical examination (V70.0–70.4)
Use additional code(s) to identify any special screening examination(s) performed (V73.0–V82.9)
For additional information concerning reporting examinations with collection of Pap smears, see Appendix B.
V72.3 Gynecological examination
Excludes: cervical Papanicolaou smear without general gynecological examination (V76.2)
routine examination in contraceptive management (V25.40–V25.49)

V72.31 Routine gynecological examination
General gynecological examination with or without
Papanicolaou cervical smear
Pelvic examination (annual) (periodic)
Use additional code to identify:
 human papillomavirus (HPV) screening (V73.81)
 routine vaginal Papanicolaou smear (V76.47)
V72.32 Encounter for Papanicolaou cervical smear to confirm
findings of recent normal smear following initial abnormal
smear
V72.4 Pregnancy examination or test
V72.40 Pregnancy examination or test, pregnancy unconfirmed
Possible pregnancy, not (yet) confirmed
V72.41 Pregnancy examination or test, negative result
V72.42 Pregnancy examination, positive result
V72.5 Radiological examination, not elsewhere classified
Routine chest X-ray
V72.6 Laboratory examination
Encounters for blood and urine testing
V72.60 Laboratory examination, unspecified
V72.61 Antibody response examination
Immunity status testing
Excludes: encounter for allergy testing (V72.7)
V72.62 Laboratory examination ordered as part of a routine general
medical examination
Blood tests for routine general physical examination
V72.63 Pre-procedural laboratory examination
Blood tests prior to treatment or procedure
Pre-operative laboratory examination
V72.69 Other laboratory examination

V72.7 Diagnostic skin and sensitization tests
V72.8 Other specified examinations
Excludes: pre-procedural laboratory examinations (V72.63)
V72.83 Other specified preoperative examination
Examination prior to chemotherapy
V72.84 Preoperative examination, unspecified
V72.85 Other specified examination
V72.86 Encounter for blood typing
V72.9 Unspecified examination

V73 Special screening examination for viral and chlamydial diseases
V73.2 Measles
V73.3 Rubella
V73.8 Other specified viral and chlamydial diseases

V73.81 Human papillomavirus (HPV)
V73.88 Other specified chlamydial diseases
V73.89 Other specified viral diseases
V73.9 Unspecified viral and chlamydial disease
V73.98 Unspecified chlamydial disease
V73.99 Unspecified viral disease

V74 Special screening examination for bacterial and spirochetal diseases
Includes: diagnostic skin tests for these diseases
V74.1 Pulmonary tuberculosis
V74.5 Venereal disease
Screening for bacterial and spirochetal sexually transmitted diseases
Screening for sexually transmitted diseases NOS
Excludes: special screening for nonbacterial sexually transmitted diseases (V73.81–V73.89, V75.4, V75.8)

V76 Special screening for malignant neoplasms
V76.1 Breast
V76.10 Breast screening, unspecified
V76.11 Screening mammogram for high-risk patient
V76.12 Other screening mammogram
V76.19 Other screening breast examination
V76.2 Cervix
Routine cervical Papanicolaou smear
Medicare patient not high risk
Excludes: that as part of a general gynecological examination (V72.31)
special screening for human papillomavirus (V73.81)
V76.4 Other sites
V76.41 Rectum
V76.43 Skin
V76.46 Ovary
V76.47 Vagina
Vaginal pap smear status—post hysterectomy for nonmalignant condition
Medicare patient not high risk
Use additional code to identify acquired absence of uterus (V88.01–V88.03)
Excludes: vaginal pap smear status—post hysterectomy for malignant condition (V67.01)
V76.49 Other sites
Fallopian tubes
V76.5 Intestine
V76.50 Intestine, unspecified
V76.51 Colon
Excludes: rectum (V76.41)
V76.52 Small intestine

V77 **Special screening for endocrine, nutritional, metabolic, and immunity disorders**
V77.0 Thyroid disorders
V77.1 Diabetes mellitus
V77.8 Obesity
V77.9 Other and unspecified endocrine, nutritional, metabolic, and immunity disorders
    V77.91 Screening for lipoid disorders
           Screening cholesterol level
           Screening for hypercholesterolemia
           Screening for hyperlipidemia

V78 **Special screening for disorders of blood and blood-forming organs**
V78.0 Iron deficiency anemia
V78.1 Other and unspecified deficiency anemia
V78.2 Sickle-cell disease or trait
V78.3 Other hemoglobinopathies
V78.8 Other disorders of blood and blood-forming organs
V78.9 Unspecified disorder of blood and blood-forming organs

V79 **Special screening for mental disorders and developmental handicaps**
V79.0 Depression
V79.1 Alcoholism

V81 **Special screening for cardiovascular, respiratory, and genitourinary diseases**
V81.1 Hypertension
V81.5 Nephropathy
       Screening for asymptomatic bacteriuria
V81.6 Other and unspecified genitourinary conditions

V82 **Special screening for other conditions**
V82.4 Maternal postnatal screening for chromosomal anomalies
     Excludes: antenatal screening by amniocentesis (V28.0)
V82.7 Genetic screening
     Excludes: genetic testing for procreative management (V26.31–V26.39)
    V82.71 Screening for genetic disease carrier status
    V82.79 Other genetic screening
V82.8 Other specified conditions
    V82.81 Osteoporosis
        Use additional code to identify:
        hormone replacement therapy (postmenopausal) status (V07.4)
        postmenopausal (natural) status (V49.81)

GENETICS **(V83–V84)**

V83 **Genetic carrier status**
V83.0 Hemophilia A carrier

V83.01 Asymptomatic hemophilia A carrier
V83.8 Other genetic carrier status
V83.81 Cystic fibrosis gene carrier
V83.89 Other genetic carrier status

V84 Genetic susceptibility to disease
Includes: confirmed abnormal gene
Use additional code, if applicable, for any associated family history of the disease (V16–V19)
V84.0 Genetic susceptibility to malignant neoplasm
Code first, if applicable, any current malignant neoplasms (150–195.8, 200.0, 230.3–234.9)
Use additional code, if applicable, for any personal history of malignant neoplasm (V10.0–V10.8)
V84.01 Genetic susceptibility to malignant neoplasm of breast
V84.02 Genetic susceptibility to malignant neoplasm of ovary
V84.04 Genetic susceptibility to malignant neoplasm of endometrium
V84.09 Genetic susceptibility to other malignant neoplasm
V84.8 Genetic susceptibility to other disease
V84.81 Genetic susceptibility to multiple endocrine neoplasia (MEN)
V84.89 Genetic susceptibility to other disease

BODY MASS INDEX (V85)
V85 Body Mass Index (BMI)
Kilograms per meters squared
Note: BMI adult codes are for use for persons over 20 years old
V85.0 Body Mass Index less than 19, adult
V85.1 Body Mass Index between 19–24, adult
V85.2 Body Mass Index between 25–29, adult
V85.21 Body Mass Index 25.0–25.9, adult
V85.22 Body Mass Index 26.0–26.9, adult
V85.23 Body Mass Index 27.0–27.9, adult
V85.24 Body Mass Index 28.0–28.9, adult
V85.25 Body Mass Index 29.0–29.9, adult
V85.3 Body Mass Index between 30–39, adult
V85.30 Body Mass Index 30.0–30.9, adult
V85.31 Body Mass Index 31.0–31.9, adult
V85.32 Body Mass Index 32.0–32.9, adult
V85.33 Body Mass Index 33.0–33.9, adult
V85.34 Body Mass Index 34.0–34.9, adult
V85.35 Body Mass Index 35.0–35.9, adult
V85.36 Body Mass Index 36.0–36.9, adult
V85.37 Body Mass Index 37.0–37.9, adult
V85.38 Body Mass Index 38.0–38.9, adult
V85.39 Body Mass Index 39.0–39.9, adult
V85.4 Body Mass Index 40 and over, adult

ESTROGEN RECEPTOR STATUS (V86)

V86 Estrogen receptor status
Code first malignant neoplasm of breast (174.0–174.9, 175.0–175.9)
V86.0 Estrogen receptor positive status (ER+)
V86.1 Estrogen receptor negative status (ER–)

OTHER SPECIFIED PERSONAL EXPOSURES AND HISTORY PRESENTING HAZARDS TO HEALTH (V87)

V87 Other specified personal exposures and history presenting hazards to health
V87.4 Personal history of drug therapy
Excludes: long-term (current) drug use (V58.61–V58.69)
V87.41 Personal history of antineoplastic chemotherapy
V87.42 Personal history of monoclonal drug therapy
V87.43 Personal history of estrogen therapy
V87.46 Personal history of immunosuppression therapy
V87.49 Personal history of other drug therapy

ACQUIRED ABSENCE OF OTHER ORGANS AND TISSUE (V88)

V88 Acquired absence of other organs and tissue
V88.0 Acquired absence of cervix and uterus
V88.01 Acquired absence of both cervix and uterus
Acquired absence of uterus NOS
Status post total hysterectomy
V88.02 Acquired absence of uterus with remaining cervical stump
Status post partial hysterectomy with remaining cervical stump
V88.03 Acquired absence of cervix with remaining uterus

OTHER SUSPECTED CONDITIONS NOT FOUND (V89)

V89 Other suspected conditions not found
V89.0 Suspected maternal and fetal conditions not found
Excludes: known or suspected fetal anomalies affecting management of mother, not ruled out (655.00–655.93, 656.00–656.93, 657.00–657.03, 658.00–658.93)
V89.01 Suspected problem with amniotic cavity and membrane not found
Suspected oligohydramnios not found
Suspected polyhydramnios not found
V89.02 Suspected placental problem not found
V89.03 Suspected fetal anomaly not found
V89.04 Suspected problem with fetal growth not found
V89.05 Suspected cervical shortening not found
V89.09 Other suspected maternal and fetal condition not found

EXTERNAL CAUSES OF INJURY AND POISONING (E800–E999)

The alphabetic index to the E codes is organized by main terms, which describe the accident, circumstance, event, or specific agent that caused the injury or other adverse effect. These codes are rarely reported by obstetrician–gynecologists. For the complete list, see the ICD-9-CM book.

ALPHABETIC INDEX TO EXTERNAL CAUSES OF INJURY

Abuse, (alleged) (suspected)
adult by
child E967.4
ex-partner E967.3
ex-spouse E967.3
father E967.0
grandchild E967.7
grandparent E967.6
mother E967.2
nonrelated caregiver E967.8
other relative E967.7
other specified person E967.1
partner E967.3
sibling E967.5
spouse E967.3
stepfather E967.0
stepmother E967.2
unspecified person E967.9
child by
boyfriend of parent or guardian E967.0
child E967.4
father E967.0
female partner of parent or guardian E967.2
girlfriend of parent or guardian E967.2
grandchild E967.7
grandparent E967.6
male partner of parent or guardian E967.0
mother E967.2
nonrelated caregiver E967.8
other relative E967.7
other specified person(s) E967.1
sibling E967.5
stepfather E967.0
stepmother E967.2
unspecified person E967.9
Accident, caused by, due to
motor vehicle (on public highway) (traffic) E819
involving collision (*see also* Collision, motor vehicle) E812
not involving collision—*see* category E816

Adverse effect, drug
in therapeutic use, ovarian hormones and synthetic substitutes
Assault (homicidal) (by) (in)
brawl (hand) (fists) (foot) E960.0
cut, any part of body E966
fight (hand) (fists) (foot) E960.0
with weapon E968.9
cutting or piercing E966
firearm(s)—*see* Shooting, homicide
injury NEC E968.9
rape E960.1
shooting—*see* Shooting, homicide
stab, any part of body E966
violence NEC E968.9
weapon E968.9
firearm—*see* Shooting, homicide
wound E968.9
cutting E966
gunshot—*see* Shooting, homicide
Battered
baby or child (syndrome)—*see* Abuse, child; category E967
person other than baby or child—*see* Assault
Brawl (hand) (fists) (foot) E960.0
Collision (accidental)
motor vehicle (on public highway) (traffic accident) E812
after leaving, running off, public highway (without antecedent collision) (without re-entry) E816
with antecedent collision on public highway—*see* categories E811–E815
with re-entrance collision with another motor vehicle E811
and
abutment (bridge) (overpass) E815
another motor vehicle (abandoned) (disabled) (parked) (stalled) (stopped) E812
with, involving re-entrance (on same roadway) (across median strip) E811

Collision *(continued)*
motor vehicle *(continued)*
and *(continued)*
any object, person, or vehicle off the
public highway resulting
from a noncollision motor
vehicle nontraffic accident
E816
bicycle (pedal cycle) E813
boundary fence E815
culvert E815
fallen stone or tree E815
guard post or guard rail E815
inter-highway divider E815
machinery (road) E815
pedestrian (conveyance) E814
person (using pedestrian conveyance) E814
post or pole (lamp) (light) (signal)
(telephone) (utility)
E815
traffic signal, sign, or marker (tem-
porary) E815
tree E815
bicycle E826
and
another bicycle (pedal cycle) E826
object (fallen) (fixed) (movable)
(moving) E826
pedestrian (conveyance) E826
person (using pedestrian conveyance) E826
pedestrian(s) (conveyance)
with fall E886.9
in sports E886.0
vehicle, motor—*see* Collision, motor
vehicle
Crash
motor vehicle—*see* Accident, motor
vehicle
Cut, cutting (any part of body)
(accidental)
homicide (attempt) E966
Entry of foreign body, material, any—*see*
Foreign body
Fall, falling (accidental) E888.9
down, from, off
bicycle (pedal cycle) E826
high place NEC E884.9
stated as undetermined whether
accidental or intentional—*see*
Jumping, from, high place

Fall, falling (accidental) *(continued)*
down, from, off *(continued)*
one level to another 884.9
pushing 886.9
same level 886.9
shoving 886.9
slipping 885.9
stairs 880.9
stumbling 885.9
tripping 885.9
other falls 888.9
Fell or jumped from high place, so
stated—*see* Jumping, from,
high place
Fight (hand) (fist) (foot) (*see also* Assault,
fight) E960.0
Foreign body, object or material (entrance
into, accidental) E915
Hit, hitting (accidental) by
bicycle (pedal cycle) E826
motor vehicle (on public highway) (traffic accident) E814
shot—*see* Shooting
vehicle NEC—*see* Accident, vehicle
NEC
Homicide, homicidal (attempt) (justifi-
able) (*see also* Assault)
E968.9
Injury, injured (accidental[ly])
by, caused by, from
assault (*see also* Assault) E968.9
bullet—*see* Shooting
foreign body—*see* Foreign body
homicidal (*see also* Assault) E968.9
in, on
fight E960.0
public highway E819
inflicted by other person, injury stated as
homicidal, intentional—*see* Assault
undetermined whether accidental or
intentional—*see* Injury, stated
as undetermined
purposely (inflicted) by other person(s)—
see Assault
Jumping from
building—*see* Jumping, from, high place
high place, in accidental circumstances or
in sport E884.9
Justifiable homicide—*see* Assault
Kicked by person(s) (accidentally)
with intent to injure or kill E960.0
in fight E960.0

Loss of control of motor vehicle (on
    public highway) (without
    antecedent collision)
    E816
  with antecedent collision on public high-
    way—*see* Collision, motor
    vehicle
  involving any object, person or vehicle
    not on public highway
    E816
  on public highway—*see* Collision,
    motor vehicle
Manslaughter (nonaccidental)—*see*
    Assault
Murder (attempt) (*see also* Assault) E968.9
Overturning (accidental) motor vehicle
    E816 (*see also* Loss of con-
    trol, motor vehicle)
  with antecedent collision on public high-
    way—*see* Collision, motor
    vehicle
  bicycle (pedal cycle) E826
  vehicle NEC—*see* Accident, vehicle NEC

Rape E960.1
Running off roadway
  bicycle (pedal cycle) E826
  motor vehicle (without antecedent colli-
    sion) E816
Shooting, shot (accidental[ly])
  homicide (attempt) E965.4
  specified firearm E965.4
  stated as
    intentional, homicidal E965.4
Slipping (accidental)
  on
    ice E885.9
    snow E885.9
    surface (slippery, wet) E885.9
Sodomy (assault) E960.1
Stab, stabbing E966
Syndrome, battered
  baby or child—*see* Abuse, child
  wife—*see* Assault
Traffic accident NEC E819
Violence, nonaccidental (*see also* Assault)
    E968.9

SUPPLEMENTARY CLASSIFICATION OF EXTERNAL CAUSES OF INJURY
AND POISONING

The Supplementary Classification of External Causes of Injury and Poisoning (E
Codes) are used to report an environmental event, circumstance, or condition that
resulted in an injury, poisoning, or other adverse effects, such as a fall or a motor
vehicle accident. These codes are never reported as a primary diagnosis.

E codes are not often used by obstetrician–gynecologists, but there may be state
or insurer rules requiring use of these codes. Obstetrician–gynecologists might
report these codes for a rape victim (E960.1) or for a pregnant patient who is seen
because of a fall down stairs (E880.9).

Motor Vehicle Traffic Accidents

The following fourth-digit subdivisions are for use with categories E811–E826 to
identify the injured person:

0   Driver of motor vehicle other than motorcycle
1   Passenger in motor vehicle other than motorcycle
2   Motorcyclist
3   Passenger on motorcycle
6   Bicyclist (Pedal cyclist)
7   Pedestrian
8   Other specified person
9   Unspecified person

E811   **Motor vehicle traffic accident involving re-entrant collision with
another motor vehicle**
Requires fourth digit. See above list to select appropriate digit.

E812   **Other motor vehicle traffic accident involving collision with motor
vehicle**
Requires fourth digit. See above list to select appropriate digit.

E813   **Motor vehicle traffic accident involving collision with other vehicle**
Requires fourth digit. See above list to select appropriate digit.

E814   **Motor vehicle traffic accident involving collision with pedestrian**
Requires fourth digit. See above list to select appropriate digit.

E815   **Other motor vehicle traffic accident involving collision on the highway**
Requires fourth digit. See above list to select appropriate digit.
Includes: Collision with object, guard rail, or wall.

E816   **Motor vehicle traffic accident due to loss of control, without collision
on the highway**
Requires fourth digit. See above list to select appropriate digit.
Includes: Loss of control due to blowout, driver falling asleep, or excessive
speed.

E826   Bicycle (pedal cycle) accident
Requires fourth digit. See above list to select appropriate digit.

Accidental Falls

E880.9 Fall on or from stairs or steps

E884.9 Fall from one level to another

E885.9 Fall on same level from slipping, tripping, or stumbling

E886   Fall on same level from collision, pushing, or shoving, by or with other person
E886.0 In sports
          Tackles in sports
E886.9 Other and unspecified

E888.9 Other and unspecified fall

Drugs, Medicinal and Biological Substances Causing Adverse Effects in Therapeutic Use

E932 Hormones and synthetic substitutes
E932.2 Ovarian hormones and synthetic substitutes
          Contraceptives, oral
          Estrogens
          Estrogens and progestogens combined
          Progestogens

Homicide and Injury Purposely Inflicted by Other Persons

Includes: Injuries inflicted by another person with intent to injure or kill, by any means

E960   Fight, brawl, rape
E960.0 Unarmed fight or brawl
          Beatings NOS
          Brawl or fight with hands, fists, feet
          Injured or killed in fight NOS
E960.1 Rape
E965.9 Assault by firearms

E966   Assault by cutting and piercing instrument
No fifth digit required.

E967   Perpetrator of child and adult abuse
E967.0 By father, stepfather, or boyfriend
          Male partner of child's parent or guardian
E967.1 By other specified person

E967.2 By mother, stepmother, or girlfriend
Female partner of child's parent or guardian
E967.3 By spouse or partner
Abuse of spouse or partner by ex-spouse or ex-partner
E967.4 By child
E967.5 By sibling
E967.6 By grandparent
E967.7 By other relative
E967.8 By non-related caregiver
E967.9 By unspecified person

968.9 Assault by other means

APPENDIX A
DIAGNOSTIC CODING FOR
TERMINATION OF PREGNANCY

ACOG's Committee on Coding and Nomenclature has defined the following terms:

First trimester = First day of last menstrual period (day 0) to less than 14 weeks

Second trimester = 14 weeks 0 days to 28 weeks 0 days

Third trimester = 28 weeks or more

Note that some state legislatures have legally defined the difference between a miscarriage and a stillbirth by the number of weeks gestation or by gram weight of the fetus. This legal definition may determine which CPT code is reported.

Missed abortion: An empty gestational sac, blighted ovum, or a fetus or fetal pole without a heartbeat prior to completion of 20 weeks 0 days gestation. Note that ICD-9-CM defines missed abortion as any fetal death prior to completion of 22 weeks gestation.

Incomplete abortion: The expulsion of some products of conception with the remainder evacuated surgically.

When reporting a global delivery code, it may be appropriate to add a modifier 52 (reduced services) if the number of antepartum visits was substantially less than 13. The following tables provide the diagnosis and procedure codes to use for various types of abortions.

Table A-1. Missed Abortion/Fetal Demise (In Utero)

Diagnostic Codes	Description	Procedure Codes	Description
632	Missed Abortion or early fetal death, prior to 22 weeks 0 days or	59820	Surgical abortion, prior to 14 weeks 0 days
656.41	Intrauterine Fetal Demise, after 22 weeks 0 days	59821	Surgical abortion, 14 weeks 0 days up to 20 weeks 0 days
		59850, 59851, or 59852	Non-surgical abortion, by injections, prior to 20 weeks 0 days
	Also report a code from 639 series for a complication if appropriate	Delivery Code	Non-surgical abortion, by injections, after 20 weeks 0 days
		59855-59857	Non-surgical abortion, by suppositories, prior to 20 weeks 0 days
		Delivery code	Non-surgical abortion, by suppositories, after 20 weeks 0 days
		E/M code	Spontaneous/other medical abortion, prior to 20 weeks 0 days
		Delivery code	Spontaneous/other medical abortion, after 20 weeks 0 days
		E/M code + 59414	Spontaneous abortion + delivery of placenta, prior to 20 weeks 0 days
		Delivery code	Spontaneous abortion + delivery of placenta, after 20 weeks 0 days

Table A-2. Coding Spontaneous (Complete) Abortion

Diagnostic Codes	Description	Procedure Codes	Description
634.X2	Spontaneous abortion any trimester Use fourth digit to indicate complication	E/M code	Prior to 20 weeks 0 days
		Delivery code	After 20 weeks 0 days

Table A-3. Coding Spontaneous (Incomplete) Abortion

Diagnostic Codes	Description	Procedure Codes	Description
634.X1	Spontaneous abortion any trimester Use fourth digit to indicate complication	59812	Prior to 20 weeks 0 days
		Delivery code	20 weeks 0 days or more

Table A–4.   Coding Induced Abortion

Diagnostic Codes	Description	Procedure Codes	Description
635.XX	Legally induced abortion any trimester	59840	By D&C, any trimester
		59841	By D&E, 14 weeks 0 days up to 20 weeks 0 days
	Use fourth digit to indicate complication	59841–22	By D&E, 20 weeks 0 days or more
		59850, 59852, or 59851	By injections, prior to 20 weeks 0 days
	Use fifth digit to indicate complete or incomplete abortion	59855–59857	By suppositories, prior to 20 weeks 0 days
		Delivery code	By suppositories, after 20 weeks 0 days
	Also report a code for a complication if appropriate, eg, 642.XX, 648.XX, 651.XX, 655.XX, 656.XX, 659.XX	E/M code	Spontaneous or other medical abortion, prior to 20 weeks 0 days
		Delivery codes	Spontaneous or other medical abortion, after 20 weeks 0 days
		E/M code + 59414	Spontaneous abortion + delivery of placenta, prior to 20 weeks 0 days
		Delivery code	Spontaneous abortion, after 20 weeks 0 days

APPENDIX B
DIAGNOSTIC CODING FOR CERVICAL PAP SMEAR FOLLOW-UP VISITS

In 2003, codes for cervical carcinoma in situ/dysplasia/abnormal Pap smears were modified and new codes were added to more clearly differentiate between abnormal pap smear results and histological findings of dysplasia. In addition, the terminology was modified to use the terminology from the most recent revision of the Bethesda System.

Physicians should report a diagnosis for the reason the patient was seen. That is, if she is being seen for a routine pap smear, then report code V72.31, even if the results for the Pap smear indicate an abnormality. When she returns for a follow-up visit following an abnormal result, the diagnostic code should reflect the abnormal results found previously.

The following flow chart indicates correct diagnostic coding for a number of different scenarios.

Coding for Abnormal Cervical Pap Test Follow-up Visits

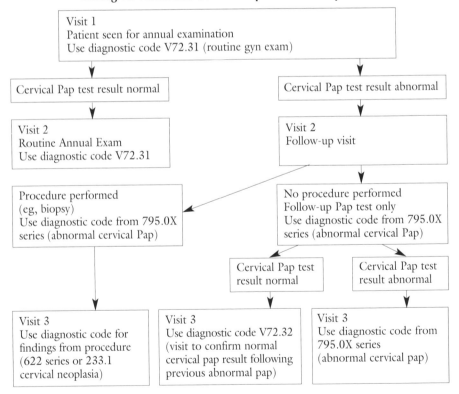

APPENDIX C
DIAGNOSTIC CODING FOR
OBSTETRIC ULTRASOUND PROCEDURES

Diagnoses for ultrasound procedures are selected as follows:

- If the condition is known to be present and is complicating the current pregnancy, report a code from the pregnancy chapter of ICD-9-CM.

- If the condition is known to be present but is not complicating the pregnancy at this time, report an appropriate V code or a code from one of the nonobstetric chapters of ICD-9-CM.

- If the physician is performing an ultrasound examination to see if a specific condition is present, report an appropriate V code. This applies to a patient who is considered "high risk" (that is, she has a personal history of a specific problem in a past pregnancy) but does not currently have a problem in this pregnancy.

- If the physician performs an ultrasound examination for a suspected maternal or fetal condition that is suspected but not found, report an appropriate code from the V89.0 category (Suspected maternal and fetal conditions not found). In some cases, the maternal or fetal condition is suspected because of an abnormal test result. These codes should not be used when the condition is confirmed. In those cases, the confirmed condition should be coded. Additionally, these codes should not be used if an illness, sign/symptom, or problem related to the suspected condition is present. In such cases the diagnosis/symptom code is assigned. These codes should be used in limited circumstances on a maternal record. Further, these codes may not be used for antenatal screening.

Following are tables with ACOG's recommendations. In the table, many of the codes from the pregnancy chapter have an X in place of a fifth digit. The X should be replaced with the correct fifth digit, depending on the episode of care.

Table C-1. Diagnoses for Ultrasound Examination Performed Because of Known or Possible Fetal Problems

Condition	Diagnostic Code	
Alphafetoprotein, abnormal serum value	V28.3	Screening for malformation using ultrasonics
	796.4	Other abnormal clinical findings
	V28.1	Screening for raised alphafetoprotein levels in amniotic fluid
Biophysical evaluation of fetus	V28.81	Encounter for fetal anatomic survey
	656.3X	Fetal distress
	656.9X	Unspecified fetal and placental problem
	656.8X	Other specified fetal and placental problems
Decreased fetal movement	V28.89	Other specified antenatal screening
	655.7X	Decreased fetal movement
	656.8X	Other known or suspected fetal abnormality
Decreased triple marker History of congenital anomaly (in previous pregnancy)	V72.85	Other specified examination
	655.8X	Other known or suspected fetal abnormality
	V28.3	Encounter for routine screening for malformation using ultrasonics
	V23.4	Pregnancy with poor obstetric history
	655.2X	Hereditary disease in family possibly affecting fetus
Determination of fetal presentation	V28.89	Other specified antenatal screening
	652.XX	Malposition or malpresentation of fetus
Estimation of fetal weight or presentation in premature rupture of membranes or premature labor	644.2X	Early onset of delivery
	644.0X	Threatened premature labor
Evaluation of fetal condition for late registrants for prenatal care	V23.7	Insufficient prenatal care
Fetal death, suspected	632	Missed abortion
	656.4X	Intrauterine death
		Code also symptoms
Follow-up to known fetal anomaly (in current pregnancy)	655.XX	Code for specific fetal anomaly
IUD, suspected fetal problem due to presence	V25.42	Surveillance of intrauterine contraceptive device
	655.8X	Suspected fetal abnormalities from IUD
IUGR, Intrauterine growth retardation	V28.4	Screening for fetal growth retardation using ultrasonics
Macrosomia	V28.89	Other specified antenatal screening Code also symptoms (eg, maternal diabetes, obesity, postdates)
Multiple gestation, serial evaluation of fetal growth	V28.4	Screening for fetal growth retardation using ultrasonics
	651.XX	Multiple gestation

(continued)

Table C–1. Diagnoses for Ultrasound Examination Performed Because of Known or Possible Fetal Problems (*continued*)

Condition	Diagnostic Code	
Multiple gestation	V28.89	Other specified antenatal screening
	651.XX	Multiple gestation
Uterine size/clinical dates discrepancy	649.6	Uterine size/date discrepancy
	656.6X	Excessive fetal growth
	656.5X	Poor fetal growth
	793.6	Abnormal findings by ultrasound of abdominal area

Table C–2. Diagnoses for Ultrasound Examinations Performed Because of Known or Possible Maternal Problems

Condition	Diagnostic Code	
Adjunct to placement of cerclage	654.5X	Cervical incompetence
Cervical insufficiency	649.7X	Cervical shortening
	V89.05	Suspected cervical shortening not found
Ectopic pregnancy, suspected	633.X	Ectopic pregnancy
		Code symptoms
Hydatidiform mole, suspected	V23.1	Pregnancy with history of trophoblastic disease
	630	Hydatidiform mole
	V89.09	Other suspected maternal and fetal condition not found
		Code symptoms
Pelvic mass	654.1X	Tumors of body of uterus
	654.9X	Other/unspecified abnormality of organs/ soft tissues of pelvis
	789.3X	Pelvic mass (specify site)
	793.6	Abnormal findings by ultrasound of abdominal area
Uterine abnormality, suspected	654.0X	Congenital abnormalities of uterus
	654.1X	Tumors of body of uterus
	654.3X	Retroverted and incarcerated gravid uterus
	654.4X	Other abnormalities in shape/position of gravid neighboring structures
	793.6	Abnormal findings by ultrasound of abdominal area
Vaginal bleeding of undetermined etiology	641.9X	Unspecified antepartum hemorrhage
	640.9X	Unspecified hemorrhage in early pregnancy

Table C–3. Diagnoses for Ultrasound Examinations Performed Because of Other Problems

Condition	Diagnostic Code	
Abruptio placentae, suspected	641.2X	Premature separation of placenta
	793.9	Abnormal placental findings by ultrasound
	V89.02	Suspected placental problem not found
Adjunct to external version	652.1X	Breech or other malpresentation successfully converted to cephalic presentation
	660.0X	Obstruction caused by malposition of fetus at onset of labor
	652.2X	Breech presentation
Adjunct to amniocentesis		Code reason for amniocentesis
		If a complete ultrasound also performed, report as appropriate:
	V28.2	Other screening based on amniocentesis
	V28.0	Screening for chromosomal anomalies by amniocentesis
Adjunct to other specific procedures		Code for reason for specific procedure
Confirm dates/unknown gestational age or last menstrual period	V28.89	Other specified antenatal screening
Follow-up evaluation for known placenta previa	641.0X	Placenta previa without hemorrhage
	641.1X	Hemorrhage from placenta previa
Observation of intrapartum events	V71.89	Observation for suspected condition not found
		Code for intrapartum events
Polyhydramnios or oligohydramnios, suspected	657.0X	Polyhydramnios
	658.0X	Oligohydramnios
	V89.01	Suspected problem with amniotic cavity and membrane not found
Post-term/prolonged pregnancy	645.1X	Pregnancy over 40 weeks to 42 weeks gestation
	645.2X	Pregnancy advanced beyond 42 weeks gestation

Appendix D
ICD-10-CM Implementation
in the United States

The International Classification of Diseases, 10th Revision, Clinical Modification (ICD-10-CM) is currently being used in most countries but not in the United States. However, the U.S. Department of Health and Human Services (HHS) has initiated the process necessary for implementation of ICD-10-CM for use in this country. The implementation date for ICD-10-CM is set for October 1, 2013. After September 30, 2013, the ICD-9-CM codes will not be reportable. This date allows three to four years for preparation to begin using the new coding system.

ICD-10-CM contain 21 chapters listing three to seven digit alphanumeric codes. In 2009, there were approximately 68,000 ICD-10-CM diagnosis codes, which totaled 54,000 more codes than in ICD-9-CM. ICD-10-CM allows coding for increased specificity in the reporting of diseases and recently recognized conditions. Further, ICD–10–CM provides noteworthy improvements over ICD–9–CM in coding primary care encounters, external causes of injury, mental disorders, neoplasms, and preventive health. The ICD–10–CM code set reflects advances in medicine and medical technology, permits the capture of more socioeconomics details, ambulatory care condition information, problems related to lifestyle, and the results of screening tests. It also provides many ICD-10-CM improvements that benefit obstetrics and gynecology coding. One of the most notable enhancements is that ICD-10-CM allows the trimester of pregnancy to be designated. Here is an example of the difference:

ICD-9-CM	ICD-10-CM
649.53 Spotting complicating pregnancy, antepartum	O26.851 Spotting complicating pregnancy, first trimester O26.852 Spotting complicating pregnancy, second trimester O26.853 Spotting complicating pregnancy, third trimester O26.859 Spotting complicating pregnancy, unspecified trimester

Note, the ICD-10-CM diagnostic codes for obstetrical conditions begins with the letter "O".

The National Center for Health Statistics (NCHS) has developed a mapping program between ICD-9-CM and ICD-10-CM to assist users with locating the corresponding diagnosis codes within the two code sets. This guide will be updated every year to include the new diagnosis codes. To view the mapping program, visit the NCHC webpage at: http://www.cdc.gov/nchs/about/otheract/icd9/icd10cm.htm

In 2012, ACOG will begin providing ob/gyn specialty driven ICD-10-CM training at the ACOG Coding Workshops and Coding Webcasts. ACOG feels most physicians, coders and other health care professionals are unlikely to remember the new ICD-10-CM coding rules if taught sooner than the year before implementation.